Updates in Clinical Dermatology

Series Editors

John Berth-Jones, University Hospitals Coventry & Warwickshire, NHS Trust
Coventry, UK

Chee Leok Goh, National Skin Centre
Singapore, Singapore

Howard I. Maibach, Department of Dermatology
University of California San Francisco Department of Dermatology
ALAMEDA, CA, USA

Updates in Clinical Dermatology aims to promote the rapid and efficient transfer of medical research into clinical practice. It is published in four volumes per year. Covering new developments and innovations in all fields of clinical dermatology, it provides the clinician with a review and summary of recent research and its implications for clinical practice. Each volume is focused on a clinically relevant topic and explains how research results impact diagnostics, treatment options and procedures as well as patient management. The reader-friendly volumes are highly structured with core messages, summaries, tables, diagrams and illustrations and are written by internationally well-known experts in the field. A volume editor supervises the authors in his/her field of expertise in order to ensure that each volume provides cutting-edge information most relevant and useful for clinical dermatologists. Contributions to the series are peer reviewed by an editorial board.

Ana M. Giménez-Arnau
Howard I. Maibach

Editors

Handbook
of Occupational
Dermatoses

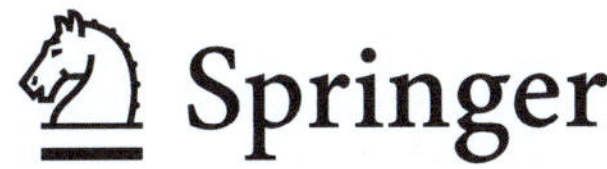

Springer

Editors
Ana M. Giménez-Arnau
Department of Dermatology
Universitat Autònoma and Universitat
Pompeu Fabra de Barcelona
Barcelona, Spain

Howard I. Maibach
Department of Dermatology
UCSF Medical Center
San Francisco, CA, USA

ISSN 2523-8884   ISSN 2523-8892   (electronic)
Updates in Clinical Dermatology
ISBN 978-3-031-22729-5   ISBN 978-3-031-22727-1   (eBook)
https://doi.org/10.1007/978-3-031-22727-1

© The Editor(s) (if applicable) and The Author(s), under exclusive license to Springer Nature Switzerland AG 2023
This work is subject to copyright. All rights are solely and exclusively licensed by the Publisher, whether the whole or part of the material is concerned, specifically the rights of translation, reprinting, reuse of illustrations, recitation, broadcasting, reproduction on microfilms or in any other physical way, and transmission or information storage and retrieval, electronic adaptation, computer software, or by similar or dissimilar methodology now known or hereafter developed.
The use of general descriptive names, registered names, trademarks, service marks, etc. in this publication does not imply, even in the absence of a specific statement, that such names are exempt from the relevant protective laws and regulations and therefore free for general use.
The publisher, the authors, and the editors are safe to assume that the advice and information in this book are believed to be true and accurate at the date of publication. Neither the publisher nor the authors or the editors give a warranty, expressed or implied, with respect to the material contained herein or for any errors or omissions that may have been made. The publisher remains neutral with regard to jurisdictional claims in published maps and institutional affiliations.

This Springer imprint is published by the registered company Springer Nature Switzerland AG
The registered company address is: Gewerbestrasse 11, 6330 Cham, Switzerland

Contents

Occupational and Work-Related Dermatosis: Definition and Classification

Felipe Heras-Mendaza
and Luis Conde-Salazar Gómez

Definition

There are various definitions for occupational dermatosis. A concise and clear one was stated by a co-operative approach to industrial dermatologic problems undertaken in 1936 between the American Medical Association and the American Dermatological Association: an occupational dermatosis is "a pathological condition of the skin for which occupational exposure can be shown to be a major causal or contributory factor" [1]. Other definitions include the possible alterations in mucosa and annexes [2] or the need that the occupational disease affects certain groups of individuals to a significantly greater extent (at least with a twofold relative risk) than the general population [3].

But not always an occupational skin disease from a medical point of view is considered as such from a juristic perspective, with consequences in social and economic compensation for the patient. The legislation about what is an occupational dermatosis varies greatly from one country to another, and of course it also varies the compensation. The legal requisites to consider a skin disease as occupational depend finally on political decisions. Thus, we can conclude that, from a legal point of view, an occupational skin disease is that one recognized in the legislation of the country where the patient is working.

The distinction between work-related diseases and occupational diseases is not always clear and stands a matter of discussion. Occupational diseases are considered as having a specific or a strong relation to occupation, generally with only one causal agent, and recognized as such. Nevertheless, work-related diseases have a complex etiology, with multiple causal agents, where factors in the work environment may play a role in the development of such diseases, together with other risk factors [4].

Work-related dermatoses are then defined as those diseases that have multiple causes, including factors of the work environment [5]. This concept entails a theoretical and legislative discussion that is not always clear and varies from one country to another. In this chapter we will refer to all these conditions as occupational dermatoses, but conceptually some of the entities discussed could be considered as work-related dermatoses.

The recognition of a disease as occupational is of such importance for the worker and other sectors of society (company, health insurance, and compensation systems) that it can be helpful following some criteria to define the disease in the most objective way possible. In view that contact dermatitis accounts for more than 90% of all

F. Heras-Mendaza (✉)
Department of Dermatology, Fundación Jiménez Díaz, Madrid, Spain

L. C.-S. Gómez
Former Department of Occupational Dermatology, Instituto de Salud Carlos III, Madrid, Spain

© The Author(s), under exclusive license to Springer Nature Switzerland AG 2023
A. M. Giménez-Arnau, H. I. Maibach (eds.), *Handbook of Occupational Dermatoses*, Updates in Clinical Dermatology, https://doi.org/10.1007/978-3-031-22727-1_1

worker's compensation claims for occupational skin diseases, Mathias established seven criteria to assess the probability of a causal relationship with employment of a contact dermatitis. He concluded that if the answer to at least four criteria should be "yes," the contact dermatitis is probably caused by a workplace exposure [6]:

1. Is the clinical appearance consistent with contact dermatitis?
2. Are there workplace exposures to potential cutaneous irritants or allergens?
3. Is the anatomic distribution of dermatitis consistent with cutaneous exposure in relation to the job task?
4. Is the temporal relationship between exposure and onset consistent with contact dermatitis?
5. Are non-occupational exposures excluded as probable causes?
6. Does dermatitis improve away from work exposure to the suspected irritant or allergen?
7. Do patch or provocation tests implicate a specific workplace exposure?

These criteria should be used with caution, as a guide, knowing that sometimes they could give false positives and negatives results. The core message is that the definition of an occupational skin disease resides on a detailed history, a clear temporal relationship of the onset of the skin disease and the job, relevant positive patch tests in the case of allergic contact dermatitis, and usually confirmation of the resolution when the causative agent is avoided.

Besides the causes of occupational dermatoses, we must be aware of some predisposing factors. Age is one of them: occupational dermatosis is more frequent in young individuals, due to work inexperience, poor protective measures, and more contact with irritants. Other factors are pre-existing dermatosis (such as atopic dermatitis and psoriasis), cold and hot temperature, low and high humidity, and difficulty accessing to hygiene and medical services.

Classification

There does not exist a universal accepted classification for occupational dermatosis. The most common classification is based on the external factors that cause these diseases (mechanical, physical, biologic, and chemical) [7–9]. However, this classification is sometimes confusing, because separating chemical from physical or mechanical causes is not always obvious.

A better classification of occupational skin diseases would be by professions (dermatosis in construction workers, metalworkers, hairdressers, etc.). But the great variety of professions is such that it would not be a good schematic organization. Furthermore, it would not be entirely correct, since within the different professions there are various jobs or workplaces, with their specific risks. In fact, in some professions each workplace has its own special problems.

Although the true frequencies of occupational dermatosis are unknown, the great majority of them correspond to contact dermatitis to different chemicals that are present at workplace (70–90% of all occupational dermatosis, depending on different studies [10–12]). The resting 10–30% of occupational dermatosis are a heterogeneous group of different entities (acne, urticaria, infections, etc.). Besides being contact dermatitis so frequent in occupational dermatology, allergic contact dermatitis is the main cause of work inability, with the very important personal, social, and economic consequences that it produces.

Taking these arguments together we have preferred a division of occupational dermatosis in two groups: contact dermatitis and non-contact dermatitis. Table 1.1 shows this classification, although not exhaustive, but containing the main entities in occupational dermatology.

Table 1.1 Classification of occupational dermatosis

1. Contact dermatitis	
Allergic contact dermatitis	Multiple allergens. Clinical patterns: localized eczema, airborne, lichenoid, lymphomatoid, photocontact allergic dermatitis…
Irritant contact dermatitis	Acute; acute delayed; cumulative; traumatic; pustular; phototoxicity…
2. Non-contact dermatitis	
Urticaria	Immunological contact urticaria; no immunological contact urticaria; protein contact dermatitis.
Acne	Oil acne; coal tar acne; acne mechanica; chloracne; cosmetic acne; other forms of acne.
Pressure- and friction-induced disorders	Callus; blisters; fissures; hemorrhages; abrasions; nodules; Koebner isomorphic phenomenon (psoriasis, lichen planus, vitiligo, eczema…).
Vibration-associated disorders	Raynaud's phenomenon (traumatic vasospastic disease or hand-arm vibration syndrome).
Foreign body granulomas	Cobalt; beryllium; aluminum; zirconium; hair; others.
Pigmentary disorders	Post-inflammatory hyper- and hypopigmentation; hyperpigmentation from tattoos and chemicals; chemical leukoderma.
Low humidity-induced disorders	Pruritus; urticaria; eczema; semicircular lipoatrophy.
Heat-associated disorders	Miliaria; intertrigo; hyperhidrosis; erythema ab igne; thermal burns.
Cold-associated disorders	Frostbites; perniosis; acrocyanosis; cold panniculitis; Raynaud's phenomenon.
Skin cancer	Arsenic; polycyclic aromatic hydrocarbons (coal tar); ultraviolet light; ionizing radiation.
Infections and infestations	Virus (warts, herpes simplex, orf, milker's nodules…); bacteria (staphylococci, streptococci, anthrax, brucellosis, erysipeloid, tularemia, leptospirosis, mycobacteria, tick-borne diseases…); fungi (tinea pedis, candida infections, sporotrichosis…); scabies, etc.
Others	Radiodermatitis (acute and chronic); scleroderma-like disease (vinyl chloride, organic solvents); nail disorders (paronychia, dyschromia, onycholysis…); self-induced dermatosis (dermatitis artefacta); others.

Occupational Contact Dermatitis

Contact dermatitis is the main problem in occupational dermatology. Although it will be treated in extension in other chapters, its key aspects will be highlighted below.

Contact dermatitis is a skin reaction (normally eczematous) caused by a chemical insult to the skin. There are numerous substances capable of producing a contact dermatitis in different jobs. It is subdivided into irritant contact dermatitis (ICD) and allergic contact dermatitis (ACD). In ACD there exists a delayed hypersensitivity reaction (type IV hypersensitivity), which is not present in ICD.

The incidence of occupational contact dermatitis is determined by the degree of socioeconomic and industrial development in an area, resulting in a lot of geographical variation [11–15]. In general, ICD is responsible for at least of 80% of occupational contact dermatitis, while the remainder are ACD. This ratio varies among occupations, but ICD is always much more frequent than the allergic one. Anyway, ICD is not always declared, because normally it tends to present as mild dermatitis and resolves without specific treatment.

Most of the occupational contact dermatitis occur on the hands, due to the manipulation of many substances (Fig. 1.1). Other localizations may exist, depending on the contact with the offending substance. For example, when an airborne mechanism exists, dermatitis tends to affect the face, neck, and other areas exposed to the air (Fig. 1.2).

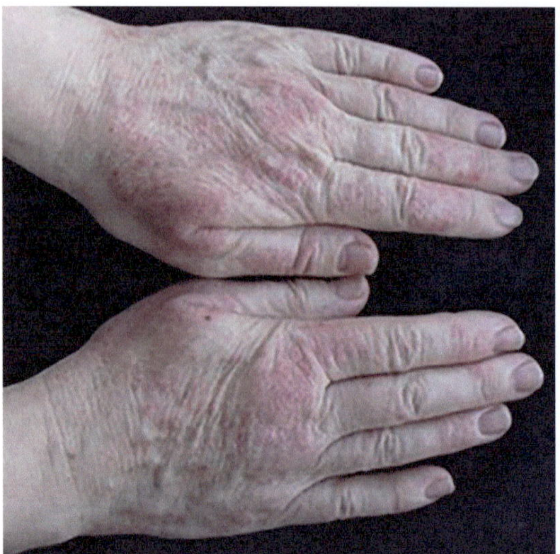

Fig. 1.1 Allergic contact dermatitis to epoxy resin in a floor layer worker

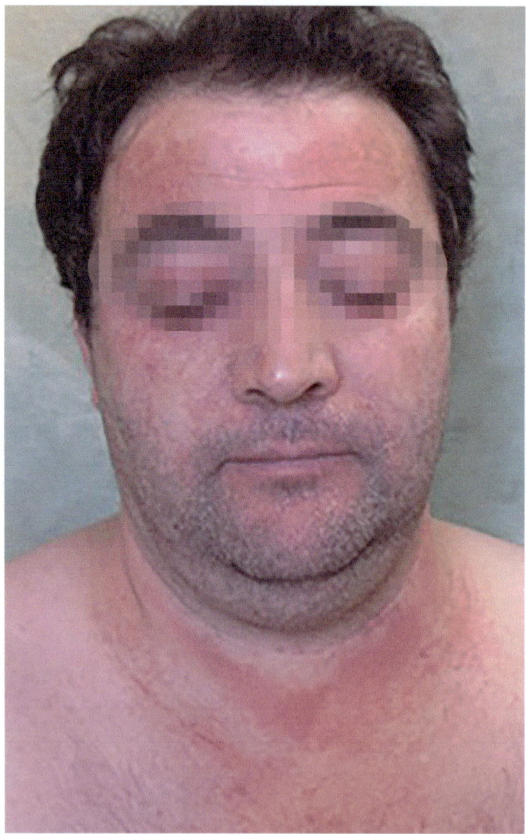

Fig. 1.2 Airborne allergic contact dermatitis to an intermediate compound in the synthesis of omeprazole in a pharmaceutical industry worker

It is very frequent to encounter an overlap between irritant and sensitizing reactions. For example, cement can cause an ICD due to the corrosive action of cement and/or an ACD from chromates. Soaps cause ICD due to surfactants and its capacity to modify the pH of the skin, but can also generate ACD from preservatives and fragrances.

A careful history and exploration are needed to achieve a correct diagnosis of contact dermatitis. Some symptoms and signs point toward one or another. For example, erythema, burning, and stinging immediately after contact with a substance suggest an irritant reaction whereas intense pruritus may support ACD [16].

In the study of these patients, we must know the irritant and allergic potential of the products managed at work, as well as the way they handle them. It is crucial to investigate the temporal relationship of the dermatitis with work periods, and the hobbies or other products that are in contact outside job. In general, occupational ACD tends to worsen more rapidly than ICD on return to work. The recovery period in ACD is normally longer (2–4 weeks) than in ICD (1–3 days in most of cases).

ACD generally presents as eczema, although rare variants exist (lichenoid, lymphomatoid, etc.). In contrast, ICD is more polymorphous. Some variants of ICD are acute ICD, acute delayed ICD, cumulative ICD, traumatic ICD, or pustular/acneiform ICD. As an example of this variability, fiberglass dermatitis is a special form of ICD that normally presents with a papular eruption that is very pruritic (Fig. 1.3). This pruritus associated with fiberglass exposure is typically sudden and intense [7]. Fiberglass is used in many industrial applications and workers often complain of pruritus on the neck, antecubital and popliteal fossae, forearms, wrists, and frictional sites, such as the belt and sock lines.

Patch tests are needed to diagnose contact dermatitis. They are positive in ACD and negative in ICD. It is essential to correctly interpret these patch test reactions, to differentiate between irritant and allergic reactions, and to search the relevance of each positive response.

Photocontact dermatitis is a variant of contact dermatitis where a substance needs ultraviolet

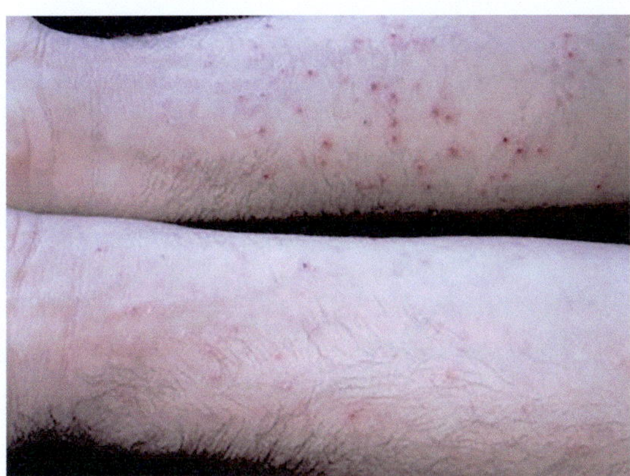

Fig. 1.3 Fiberglass irritant contact dermatitis in a worker who manufactured insulating panels without adequate protection

(UV) light to produce a contact dermatitis. This can be an irritant reaction (phototoxicity, for example in the association of furocoumarins and UV light) or it can be an allergic reaction (photo-contact allergic reaction, as can occur in the association of topical non-steroidal anti-inflammatory drugs and UV light).

Phototoxic dermatitis typically appears as a first- or second-degree sunburn, rather than as eczema. Hyperpigmentation frequently develops. In contrast, photoallergic dermatitis has eczematous morphologic features [17]. The diagnosis of allergic photocontact reaction can be made with proper photopatch tests.

Other entities can be present with or simulate contact dermatitis. Hence the importance of knowing endogenous eczematous diseases (atopic dermatitis, dyshidrotic eczema, seborrheic dermatitis…), as well as psoriasis, lichen planus, mycosis fungoides and in general the spectrum of skin diseases. A diagnostic of occupational contact dermatitis can open a litigating period with even judicial implications; so all efforts must be done in making a correct diagnosis.

Occupational Non-contact Dermatitis

A heterogenous group of entities are responsible for occupational non-contact dermatitis (Table 1.1). These problems are found less frequently than contact dermatitis in the occupational setting. We present below the main pictures.

Urticaria

Occupational contact urticaria can be immunological (IgE-mediated) or non-immunological. The clinical picture is that of wheals/redness/pruritus that appears suddenly, usually within 30 min after contact with the causative agent. It clears completely within hours and can be caused by a multitude of substances, from low molecular weight chemicals to proteins [18, 19].

Occupations at risk of developing contact urticaria are specially those who manage protein sources, as fruits, vegetables, spices, plants, animal tissues, grains, and enzymes [18–20]. Natural rubber latex emerged in the 1980s as a major cause of occupational contact urticaria, but fortunately the incidence has declined with different efforts, mainly the use of latex-free gloves and low-protein rubber gloves [21, 22].

Protein contact dermatitis is a special type of initially contact urticaria involved in the contact urticaria syndrome that appears on previously damaged skin with eczema. On this dermatitis areas, wheals or even a vesicular exacerbation can be noted a few minutes after contact with the causal protein [18, 23].

An atopic predisposition is the most important risk factor for contact or systemic urticaria caused by immediate hypersensitivity. The main complementary tool for the diagnosis is the prick test, although other diagnostic tests can be useful (measurement of specific IgE, basophil activation test, rubbing test, etc.).

Acne

Occupational acne can be seen in different workers, but especially those who are in contact with greasy and oily products. It may affect any follicle of the body, and not just the face or the typical localizations of acne vulgaris. People with predisposition to acne are at risk of developing occupational acne, but it also affects those without this predisposition. It has been described different types of occupational acne. The most important forms are oil acne, coal tar acne, acne mechanica, and chloracne.

Oil acne is the most common form of occupational acne, and it is caused mainly by greases and insoluble oils, that are comedogenic. Its incidence has declined in the past decades, due to the decreased use of pure cutting fluids and the improved hygienic conditions. Machine tool operators, mechanics, roofers, petroleum refiners, rubber workers, textile mill workers, and road pavers are workers at risk of developing oil acne [24].

Oil acne is more common in areas where contact with oil takes place, such as dorsa of the hands and fingers, arms, forearms, and abdomen, presenting as follicular papules, pustules, and sometimes nodules (Fig. 1.4). Other localizations are possible, according to the contact with the oil and the occlusion. For example, acne on buttocks when the worker is seated on a contaminated seat or on thighs due to hand transportation. Avoiding oil acne includes good hygiene measures, isolation of the machinery, and frequent work clothes changes.

Certain coal tars are also responsible for occupational acne, due to obstruction of the sebaceous glands by the mixture, forming black plugs. Coal tar is used in many industries: in aluminum production, steel and iron foundries, tar refineries, road paving, roof insulation, pavement sealcoat, and wood surfaces painting. These workers are exposed mainly through inhalation and dermal contact. Lesions in coal tar acne tend to affect the face, suggesting an airborne distribution [25].

Acne mechanica refers to a form of acne vulgaris aggravated by different traumas to the skin. This is sometimes the case of an occupational factor. The stressors provoking acne mechanica are diverse, as protracted pressure from tight clothing, helmets, packs, seats, resting the head in the hands in a particular way, friction, tension, or rubbing [26].

A type of acne mechanica is the one caused by the prolonged use of face masks, a current topic during the COVID-19 pandemic ("maskne"). This acneiform eruption is associated with prolonged wear and occlusion of masks, especially in healthcare workers. It must be differentiated from irritant contact dermatitis, which is another common issue due to masks, affecting the cheeks and nasal bridge due to pressure and friction, especially in association with personal history of atopic dermatitis. Masks are also responsible for allergic contact dermatitis to the elastic straps, glue, nickel [27], and formaldehyde released from the mask [28]. In summary, occupational acne due to masks must be differentiated from contact dermatitis and worsening of other processes, such as seborrheic dermatitis and rosacea [29].

Chloracne is a distinctive and often severe form of occupational acne caused by exposure to various chlorinated compounds, which may also be toxic to other organs, such as the liver and the neurologic system. Nowadays is rare, but still possible to encounter in some workers during chemical manufacturing. In the past chloracne was sometimes related to accidents, as the explosion of a reactor involved in trichlorophenol synthesis in Seveso (Italy) in 1969 [24, 30].

Chloracne may be caused both by contact of the skin with the implicated substance and by ingestion and/or inhalation of fumes. Malar region and behind the ears are the most common sites of chloracne. Lesions tend to be monomorphic, with multiple closed comedones and micro-

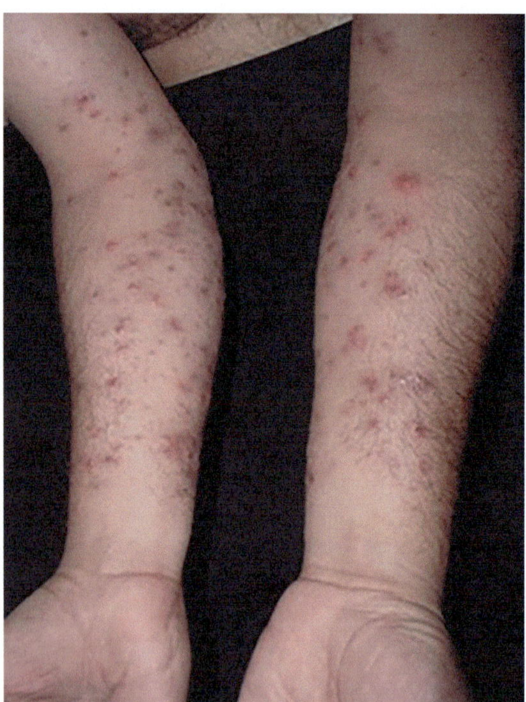

Fig. 1.4 Oil acne in a metalworker of a small workshop. An outbreak was observed in several workers due to poor hygiene and the lack of preventing measures against cutting fluids

cysts. Inflammatory lesions can occur but are less frequent. Associated with acne lesions, xerosis, hypertrichosis, melanosis, and frequent itching can be seen in chloracne [24, 30]. A special attention should be paid to possible involvement of internal organs if chloracne is suspected.

Other forms of occupational acne may be seen. Cosmetic acne presents in actors, actresses, and cosmetologists who use oily cosmetics for prolonged periods of time, causing mainly comedonal lesions on the face. Occupational acne may also appear in pharmaceutical synthesis of steroids and other medications. Sometimes acne also affects kitchen workers exposed to grease [24]. Finally, Favre-Racouchot disease presents with comedones and epidermal cysts mainly in periorbital regions. It is due to UV-light damage and can be considered also a form of occupational acne in sun-exposed workers.

Pressure- and Friction-Induced Disorders

Many jobs lead to localized pressure and friction, with the subsequent formation of callus, blisters, fissures, or hemorrhages. Normally this is solved with an appropriate protection and reducing repetitive tasks.

Athletes have dermatoses due to trauma, mainly on feet. Repeated trauma can cause erythema, edema, and separation of toenail ("jogger's toe"), hyperkeratotic patches on heel from running, splinter hemorrhages of toenails ("tennis toe"), punctate hemorrhages on heels ("black heel" in sports as basketball), blisters from friction, shin abrasions and erosions ("skier's shins"), or subcutaneous masses ("surfer's nodules") [7].

During the COVID-19 pandemic it has been observed an increased number of cases of erythema and desquamation in areas of more contact with masks and goggles, due to maintained pressure and friction of these protective equipment [29, 31].

The Koebner (isomorphic) phenomenon from occupational trauma in workers with psoriasis is very common. In fact, psoriasis on sites of trauma or friction can be the first appearance of psoriasis in a previously unaffected individual. Work-related psoriasis lesions appear very frequently

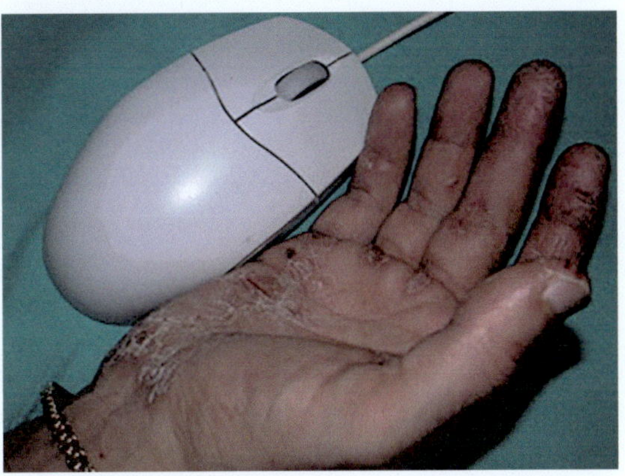

Fig. 1.5 Koebner phenomenon in an informatic with mild psoriasis elsewhere. Psoriasis was intense in areas of friction with the computer mouse

on skin of palmar surfaces where the worker applies a repetitive pressure (Fig. 1.5). Many dermatologists may overlook the cause of such lesions, and treatments tend to fail if a Koebner phenomenon is not suspected. Preventive measures for such cases include use of padded gloves and alternative methods to realize the repetitive task that is responsible for the isomorphic phenomenon. Other dermatologic diseases, such as lichen planus, vitiligo, or even eczema (post-traumatic eczema [32]), can manifest as isomorphic reactions from work-related traumas, although less frequently than psoriasis.

Vibration-Associated Disorders

A picture similar to Raynaud's phenomenon can occur in workers who manage vibrating tools, like chain saws, pneumatic hammers, and chipping tools. This entity is also known as traumatic vasospastic disease, vibration white finger, or the hand-arm vibration syndrome [17, 33]. It is characterized by paroxysmal vasospasm of the hands, with blanching accompanied by numbness and reduced sensitivity, particularly in winter. Attacks may last 1–60 min and generally resolve rewarming the hands, accompanied by hyperemia and pain. Continued vibration exposure, the attacks become more frequent, also more prolonged and in all seasons. Ultimately, ulcers can occur. Besides this vasospastic symptoms, neurological symptoms can exist (sensory and motor changes).

There is a controversy about possible carpal tunnel syndrome, bone and joint pathology associated with this syndrome [33].

The hand-arm vibration syndrome may be unilateral but is otherwise clinically indistinguishable from Raynaud's phenomenon. It is not associated with an underlying systemic connective tissue disorder [17]. There exists a latent period between the onset of exposure to vibration and the beginning of symptoms. This period is variable and is dependent upon factors, including tool vibration frequencies, total vibration exposure, hand grip strength, climatic conditions, individual susceptibility, and smoking habit [33]. Although this syndrome appears more frequently in workers managing vibrating tools in cold environments, it also exists in temperate climates [34].

Foreign Body Granulomas

The introduction through the skin of substances or products used at work can generate nodules with occasional inflammatory reaction and fistulation. Various metals can produce granulomas, such as cobalt, beryllium, aluminum, or zirconium. Barbers and hairdressers suffer sometimes this granulomatous reaction due to a cut hair, normally present in an interdigital space (Fig. 1.6) [35].

Pigmentary Disorders

Post-inflammatory hyperpigmentation due to work-related traumas, burns, or inflammatory diseases is quite often. Hyperpigmentation can result also from tattoos following injuries with coal dust, dyes, and various metals. Post-inflammatory hypopigmentation is less frequent, but it can also follow various traumas and skin diseases from work.

There are numerous chemicals that affect pigment cells, resulting in hyper- or hypopigmentation. A special concern is chemical leukoderma because it mimics idiopathic vitiligo. Most chemicals that produce this leukoderma are aromatic or aliphatic derivatives of phenols and catechols, but also mercury, arsenics, cinnamic aldehyde, p-phenylenediamine, corticosteroids, and other substances. Occupations at risk are workers in contact with glues, paints, oils, dyes,

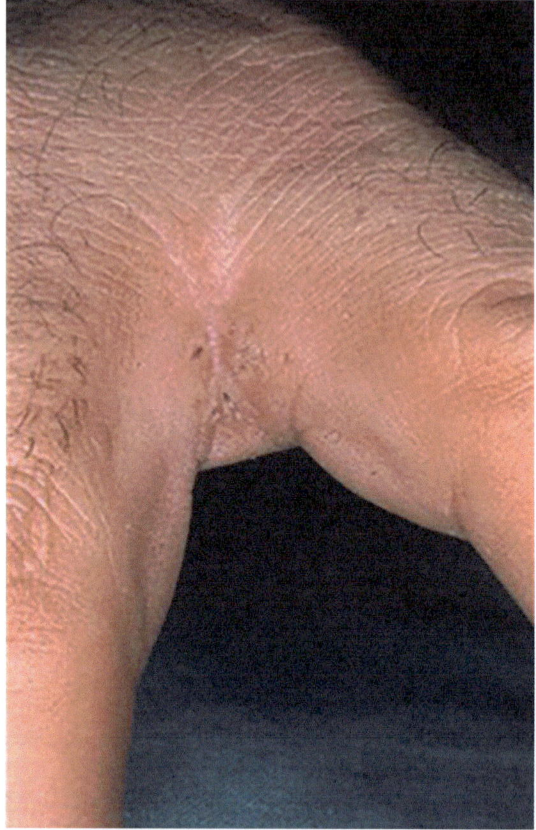

Fig. 1.6 Diverse fistulas due to hairs in the interdigital space of a dog groomer worker

and antioxidants, among others. The differentiation of chemical leukoderma from vitiligo is very important, because avoidance of the offending chemical shows a better outcome than vitiligo [36, 37].

Low Humidity-Induced Disorders

Low humidity occupational dermatosis occurs in environments of low relative humidity (35% approximately), particularly if the temperature is high. Symptoms include pruritus, urticaria, and mild eczema in different locations. The problem is solved when the average relative humidity is raised to approximately 50% [38].

Semicircular lipoatrophy could be considered a special low humidity disorder, at least indirectly. This entity presents as a subcutaneous atrophy mainly on the anterior thighs of women who work in offices and other enclosed buildings. Several hypotheses have been suggested, but the increase of electrostatic energy could be an important factor. Enclosed buildings with cooling systems generate low levels of relative humidity, and this favors the presence of an increase in electrostatic energy. Women wearing synthetic clothes are at risk, because clothing discharge is produced through the area where the pressure is highest, which usually coincides with the anterior region of the thighs. Removing electrostatic charge generation in the workplace leads to resolution of lesions [39].

Heat-Associated Disorders

Workers exposed to heat may develop different skin lesions. Miliaria can appear, especially with hot and humid environments, such as tropical climates. Intertrigo and hyperhidrosis can occur from work practice that requires safety shoes and a great deal of foot activity. Occluded feet in hot and wet environment can cause whitening and wrinkling of the sole with pain or altered sensation, fissure-like grooves, severe maceration between and under the toes, and erosions. Military combat personnel operating in tropical areas are at special risk, but these changes can appear in other workers with continuous water contact [7].

Erythema ab igne is caused by infrared radiation emitted by a heat source. It was more frequent in the past in bakers, fire fighters, and other workers with a history of chronic heat exposure. The condition is found predominantly on the inner and outer aspects of the shins [7]. Different localizations may exist if the source of heat affects other body areas. For example, working with laptops in contact with the body is a current cause of erythema ab igne on thighs, abdomen, or breasts, depending on where workers place them extensively [40]. Erythema ab igne has a potential to develop malignant lesions after many years, so prudent avoidance of triggers and follow-up in developed cases must be done.

Burns can result from different insults to the skin, like heat (thermal burns), chemicals, electricity, or radiation. Thermal burns account for almost 30% of all work-related burns. Hands, arms, and face are the most frequently affected areas. These burns are normally due to accidents in heating, cleaning machinery like grills and ovens, and hanging power tools, like torches [41]. They also can be seen on the legs from hot asphalt used by road workers [7]. Prognosis of thermal burns depends on different factors, such as the depth of the burn (first/second/third degree), the localization, the total body surface area affected, the age, or the associated inhalational injury [42].

Cold-Associated Disorders

Workers who spend long periods of time outdoors in cold climates or those who work in refrigerated rooms are prone to cold injuries, such as frostbites, perniosis, acrocyanosis, cold panniculitis, or Raynaud's phenomenon [7]. Some of these entities have a genetic background and collagen-associated diseases that must be evaluated.

Skin Cancer

Skin cancer from occupational origin may develop due to some chemicals, ultraviolet (UV) light, and ionizing radiation. It is widely suspected that the true incidence of occupational skin cancer is underreported [43]. Its etiologic factors need a chronic exposure and have a long latent period until the malignancy develops, hindering the diagnostic of occupational origin and emerging doubts on recreative activities and other non-occupational exposures.

Workers exposed to arsenic may develop skin cancer. Arsenic is used in the production of glass, the making of semiconductors, in the manufacture of insecticides and herbicides, in smelting and mining [44]. These workers may develop arsenical keratoses that are well-circumscribed keratotic papules on palms and soles. These arsenical keratoses may progress to squamous cell carcinoma. Induration, inflammation, and ulceration occur when the lesion becomes malignant [7]. Intra-epidermal carcinoma or multiple basal cell carcinomas may also be associated with arsenic exposure [44].

Polycyclic aromatic hydrocarbons are also associated with pre-malignant lesions, basal cell carcinomas, keratoacanthomas, and squamous cell carcinomas. Industries in which these chemicals are produced include gas production from coal, coke plants, aluminum production, steel and iron foundries, and exposure to diesel engine exhaust fumes [44]. Cancer as an effect of coal tar on skin has been extensively investigated. Many studies support the tumorigenic potential of coal tar but indicate the necessity for chronic exposure. Now many countries have a strict regulation about its use. Nevertheless, significant sources of exposure still exist [25]. Occurrence of squamous cell carcinoma on skin that is not chronically exposed to sunlight should raise suspicion of work-related chemical carcinogen exposure [17].

UV-light exposure occurs mainly in outdoor workers, such as farmers, sailors, or construction workers. Besides the sun, other sources of UV-light exposure must be considered, as welding [45]. Legislation about contemplating a UV-light skin cancer as an occupational disease varies from one country to another. For example, in Germany, squamous cell carcinoma or multiple actinic keratoses have been recognized as an occupational disease since 2015, but they must meet certain requirements, such as the absence of other non-occupational risk factors or the additional UV exposure of at least 40% at work [3].

Ionizing radiation is well-recognized as having the potential to cause squamous cell carcinoma and pre-malignant changes from the experiences of the first scientists and physicians to use X-rays and other radiation sources [44]. Zometimes an occupational disease, and it is important to be aware of its cancerogenic potential [46].

Skin cancer can also arise from chronic scars due to occupational accidents. Its recognition is also important for the worker, in terms of possible compensations [47].

Infections

The variety of infections that can be acquired at work is enormous, and in general parallel those acquired in the non-occupational setting. Nevertheless, some infections are characteristic of certain occupational activities and must be known by the physician.

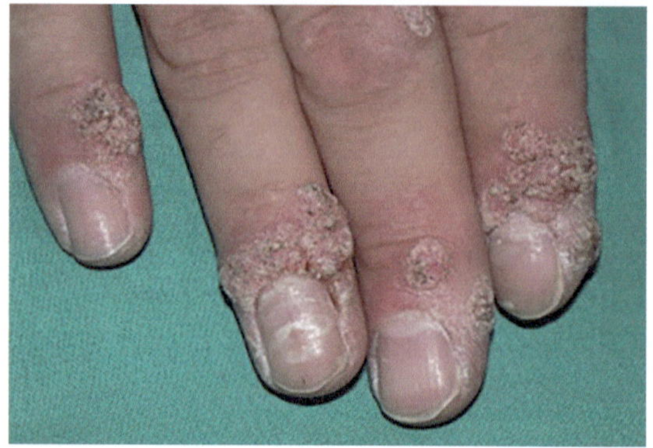

Fig. 1.7 Worker of a slaughterhouse affected with numerous viral warts during an outbreak in several workers manipulating lambs

Viral warts can be seen in meat and fish handlers (butcher's warts), sometimes with several workers affected in a workplace (Fig. 1.7). Viral warts may also appear in healthcare workers following laser surgery or cryotherapy, due to contamination [48]. Healthcare workers are also at risk of herpes simplex virus infections. Orf (ecthyma contagiosum) is caused by poxviruses that through the infection of goats and sheep can infect farmers, veterinarians, and shepherds. With clinical similarities to orf, milker's nodules are transmitted from cows.

Bacterial infections can be caused by staphylococci and streptococci acquired at workplace from diverse injuries. Anthrax, brucellosis, erysipeloid, tularemia, leptospirosis, and some mycobacteria infections can affect workers exposed to animals. Tick-borne diseases, such as Lyme disease and Rocky Mountain spotted fever, can affect outdoor and forestry workers.

Fungal infections may also have an occupational origin. Tinea pedis is more frequent with high humidity and occlusive footwear: miners, sailors, farmers, construction workers, and sportsmen are at increased risk. Candida colonization can contribute to chronic paronychia in workers exposed to water, cooking and irritants, such as dishwashing, bar work, laundering, food handling, and exposure to cutting oils [49]. Sporotrichosis occurs in miners, florists, and nurserymen. Coccidioidomycosis, mycetoma, and chromoblastomycosis may appear in agricultural and farm workers in some regions [7].

Conclusion

The study of occupational dermatosis requires a broad knowledge of general dermatology, but particularly of contact dermatitis conditions and other eczematous entities with which its differential diagnosis is usually made. The existence of a temporal relationship between work and the appearance of an occupational dermatosis is key to establishing the diagnosis. Complementary tests (mainly patch- and prick-tests) must be carried out with the allergens to which the worker is exposed. It is essential the correct differentiation between irritant and allergic responses, as well as the establishment of the relevance of the sensitizations. It should not be forgotten that other entities, such as some forms of acne, psoriasis, or vitiligo, are many times caused or aggravated by work.

References

1. Noojin RO. Brief history of industrial dermatology. AMA Arch Derm Syphilol. 1954;70:723–31.
2. Alchorne Ade O, Alchorne MM, Silva MM. Occupational dermatosis. An Bras Dermatol. 2010;85:137–47.
3. Diepgen TL. New developments in occupational dermatology. J Dtsch Dermatol Ges. 2016;14:875–89.
4. Work-related Diseases and Occupational Diseases: The ILO International List. https://www.iloencyclopaedia.org/part-iii-48230/topics-in-workers-compensation-systems/item/355-work-related-diseases-and-occupational-diseases-the-ilo-international-list. Accessed 3 Oct 2021.
5. Alfonso JH, Bauer A, Bensefa-Colas L, Boman A, Bubas M, Constandt L, et al. Minimum standards on prevention, diagnosis and treatment of occupational and work-related skin diseases in Europe - position paper of the COST Action StanDerm (TD 1206). J Eur Acad Dermatol Venereol. 2017;31(Suppl 4):31–43.
6. Mathias CG. Contact dermatitis and workers' compensation: criteria for establishing occupational causation and aggravation. J Am Acad Dermatol. 1989;20:842–8.
7. Samitz MH. Occupational dermatoses. Clin Dermatol. 1983;1:25–34.
8. Géraut C. Les dermatoses professionnelles [Occupational dermatoses]. Rev Prat. 1987;37:2079–91.
9. Beltrani VS. Occupational dermatoses. Curr Opin Allergy Clin Immunol. 2003;3:115–23.
10. Nicholson PJ, Llewellyn D, English JS; Guidelines Development Group. Evidence-based guidelines for the prevention, identification and management of occupational contact dermatitis and urticaria. Contact Dermatitis 2010;63:177–186.
11. Aalto-Korte K, Koskela K, Pesonen M. 12-year data on dermatologic cases in the Finnish Register of Occupational Diseases I: distribution of different diagnoses and main causes of allergic contact dermatitis. Contact Dermatitis. 2020;82:337–42.
12. DeKoven JG, DeKoven BM, Warshaw EM, Mathias CGT, Taylor JS, Sasseville D et al. Occupational contact dermatitis: retrospective analysis of North American Contact Dermatitis Group Data, 2001 to 2016. J Am Acad Dermatol. 2021. https://doi.org/10.1016/j.jaad.2021.03.042.
13. Santarossa M, Mauro M, Belloni Fortina A, Corradin MT, Larese FF. Occupational contact dermatitis in Triveneto: analysis of patch test data of the North Eastern Italian Database from 1996 to 2016. Contact Dermatitis. 2020;82:370–9.
14. Bensefa-Colas L, Telle-Lamberton M, Paris C, Faye S, Stocks SJ, Luc A, Momas I, French National Network of Occupational Disease Vigilance Prevention (RNV3P), et al. Occupational allergic contact dermatitis and major allergens in France: temporal trends for the period 2001–2010. Br J Dermatol. 2014;171:1375–85.
15. Bhatia R, Sharma VK. Occupational dermatoses: an Asian perspective. Indian J Dermatol Venereol Leprol. 2017;83:525–35.
16. Clark SC, Zirwas MJ. Management of occupational dermatitis. Dermatol Clin. 2009;27:365–83.
17. Mathias CG. Occupational dermatoses. J Am Acad Dermatol. 1988;19:1107–14.
18. Amaro C, Goossens A. Immunological occupational contact urticaria and contact dermatitis from proteins: a review. Contact Dermatitis. 2008;58:67–75.
19. Gimenez-Arnau A, Maurer M, De La Cuadra J, Maibach H. Immediate contact skin reactions, an update of Contact Urticaria, Contact Urticaria Syndrome and Protein Contact Dermatitis -- "A Never Ending Story". Eur J Dermatol. 2010;20:552–62.
20. Pesonen M, Koskela K, Aalto-Korte K. Contact urticaria and protein contact dermatitis in the Finnish Register of Occupational Diseases in a period of 12 years. Contact Dermatitis. 2020;83:1–7.
21. Doutre MS. Occupational contact urticaria and protein contact dermatitis. Eur J Dermatol. 2005;15:419–24.
22. Raulf M. Current state of occupational latex allergy. Curr Opin Allergy Clin Immunol. 2020;20:112–6.
23. Hjorth N, Roed-Petersen J. Occupational protein contact dermatitis in food handlers. Contact Dermatitis. 1976;2:28–42.
24. Kokelj F. Occupational acne. Clin Dermatol. 1992;10:213–7.
25. Moustafa GA, Xanthopoulou E, Riza E, Linos A. Skin disease after occupational dermal exposure to coal tar: a review of the scientific literature. Int J Dermatol. 2015;54:868–79.

26. Mills OH Jr, Kligman A. Acne mechanica. Arch Dermatol. 1975;111:481–3.

27. Schwensen JFB, Simonsen AB, Zachariae C, Johansen JD. Facial dermatoses in health care professionals induced by the use of protective masks during the COVID-19 pandemic. Contact Dermatitis. 2021. https://doi.org/10.1111/cod.13948.

28. Yu J, Chen JK, Mowad CM, Reeder M, Hylwa S, Chisolm S, et al. Occupational dermatitis to facial personal protective equipment in health care workers: a systematic review. J Am Acad Dermatol. 2021;84:486–94.

29. Ferguson FJ, Street G, Cunningham L, White IR, McFadden JP, Williams J. Occupational dermatology in the time of the COVID-19 pandemic: a report of experience from London and Manchester, UK. Br J Dermatol. 2021;184:180–2.

30. Wattanakrai P, Taylor JS. Occupational and environmental acne. In: Rustemeyer T, Elsner P, John SM, Maibach HI, editors. Kanerva's occupational dermatology. 2nd ed. Berlin, Heidelberg: Springer-Verlag; 2012. p. 333–48.

31. Lan J, Song Z, Miao X, Li H, Li Y, Dong L, et al. Skin damage among health care workers managing coronavirus disease-2019. J Am Acad Dermatol. 2020;82:1215–6.

32. Mathias CG. Post-traumatic eczema. Dermatol Clin. 1988;6:35–42.

33. Chetter IC, Kent PJ, Kester RC. The hand arm vibration syndrome: a review. Cardiovasc Surg. 1998;6:1–9.

34. Wei N, Lin H, Chen T, Xiao B, Yan M, Lang L, et al. The hand-arm vibration syndrome associated with the grinding of handheld workpieces in a subtropical environment. Int Arch Occup Environ Health. 2021;94:773–81.

35. Alomar A, Conde-Salazar L, Heras F. Barbers' dermatoses (Barber's hair sinus). In: Rustemeyer T, Elsner P, John SM, Maibach HI, editors. Kanerva's occupational dermatology. 2nd ed. Berlin, Heidelberg: Springer-Verlag; 2012. p. 1277–9.

36. Ghosh S, Mukhopadhyay S. Chemical leucoderma: a clinico-aetiological study of 864 cases in the perspective of a developing country. Br J Dermatol. 2009;160:40–7.

37. Bonamonte D, Vestita M, Romita P, Filoni A, Foti C, Angelini G. Chemical leukoderma. Dermatitis. 2016;27:90–9.

38. Rycroft RJ, Smith WD. Low humidity occupational dermatoses. Contact Dermatitis. 1980;6:488–92.

39. Linares-García Valdecasas R, Cuerda-Galindo E, Bargueño JR, Naranjo Garcia P, Vogelfrang-Garncarz D, Palomar-Gallego MA. Semicircular lipoatrophy: an electrostatic hypothesis. Dermatology. 2015;230:222–7.

40. Lewis P, Wild U, Erren TC. Working from home during and after COVID-19: watch out for erythema ab igne when using laptops. Br J Gen Pract. 2020;30(70):404.

41. Reichard AA, Konda S, Jackson LL. Occupational burns treated in emergency departments. Am J Ind Med. 2015;58:290–8.

42. Colohan SM. Predicting prognosis in thermal burns with associated inhalational injury: a systematic review of prognostic factors in adult burn victims. J Burn Care Res. 2010;31:529–39.

43. Carøe TK, Ebbehøj NE, Wulf HC, Agner T. Occupational skin cancer may be underreported. Dan Med J. 2013;60:A4624.

44. Gawkrodger DJ. Occupational skin cancers. Occup Med (Lond). 2004;54:458–63.

45. Falcone LM, Zeidler-Erdely PC. Skin cancer and welding. Clin Exp Dermatol. 2019;44:130–4.

46. Sugita K, Yamamoto O, Suenaga Y. [Seven cases of radiation-induced cutaneous squamous cell carcinoma]. J UOEH. 2000;e22:259–67.

47. Broding HC, Köllner A, Brüning T, Fartasch M. Maligne Hauttumoren in beruflich verursachten Narben [Cutaneous malignancies in occupationally-induced scars]. Hautarzt. 2011;62:757–63.

48. Nori S, Greene MA, Schrager HM, Falanga V. Infectious occupational exposures in dermatology—a review of risks and prevention measures. I. For all dermatologists. J Am Acad Dermatol. 2005;53:1010–9.

49. Harries MJ, Lear JT. Occupational skin infections. Occup Med (Lond). 2004;54:441–9.

Epidemiology and Burden of Occupational Skin Diseases

Richard Brans

R. Brans (✉)
Department of Dermatology, Environmental Medicine and Health Theory, University of Osnabrück, Osnabrück, Germany

Institute for Interdisciplinary Dermatologic Prevention and Rehabilitation (iDerm) at the University of Osnabrück, Osnabrück, Germany
e-mail: rbrans@uni-osnabrueck.de; rbrans@uos.de

Introduction

In many workplaces, the skin is exposed to various hazards causing skin disorders. Work-related skin diseases (WRSD) include any skin disorders which are wholly or partially caused or made worse by work or workplace activity. Usually, multiple causes are involved, including factors of the work environment. Occupational skin diseases (OSD) are directly caused by work and fulfil all given criteria for recognition of an occupational disease according to the official national list of occupational diseases which differ from country to country [1]. However, no official international agreement on definitions for WRSD and OSD exists and differentiation between WRSD and OSD is often not clear-cut [1]. Therefore, in the following WRSD and OSD will be referred to as OSD only.

The most relevant hazards causing OSD are presented in Table 2.1 and include wet work, exposure to irritants and/or allergens, biological hazards (e.g. bacteria, viruses, fungi, parasites) and physical factors (e.g. ultraviolet (UV) radiation, ionizing radiation, mechanical strain, heat, cold). Common OSD include contact dermatitis, contact urticaria, acne/folliculitis, pigmentation changes, skin infections, mechanical skin diseases and skin cancer. Apart from exclusively occupational dermatoses, occupational activities can also aggravate pre-existing endogenous dermatoses, including acne, atopic dermatitis and psoriasis.

Important sources of epidemiological data on OSD are occupational disease registries, administrative data, case series of patients and cross-sectional studies in one or more occupational groups. As definitions for OSD, access to health professionals as well as criteria for reporting and recognizing OSD differs in the various countries, national notification rates vary greatly which leads to incomplete epidemiological data. In addition, a large proportion of individuals suffering from mild OSD symptoms do not come to medical attention [2]. In observational studies focusing on specific occupational groups, the ascertainment of cases varies from medical examination to self-administered questionnaires which also has an impact on the accuracy of data [3]. Therefore, it is difficult to determine the true occurrence and burden of OSD. There are clear indications that underdiagnosing and underreporting are common and thus, the magnitude of the problem is underestimated.

In the following, there will be a focus on the two most common OSD: Occupational contact

© The Author(s), under exclusive license to Springer Nature Switzerland AG 2023
A. M. Giménez-Arnau, H. I. Maibach (eds.), *Handbook of Occupational Dermatoses*, Updates in Clinical Dermatology, https://doi.org/10.1007/978-3-031-22727-1_2

Table 2.1 Causes of occupational skin diseases

Cause (examples)	Skin disease (examples)
Chemicals	
• Water/moisture/occlusion.	• Irritant contact dermatitis.
	• Worsening of pre-existing dermatosis.
• Irritant chemicals.	• Irritant contact dermatitis.
	• Worsening of pre-existing dermatosis.
• Contact allergens.	• Allergic contact dermatitis.
	• Protein contact dermatitis/contact urticaria.
• Acnegenic agents (e.g. oil, halogenated aromatic hydrocarbons, coal tar).	• Acne/folliculitis.
• Tar, tar products.	• Skin cancer.
• Arsenic.	• Skin cancer.
	• Keratoderma.
	• Hyperpigmentation.
• Monobenzylether of hydroquinone, alkylphenols, catechols.	• Hypopigmentation, leukoderma.
• Polychlorinated biphenyl, dioxins, azo dyes, various metals (silver, mercury, bismuth).	• Hyperpigmentation.
Infectious pathogens	
• Sarcoptes scabiei.	• Scabies.
• Erysipelothrix rhusiopathiae.	• Erysipeloid.
• Mycobacterium marinum.	• Fish tank granuloma.
• Borrelia burgdorferi.	• Erythema chronicum migrans.
• Trichophytia verrucosa.	• Trichophytia profunda.
• Paravaccinia virus.	• Milker's nodules.
Physical factors	
• Natural UV radiation.	• Skin cancer.
	• Phototoxic/photoallergic contact dermatitis.
	• Urticaria.
	• Worsening of pre-existing dermatosis.
• Ionizing radiation.	• Radiodermatitis.
	• Skin cancer.
• Mechanical trauma, pressure, friction.	• Irritant contact dermatitis.
	• Worsening of pre-existing dermatosis.
	• Hyperkeratosis, callus.
	• Acne.
	• Urticaria.
• Heat.	• Erythema ab igne.
	• Miliaria.
• Cold.	• Perniones/frostbite.
	• Cold panniculitis.
	• Urticaria.
• Vibration.	• Raynaud's disease.

dermatitis (OCD) and non-melanoma skin cancer (NMSC) arising from occupational exposure to solar ultraviolet (UV) radiation.

Occupational Contact Dermatitis (OCD)

Epidemiology

OCD is the most common OSD accounting for 70–95% of all cases [4, 5]. In many countries, OCD ranks first among all notified occupational diseases. In 2019, of more than 80,000 notified occupational diseases in Germany, 19,883 were skin diseases (except for skin cancer and some skin infections) and consisted mainly of OCD [6]. Depending on the national criteria for recognition, OCD belongs also to the most commonly recognized occupational diseases. In Denmark, for instance, OCD is the most frequently recognized occupational disease, comprising around one-third of all recognized occupational diseases [7]. The annual incidence of registered OCD in some countries is around 5–19 cases per 10,000 full-time workers and higher in high-risk occupations [3, 4, 8–10].

Women are usually more frequently affected [3, 11]. For instance, 67.3% of all individuals with recognized OCD notified in Denmark between 2010 and 2015 were female (n = 6020) [7]. Differences between the sexes are mainly explained by their differing distribution in occupations at risk and thus, differing types and extents of exposures to skin hazards. The onset of OCD is often early in life with an average age of 25 to 36 years [10, 11]. It frequently starts during training or within the first few months of working in high-risk occupations [3, 11]. In 80–90% of cases, OCD affects the hands which are mainly exposed to skin hazards [11]. The 1-year prevalence of hand dermatitis in the general population is approximately 9% [12] and at least twice as high in high-risk occupations. Studies, e.g., in healthcare workers found point-prevalence rates of hand dermatitis varying from 20 to 31% [13, 14].

The frequency of OCD varies considerably among professions. At high risk are particularly

Table 2.2 Common high-risk occupations for occupational contact dermatitis

Cleaner
Construction worker
Dental technician
Florist
Food handler (e.g. chef, baker)
Gardener
Healthcare worker (e.g. nurse)
Hairdresser and barber
Metalworker
Motor mechanic
Painter
Printer
Tile setter
Woodworker

hairdressers, cleaners, chefs/food handlers, florists, metal workers, construction workers, dental technicians aand healthcare workers (Table 2.2) [7, 10, 11, 15, 16]. In a recent Danish study of individuals with recognized OCD notified in Denmark between 2010 and 2015, the highest annual incidence rate was found for hairdressers (136 per 10,000 workers) [7]. This was higher than the annual incidence rate of notified cases for hairdressers in Northern Bavaria between 1990 and 1999 (97.4 per 10,000 workers) [10]. High annual incidence rates in Denmark were also recorded for leather tanning and processing workers (99 per 10,000 workers), beauticians (76 per 10,000 workers), bakers (59 per 10,000 workers), florists (57 per 10,000 workers), and glue manufacture workers (52 per 10,000 workers). Other highly affected professions were healthcare workers (12 per 10,000 workers) and metalworkers (11 per 10,000) [7]. Their annual incidence rates were similar in Northern Bavaria from 1990–1999 (7.3 and 9 cases per 10,000 workers, respectively) [10]. In a tertiary referral clinic for occupational dermatology in Australia, data of 2894 patients seen between 1993 and 2010 were analysed. Occupational groups with the highest annual incidence of OSD (mainly OCD) were the hair and beauty professions (7.0 per 10,000 workers) followed by machine and plant operators (3.8 per 10,000 workers) and healthcare workers (2.1 per 10,000 workers) [16].

Irritants and allergens causing OCD are often highly specific for a particular profession. In general, irritant contact dermatitis (ICD) is more common than allergic contact dermatitis (ACD) [11]. In the Australian data set, 44% suffered from irritant contact dermatitis (ICD) and 33% from allergic contact dermatitis (ACD) [16]. In a registry study from Germany, the rate of ICD was also high (75%) [4]. Occupational ICD is mainly related to wet work, detergents, dirty work, cutting fluids and oils [17]. Occupations particularly at risk for ACD are painters and varnishers, dental technicians, construction workers, beauticians and hairdressers [10, 15]. In a study of the European Surveillance System on Contact Allergies (ESSCA) analysing patch test data from 2002 to 2010, the most common jobs affected by ACD were hairdressers, nurses, precision workers in metal and related materials, toolmakers and related trades [18]. The allergens which had at least double the risk of OCD included thiurams, epoxy resin and antimicrobials including methylchloroisothiazolinone (MCI)/methylisothiazolinone (MI), methyldibromo glutaronitrile, and formaldehyde [18]. Also other studies confirm that common causes of occupational ACD are epoxy chemicals, rubber, preservatives/biocides, metals, (meth)acrylates and hairdressing chemicals [17, 19, 20].

Burden

The severity of OCD varies and ranges from minor to disabling major lesions. A mild degree of OCD is often accepted as normal and may not cause any relevant burden. However, severe lesions and the often relapsing, chronic course of the disease lead to considerable occupational, domestic, social and psychological implications. Studies with follow-ups over several years revealed that contact dermatitis has a poor prognosis with healing in only half or fewer than half of the patients [21]. In a Finnish study, OCD had healed in 40% of patients 7–14 years after diagnosis [22]. A recent study from Denmark found that only 19% with recognized OCD reported complete healing 4–5 years later [23]. OCD is usually complicated to cure if the affected individual remains in the professions and is persistently exposed to causative irritants and/or allergens. The prognosis additionally depends on the severity of symptoms, the period of follow-up, and the intensity of exposure. ACD is thought to be associated with a worse prognosis than ICD, but may depend on the possibilities to avoid the causative allergen [22, 24].

OCD is usually located on the hands, and thus, on a highly visible area of the body causing difficulties in social interaction. Moreover, manual work and daily life activities could be impaired. It was demonstrated that OCD frequently leads to finger joint restrictions reducing productivity [25]. All this causes a considerable adverse impact on the quality of life and the work-life of the individual [26]. It is well known that health-related quality of life is significantly impaired in patients with OCD [27–29]. In addition, a study in individuals with occupational hand dermatitis found that 20% had a positive anxiety score and 14% a positive depression score [30].

OCD has significant consequences on the work performance. Up to 50% of affected individuals lose time from work due to OCD [26]. In a study from Germany, 62.9% of 151 workers with occupational hand dermatitis reported work absenteeism because of the disease in the year before entering a tertiary prevention programme. The average amount was 76.4 days off work. 11.5% had been on sick leave for 6 months or longer [31]. In a Swedish study, 48% of individuals with OCD had been on sick leave due to OCD for at least one period of 7 days in a 12-year follow-up period [32]. About 20% of workers with recognized OCD from Denmark reported an annual work absenteeism of >5 weeks due to OCD [33]. Moreover, a considerable number of workers with OCD lose their job or change their job because of OCD, particularly those with severe and persistent disease [26]. In a Danish study, 23% of workers with recognized occupational hand dermatitis reported to have lost their job at least once during the past 12 months [33]. Another study from Denmark revealed that 4–5 years after recognition of occupational hand dermatitis/contact urticaria, 51.3% were no longer in the same profession: 32.5% had changed profession and 18.8% were no longer employed [34]. In a Finnish study, 34% of patients with occupational hand dermatitis had changed their job because of the disease according to a follow-up questionnaire 7–14 years after diagnosis [22]. Chances of remaining in the same occupation depend on the profession. Rates of leaving the profession are particularly high among hairdressers with OCD. A study from Denmark showed that 44.3% of hairdressers had left the profession after an average of 8.4 years, 45.5% because of hand dermatitis [35].

The total economic impact of OCD is considered very high. However, studies assessing the costs of OCD are scarce. The following costs must be taken into consideration: direct costs (for medical care), indirect costs (loss of productivity due to lost workdays), as well as costs for re-training, rehabilitation and worker's compensation [36]. Diepgen et al. estimated the cost of illness for 151 patients with occupational hand dermatitis in the year before entering a tertiary prevention programme in Germany [31]. Annual direct and indirect costs were calculated as €8799 per patient, of which 70% were related to indirect costs. Another German study estimated the costs in a bigger cohort of patients ($n = 1041$) with OSD (mainly OCD) entering a tertiary prevention programme. Estimated direct and indirect costs per person in the year before were €383 and €4865, respectively [37]. OCD does not only cause significant societal costs, but has also an adverse impact on the personal economic situation of affected individuals. A recent Danish study analysing data of all individuals with recognized OCD notified between 2010 and 2015 ($n = 8940$) demonstrated that the average degree of employment during the 2 years prior compared to the 2 years following notification fell from 123 to 114 workhours/month [7]. This corresponded to an average annual loss of income per worker of approximately €1570. According to a survey from Sweden, OCD caused worsening of the personal economic situation in 32% of workers. Of these, 45% reported loss of income of ≥25% [32]. Also in a Finnish study, 23% of patients with OCD reported worsening of their economic situation [22].

Non-Melanoma Skin Cancer (NMSC) Arising from Occupational Exposure to Solar Ultraviolet (UV) Radiation

Epidemiology

Non-melanoma skin cancer (NMSC) is by far the world's most frequently diagnosed cancer with an incidence of 7.7 million cases in 2017 [38], comprising about one third of the global incidence of malignancies [39, 40]. NMSC is composed of two distinct subtypes: cutaneous squamous cell carcinoma (SCC) and basal cell carcinoma (BCC). The incidence of BCC is on average double that of SCC [41]. Exposure to solar UV radiation is the most important risk factor for the development of NMSC causing higher incidence rates in fair-skinned populations [41, 42]. The relationship between SCC and cumulative sun exposure is well established. For BCC, the situation is more complex. Probably intermittent strong sun exposure is also relevant. SCC is primarily located on body sites most exposed to the sun, such as the face, ears, scalp and back of the hands. BCC is frequently located on the head and neck, but also commonly located on the trunk. The emission of UV radiation reaching the earth's surface depends among other factors on elevation, latitude, altitude and weather conditions. Thus, the incidence of NMSC varies widely by geographical location [41, 43]. Many population-based cancer registries worldwide do not report NMSC. Moreover, often only primary tumours are registered, while consecutive tumours are not. Therefore, the true incidence of NMSC is usually underestimated. In 2012, 3.3 million people in the USA were diagnosed with NMSC. However, as many of them were diagnosed with more than one NMSC, the total number of NMSC rather reached 5.8 million cases [44]. The highest incidence for NMSC is found in Australia (>1000/100000 person-years for BCC) [41]. In Europe, there are approximately 2,000,000 diagnoses of NMSC (actinic keratoses excluded) per year [44]. The incidence increases with age and thus, the majority of NMSC are diagnosed in people over 40 years old [44].

Solar radiation during outdoor work is considered to be the most common occupational exposure to carcinogens within the EU. Operational definitions of outdoor work vary between countries [43]. According to the European Agency for Safety and Health at Work are outdoor workers those who spend >75% of their working time outdoors [43]. Based on this definition, 14.5 million workers in the EU are estimated to be exposed to solar UV radiation. The majority of these (90%) is male [44, 45]. Occupational sectors with a high amount of outdoor work include agriculture, forestry, horticulture, construction, maintenance work, seafaring, fishing and public services. It is well established that outdoor workers are exposed to higher UV exposure dosages than indoor workers or the rest of the population resulting in a substantially increased risk of developing SCC and BCC [43, 45–48]. This is different for cutaneous malignant melanoma (CMM) which is a less common but more fatal type of skin cancer. Solar UV exposure is also among the most relevant risk factors for CMM. However, rather intermittent sun exposure, including repeated sunburns in early life, than high cumulative sun exposure has been associated with CMM [44]. In only a few studies, an increased risk for CMM has been found for outdoor work. Most studies show a negative or no association instead [44, 45, 49]. Hence, there is overall a lack of evidence for an association between CMM and outdoor work. Due to most outdoor workers being men, occupational NMSC is more common in men [50]. Because of the cumulative damage and the long latency period between exposure and development of NMSC, it is more common in older age groups with the highest rates in those aged 60 and above. Thus, it usually occurs in already retired workers [50].

The number of epidemiological studies focusing on NMSC in outdoor workers is still limited as many cancer registries do not report NMSC or do not include information about a patient's profession [51]. Moreover, as mentioned before, consecutive tumours are often not registered. This leads to incomplete data and results in a vast underreporting of the burden of NMSC arising from occupational solar UV radiation [51].

To date, NMSC as a result of UV radiation is a recognized occupational disease for outdoor workers only in some countries, including Australia and Canada [51]. In 2011, an estimated 5.3% of the 53,696 newly diagnosed cases of BCC and 9.2% of the 18,549 newly diagnosed cases of SCC in Canada were attributable to occupational solar UV radiation exposure [50]. In Europe, NMSC as a result of solar UV radiation is a recognized occupational disease in only seven countries. However, in many of them it is rarely reported or recognized [52]. In Denmark, for instance, only 36 cases of skin cancer had been recognized between 2000 and 2009 [53]. In 2015, solar UV-inflicted SCC (including multiple actinic keratoses and Bowen's disease) has been introduced as recognized occupational disease in Germany. Since then numbers of notifications have been very high (> 9000 reported cases per year) and have become the second most frequently recognized occupational disease in Germany [43].

Burden

NMSC is characterized by a life-long chronicity with usually abundant newly forming lesions resulting in a continuous need for treatment. As older age groups are primarily affected and life expectancies increase, burden of NMSC is likely to increase in the future [51]. Due to the chronicity of the disease, NMSC patients often undergo repeatedly surgery. Often, NMSC are located on highly visible areas, including face, ears and hands. Therefore, patients may suffer from the appearance of the disease as well as cosmetic and functional sequelae after surgical removals. Thus, NMSC patients endure a considerable reduction in quality of life [54, 55].

Risk of metastasis and related mortality is low but higher in SCC than BCC [44]. Despite rarely fatal, the burden of NMSC is significant due to the high incidence, treatment costs and adverse impact on quality of life [39]. The Global Burden of Disease project estimated that 1.3 million disability-adjusted life years lost in 2017 were attributable to NMSC [38]. The average annual cost for treatment of NMSC, regardless of its causation, in the USA between 2007 and 2011 amounted to USD $4.8 billion [56]. In Australia, NMSC comprises 75% of all cancers accounting for costs of AUD $511 million related to diagnosis, treatment and pathology in 2010 [57]. There is a lack of studies assessing the economic burden of NMSC attributable to occupational exposure to solar UV radiation. For Canada, the estimated direct and indirect costs of occupational solar UV-inflicted NMSC cases in 2011 were CAD $28.9 million [50]. 70% of costs were associated with direct costs and 30% with indirect costs. From this result, the economic burden of occupational NMSC in 2011 in the USA was estimated at CAD $1.7 billion [50]. The annual direct healthcare costs in Europe are estimated to range from €341 to €853 million per year [51].

References

1. Mahler V, Aalto-Korte K, Alfonso JH, Bakker JG, Bauer A, Bensefa-Colas L, et al. Occupational skin diseases: actual state analysis of patient management pathways in 28 European countries. J Eur Acad Dermatol Venereol. 2017;31(Suppl 4):12–30.

2. Smit HA, Burdorf A, Coenraads PJ. Prevalence of hand dermatitis in different occupations. Int J Epidemiol. 1993;22(2):288–93.

3. Diepgen TL. Occupational skin-disease data in Europe. Int Arch Occup Environ Health. 2003;76(5):331–8.

4. Dickel H, Bruckner T, Bernhard-Klimt C, Koch T, Scheidt R, Diepgen TL. Surveillance scheme for occupational skin disease in the Saarland, FRG. First report from BKH-S. Contact Dermatitis. 2002;46(4):197–206.

5. Turner S, Carder M, van Tongeren M, McNamee R, Lines S, Hussey L, et al. The incidence of occupational skin disease as reported to the health and occupation reporting (THOR) network between 2002 and 2005. Br J Dermatol. 2007;157(4):713–22.

6. Herloch V, Elsner P. The (new) occupational disease no. 5101: "severe or recurrent skin diseases". J Dtsch Dermatol Ges. 2021;19(5):720–41. https://doi.org/10.1111/ddg.14537.

7. Dietz JB, Menne T, Meyer HW, Viskum S, Flyvholm MA, Ahrensboll-Friis U, et al. Degree of employment, sick leave, and costs following notification of occupational contact dermatitis-a register-based study. Contact Dermatitis. 2021;84(4):224–35. https://doi.org/10.1111/cod.13719.

8. Kanerva L, Jolanki R, Toikkanen J, Tarvainen K, Estlander T. Statistics on occupational dermatoses in Finland. Curr Probl Dermatol. 1995;23:28–40. https://doi.org/10.1159/000424295.

9. Keegel T, Moyle M, Dharmage S, Frowen K, Nixon R. The epidemiology of occupational contact dermatitis (1990–2007): a systematic review. Int J Dermatol. 2009;48(6):571–8.

10. Dickel H, Kuss O, Blesius CR, Schmidt A, Diepgen TL. Occupational skin diseases in northern Bavaria between 1990 and 1999: a population-based study. Br J Dermatol. 2001;145(3):453–62.

11. Skoet R, Olsen J, Mathiesen B, Iversen L, Johansen JD, Agner T. A survey of occupational hand eczema in Denmark. Contact Dermatitis. 2004;51(4):159–66.

12. Quaade AS, Simonsen AB, Halling AS, Thyssen JP, Johansen JD. Prevalence, incidence, and severity of hand eczema in the general population - a systematic review and meta-analysis. Contact Dermatitis. 2021;84(6):361–74. https://doi.org/10.1111/cod.13804.

13. Nichol K, Copes R, Kersey K, Eriksson J, Holness DL. Screening for hand dermatitis in healthcare workers: comparing workplace screening with dermatologist photo screening. Contact Dermatitis. 2019;80(6):374–81. https://doi.org/10.1111/cod.13231.

14. Campion KM. A survey of occupational skin disease in UK health care workers. Occup Med (Lond). 2015;65(1):29–31. https://doi.org/10.1093/occmed/kqu170.

15. Aalto-Korte K, Koskela K, Pesonen M. 12-year data on skin diseases in the Finnish register of occupational diseases II: risk occupations with special reference to allergic contact dermatitis. Contact Dermatitis. 2020;82(6):343–9. https://doi.org/10.1111/cod.13510.

16. Cahill JL, Williams JD, Matheson MC, Palmer AM, Burgess JA, Dharmage SC, et al. Occupational skin disease in Victoria, Australia. Australas J Dermatol. 2016;57(2):108–14. https://doi.org/10.1111/ajd.12375.

17. Aalto-Korte K, Koskela K, Pesonen M. 12-year data on dermatologic cases in the Finnish register of occupational diseases I: distribution of different diagnoses and main causes of allergic contact dermatitis. Contact Dermatitis. 2020;82(6):337–42. https://doi.org/10.1111/cod.13488.

18. Pesonen M, Jolanki R, Larese Filon F, Wilkinson M, Krecisz B, Kiec-Swierczynska M, et al. Patch test results of the European baseline series among patients with occupational contact dermatitis across Europe - analyses of the European surveillance system on contact allergy network, 2002–2010. Contact Dermatitis. 2015;72(3):154–63.

19. Caroe TK, Ebbehoj N, Agner T. A survey of exposures related to recognized occupational contact dermatitis in Denmark in 2010. Contact Derma-

titis. 2014;70(1):56–62. https://doi.org/10.1111/cod.12134.

20. Bensefa-Colas L, Telle-Lamberton M, Paris C, Faye S, Stocks SJ, Luc A, et al. Occupational allergic contact dermatitis and major allergens in France: temporal trends for the period 2001–2010. Br J Dermatol. 2014;171(6):1375–85.

21. Hogan DJ, Dannaker CJ, Maibach HI. The prognosis of contact dermatitis. J Am Acad Dermatol. 1990;23(2 Pt 1):300–7.

22. Mälkonen T, Alanko K, Jolanki R, Luukkonen R, Aalto-Korte K, Lauerma A, et al. Long-term follow-up study of occupational hand eczema. Br J Dermatol. 2010;163(5):999–1006.

23. Olesen CM, Agner T, Ebbehoj NE, Caroe TK. Factors influencing prognosis for occupational hand eczema: new trends. Br J Dermatol. 2019;181(6):1280–6. https://doi.org/10.1111/bjd.17870.

24. Meding B, Swanbeck G. Consequences of having hand eczema. Contact Dermatitis. 1990;23(1):6–14.

25. Holness DL, Beaton D, Harniman E, DeKoven J, Skotnicki S, Nixon R, et al. Hand and upper extremity function in workers with hand dermatitis. Dermatitis. 2013;24(3):131–6. https://doi.org/10.1097/DER.0b013e3182910416.

26. Nicholson PJ, Llewellyn D, English JS. Evidence-based guidelines for the prevention, identification and management of occupational contact dermatitis and urticaria. Contact Dermatitis. 2010;63(4):177–86.

27. Cvetkovski RS, Zachariae R, Jensen H, Olsen J, Johansen JD, Agner T. Quality of life and depression in a population of occupational hand eczema patients. Contact Dermatitis. 2006;54(2):106–11.

28. Matterne U, Apfelbacher CJ, Soder S, Diepgen TL, Weisshaar E. Health-related quality of life in health care workers with work-related skin diseases. Contact Dermatitis. 2009;61(3):145–51.

29. Chernyshov PV, John SM, Tomas-Aragones L, Goncalo M, Svensson A, Bewley A, et al. Quality of life measurement in occupational skin diseases. Position paper of the European academy of dermatology and venereology task forces on quality of life and patient oriented outcomes and occupational skin disease. J Eur Acad Dermatol Venereol. 2020;34(9):1924–31. https://doi.org/10.1111/jdv.16742.

30. Boehm D, Schmid-Ott G, Finkeldey F, John SM, Dwinger C, Werfel T, et al. Anxiety, depression and impaired health-related quality of life in patients with occupational hand eczema. Contact Dermatitis. 2012;67(4):184–92.

31. Diepgen TL, Scheidt R, Weisshaar E, John SM, Hieke K. Cost of illness from occupational hand eczema in Germany. Contact Dermatitis. 2013;69(2):99–106.

32. Meding B, Lantto R, Lindahl G, Wrangsjo K, Bengtsson B. Occupational skin disease in Sweden—a 12-year follow-up. Contact Dermatitis. 2005;53(6):308–13.

33. Cvetkovski RS, Rothman KJ, Olsen J, Mathiesen B, Iversen L, Johansen JD, et al. Relation between diagnoses on severity, sick leave and loss of job among patients with occupational hand eczema. Br J Dermatol. 2005;152(1):93–8.

34. Caroe TK, Ebbehoj NE, Bonde JP, Agner T. Occupational hand eczema and/or contact urticaria: factors associated with change of profession or not remaining in the workforce. Contact Dermatitis. 2018;78(1):55–63. https://doi.org/10.1111/cod.12869.

35. Lysdal SH, Sosted H, Andersen KE, Johansen JD. Hand eczema in hairdressers: a Danish register-based study of the prevalence of hand eczema and its career consequences. Contact Dermatitis. 2011;65(3):151–8.

36. Diepgen TL. Occupational skin diseases. J Dtsch Dermatol Ges. 2012;10(5):297–313; quiz 4–5.

37. Andrees V, John SM, Nienhaus A, Skudlik C, Brans R, Augustin M, et al. Economic evaluation of a tertiary prevention program for occupational skin diseases in Germany. Contact Dermatitis. 2020;82(6):361–9. https://doi.org/10.1111/cod.13506.

38. Global Burden of Disease Cancer Collaboration, Fitzmaurice C, Abate D, Abbasi N, Abbastabar H, Abd-Allah F, et al. Global, regional, and National Cancer Incidence, mortality, years of life lost, years lived with disability, and disability-adjusted life-years for 29 cancer groups, 1990 to 2017: a systematic analysis for the global burden of disease study. JAMA Oncol. 2019;5(12):1749–68. https://doi.org/10.1001/jamaoncol.2019.2996.

39. Alam M, Ratner D. Cutaneous squamous-cell carcinoma. N Engl J Med. 2001;344(13):975–83. https://doi.org/10.1056/NEJM200103293441306.

40. Surdu S. Non-melanoma skin cancer: occupational risk from UV light and arsenic exposure. Rev Environ Health. 2014;29(3):255–64. https://doi.org/10.1515/reveh-2014-0040.

41. Lomas A, Leonardi-Bee J, Bath-Hextall F. A systematic review of worldwide incidence of nonmelanoma skin cancer. Br J Dermatol. 2012;166(5):1069–80. https://doi.org/10.1111/j.1365-2133.2012.10830.x.

42. Saladi RN, Persaud AN. The causes of skin cancer: a comprehensive review. Drugs Today (Barc). 2005;41(1):37–53. https://doi.org/10.1358/dot.2005.41.1.875777.

43. Loney T, Paulo MS, Modenese A, Gobba F, Tenkate T, Whiteman DC, et al. Global evidence on occupational sun exposure and keratinocyte cancers: a systematic review. Br J Dermatol. 2021;184(2):208–18. https://doi.org/10.1111/bjd.19152.

44. Modenese A, Korpinen L, Gobba F. Solar radiation exposure and outdoor work: an underestimated occupational risk. Int J Environ Res Public Health. 2018;15(10):2063. https://doi.org/10.3390/ijerph15102063.

45. Trakatelli M, Barkitzi K, Apap C, Majewski S, De Vries E, group E. Skin cancer risk in outdoor workers: a European multicenter case-control study. J Eur Acad Dermatol Venereol. 2016;30(Suppl 3):5–11. https://doi.org/10.1111/jdv.13603.

46. Schmitt J, Haufe E, Trautmann F, Schulze HJ, Elsner P, Drexler H, et al. Occupational UV-exposure is a major risk factor for basal cell carcinoma: results of

the population-based case-control study FB-181. J Occup Environ Med. 2018;60(1):36–43. https://doi.org/10.1097/JOM.0000000000001217.

47. Bauer A, Haufe E, Heinrich L, Seidler A, Schulze HJ, Elsner P, et al. Basal cell carcinoma risk and solar UV exposure in occupationally relevant anatomic sites: do histological subtype, tumor localization and Fitzpatrick phototype play a role? A population-based case-control study. J Occup Med Toxicol. 2020;15:28. https://doi.org/10.1186/s12995-020-00279-8.

48. Schmitt J, Haufe E, Trautmann F, Schulze HJ, Elsner P, Drexler H, et al. Is ultraviolet exposure acquired at work the most important risk factor for cutaneous squamous cell carcinoma? Results of the population-based case-control study FB-181. Br J Dermatol. 2018;178(2):462–72. https://doi.org/10.1111/bjd.15906.

49. Alfonso JH, Martinsen JI, Weiderpass E, Pukkala E, Kjaerheim K, Tryggvadottir L, et al. Occupation and cutaneous melanoma: a 45-year historical cohort study of 14.9 million people in five Nordic countries. Br J Dermatol. 2021;184(4):672–80. https://doi.org/10.1111/bjd.19379.

50. Mofidi A, Tompa E, Spencer J, Kalcevich C, Peters CE, Kim J, et al. The economic burden of occupational non-melanoma skin cancer due to solar radiation. J Occup Environ Hyg. 2018;15(6):481–91. https://doi.org/10.1080/15459624.2018.1447118.

51. John SM, Garbe C, French LE, Takala J, Yared W, Cardone A, et al. Improved protection of outdoor workers from solar ultraviolet radiation: position statement. J Eur Acad Dermatol Venereol. 2021;35(6):1278–84. https://doi.org/10.1111/jdv.17011.

52. Ulrich C, Salavastru C, Agner T, Bauer A, Brans R, Crepy MN, et al. The European status quo in legal recognition and patient-care services of occupational skin cancer. J Eur Acad Dermatol Venereol. 2016;30(Suppl 3):46–51. https://doi.org/10.1111/jdv.13609.

53. Caroe TK, Ebbehoj NE, Wulf HC, Agner T. Occupational skin cancer may be underreported. Dan Med J. 2013;60(5):A4624.

54. Philipp-Dormston WG, Muller K, Novak B, Stromer K, Termeer C, Hammann U, et al. Patient-reported health outcomes in patients with non-melanoma skin cancer and actinic keratosis: results from a large-scale observational study analysing effects of diagnoses and disease progression. J Eur Acad Dermatol Venereol. 2018;32(7):1138–46. https://doi.org/10.1111/jdv.14703.

55. Gaulin C, Sebaratnam DF, Fernandez-Penas P. Quality of life in non-melanoma skin cancer. Australas J Dermatol. 2015;56(1):70–6. https://doi.org/10.1111/ajd.12205.

56. Guy GP Jr, Machlin SR, Ekwueme DU, Yabroff KR. Prevalence and costs of skin cancer treatment in the U.S., 2002–2006 and 2007–2011. Am J Prev Med. 2015;48(2):183–7. https://doi.org/10.1016/j.amepre.2014.08.036.

57. Fransen M, Karahalios A, Sharma N, English DR, Giles GG, Sinclair RD. Non-melanoma skin cancer in Australia. Med J Aust. 2012;197(10):565–8. https://doi.org/10.5694/mja12.10654.

Occupational Dermatitis Due to Irritation and Allergic Sensitization

3

M.-N. Crepy ⓘ

List of Abbreviations

ACD   Allergic contact dermatitis
ICD   Irritant contact dermatitis
HE   Hand eczema

Introduction and Terminology

Occupational contact dermatitis is an inflammatory skin condition resulting from skin contact with materials found in the workplace. It can be broadly classified into irritant and allergic reactions. However, it is often multifactorial. The main localization is the hands.

Strictly speaking, the word eczema comes from the Greek for "boiling," in reference to the tiny vesicles (bubbles) that are often seen in the early acute stages of the disorder, but less often in its later chronic stages. Dermatitis means inflammation of the skin and is therefore, a broader term than eczema, including mainly environmental induced dermatitis. However, in the scientific literature, eczema and dermatitis are used as synonyms to describe an inflammatory skin disease with specific histological and clinical features [1].

Occupational Irritant Contact Dermatitis

Irritant contact dermatitis (ICD) is a skin inflammation induced by the direct effect of chemicals or physical agents on the skin barrier. It is mediated by pro-inflammatory cytokines released from keratinocytes and resident innate immune cells without specific activation of the adaptive immune system [2]. Thus it may be observed from the first exposure and can be suffered, by all people [3]. Its physiopathology is complex and not completely defined. Skin inflammation is mediated by pro-inflammatory cytokines released from keratinocytes and resident innate immune cells without specific activation of the adaptive immune system. [4].

ICD is the most common type of contact dermatitis and a major public health interest as it represents up to 80% of occupational contact dermatitis [5, 6]. It causes significant functional impairment, disruption at work and has a high impact on the quality of life. In Western countries, ICD accounts for approximately 30% of the total occupational disease burden [7, 8].

Clinical Features

ICD is not a clinical entity, but rather a spectrum of diseases, with different clinical presentations and etiological factors which depend on the type

M.-N. Crepy (✉)
Occupational and Environmental Diseases
Department Unit at Hotel-Dieu Hospital,
Paris, France

Dermatology Department Unit at Cochin Hospital,
Paris, France

© The Author(s), under exclusive license to Springer Nature Switzerland AG 2023

A. M. Giménez-Arnau, H. I. Maibach (eds.), *Handbook of Occupational Dermatoses*, Updates in Clinical Dermatology, https://doi.org/10.1007/978-3-031-22727-1_3

of irritant, its concentration, the type of exposure, environmental factors (such as humidity, temperature, mechanical pression), and the individual response [4, 9].

The clinical entities most relevant in occupational setting are: Chemical burns, Acute ICD, Chronic ICD, Irritant reactions, airborne irritant contact dermatitis and phototoxic contact dermatitis.

Chemical Burns

A chemical burn is an acute, severe irritant reaction by which the cells have been severely damaged with development of necrosis [10, 11].

The major symptoms are burning and smarting, which develop usually within minutes. Clinically, a chemical burn is characterized by erythema, blisters, erosions, and necrotic skin, limited to the exposed sites. Usually, the symptoms develop immediately or in close connection to exposure, but certain chemicals, such as hydrofluoric acid, can give delayed reactions which first appear several hours, or even a day, after the exposure [10, 11].

Strong acids and alkalis are the major causes of chemical burns. The halogenated acids are particularly dangerous because they may lead to deep continuous tissue destruction even after short skin contact. Many substances can cause chemical burns only after prolonged skin contact, particularly under occlusion form, e.g., gloves, boots, shoes, or clothes. These substances include detergents, Portland Cement (Fig. 3.1), plants, plastic monomers [4, 10, 11].

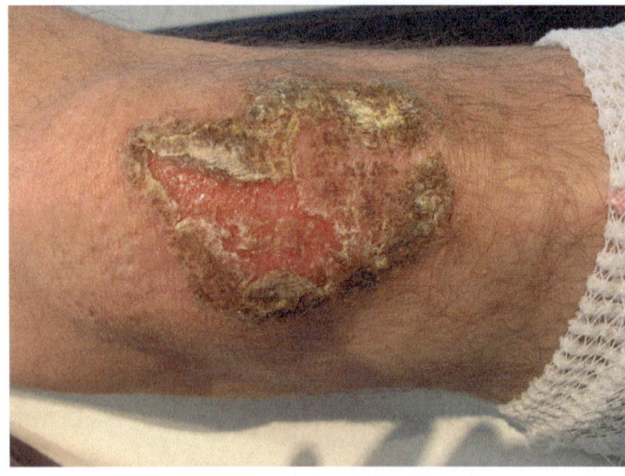

Fig. 3.1 Cement burn in a construction worker, courtesy Dr. Genillier

Acute Irritant Contact Dermatitis

Acute ICD develops upon exposure to moderate to strong irritants such as strong acids or alkaline solutions. Symptoms in the acute phase include erythema, edema, blisters, bullae, and erosions, usually accompanied by burning, stinging, or soreness of the skin [3]. The lesions are usually sharply demarcated (Fig. 3.2) and heal upon avoidance of skin irritants exposure within several days to weeks depending on the reaction's severity and individual endogenous factors. In the healing phase, crusting, scaling, and sometimes postinflammatory hyperpigmentation may appear. The lesions are usually confined to the area of exposure to the irritant and therefore, often asymmetrically distributed.

The typical situation is an accident at work and the healing is described as the decrescendo phenomenon as the irritant reaction starts immediately after the exposure, in contrast to ACD, in which there is a transient increase in the reaction before healing occurs (crescendo phenomenon) [12]. Hence, the diagnosis is easy in most cases,

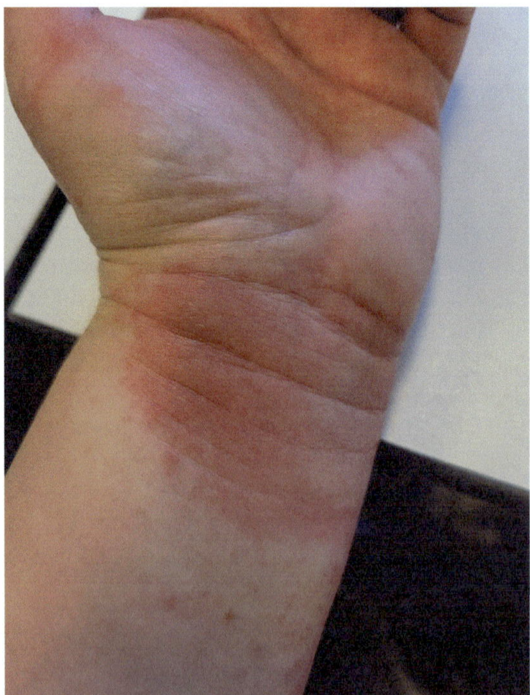

Fig. 3.2 Acute ICD in a chemist to accidental exposure to corrosive vapors chemicals

and the association between exposure and skin reaction is commonly evident.

Acute delayed ICD is characteristic for certain irritants such as benzalkonium chloride which can potentially cause a delayed inflammatory response, approximately 8–24 h or more after exposure [3]. The symptoms and clinical features are similar to acute ICD. The delayed response may lead to a misdiagnosis of ACD and then patch testing may be helpful.

Chronic Irritant Contact Dermatitis

Chronic ICD is the consequence of multiple sub-threshold damages to the skin. A detailed history usually reveals the dermatitis is not caused by a single exposure to a strong irritant, but rather by repetitive contact with water, detergents, organic solvents, irritant foods, or other known mild to moderate irritants.

It develops slowly after repeated subthreshold irritations over a period ranging from days to years. It can result of a too frequent repetition of one impairing factor, but generally it is associated with a variety of stimuli which may occur both at work and in private life. Subsequently, the link between exposure and the disease may not be obvious. It is associated with a poor prognosis [6].

In occupational settings, the main localization is on the hands. Classic symptoms are erythema, increasing dryness, followed by hyperkeratosis with frequent fissures, more frequently on the extensor and lateral surfaces of fingers, and back of hands [1]. Sometimes, the pattern is nummular on the backs of the hands. It can start in the webs and spread later to the sides and backs of the hands [4].

Irritant Reaction

It is defined as a type of subclinical irritant dermatitis for individuals exposed to wet work and other mild irritants (substances that do not cause a severe skin reaction on short contact (<1 h) [4]. The clinical picture is monomorphic rather than polymorphic and characterized by one or more of the following signs (scaling, erythema, wheals, papules). It often begins under rings.

Airborne Irritant Contact Dermatitis

It is caused by volatile chemicals, dust, and even sharp particles suspended in the air and is, therefore, mainly located on uncovered skin areas such as face, hands, and arms.

Phototoxic contact dermatitis

Phototoxic contact dermatitis is the least commonly reported form of occupational ICD. It is the result of an interaction between a photoabsorbing chemical (exogenous chromophore) in the skin and ultraviolet radiation, inducing aggression of skin cells and inflammation [10, 13].

The reaction is non-allergic and can happen to anyone exposed to the chemical in question and UV radiation. The main occupational causes are plants containing furocoumarins (Umbelliferae, Rutaceae, Moraceae) [13]. Thus phototoxicity is most commonly seen among outdoor workers and agricultural workers.

Histopathological Features

Histopathology does not reliably differentiate between ICD, ACD, and atopic dermatitis, but helps to exclude psoriasis, tinea, or T-cell lymphoma [14]. Irritant contact dermatitis reactions show much greater pleomorphism than those elicited by allergens depending on the chemical nature and/or concentration of irritants and the individual reactivity of the skin (genome) [15]. Intercellular edema or spongiosis in the epidermis is present in the vast majority of the cases. In general, spongiosis is less pronounced than that seen in allergic contact dermatitis. Histopathology comparing ICD, ACD, and atopic dermatitis found necrotic epidermal keratinocytes to be associated with ICD [14].

Causative Factors

Exogenous Factors

Occupational ICD is frequent in professions with exposure to irritant chemicals and mechanical friction (TE7007049ENC), [10, 16]. Sectors of activity and professions at high risk of irritant contact dermatitis are listed in Table 3.2.

Water and Chemicals

Irritant contact dermatitis is primarily caused by chemicals or water/moisture which damage skin structures in a direct non-allergic way. Wet work is the main cause for chronic ICD. Criteria for wet work according to German regulations include a skin exposure to liquid longer than 2 h daily, the use of occlusive gloves for longer than 2 h daily, or frequent handwashing more than 20 times daily [17]. Occupations associated with a high amount of wet work are, e.g., hairdressing, food handling, healthcare, cleaning, floristry, and metalwork [10]. It was demonstrated that the duration of wet work and in particular the frequency of handwashing correlate with the development of occupational irritant hand dermatitis [18],

Many other chemical irritants can cause chronic ICD: detergents especially industrial surfactants and detergents, disinfectants, solvents, cement, metalworking fluids, oxidizing or reducing agents [9, 10]. Substances which commonly cause ICD are listed in Tables 3.1 and 3.2 (by profession).

Physical Causes

Mechanical, thermal, and climatic influences are important contributory or sometimes even causative factors [19].

Repetitive frictional trauma to the skin can produce dermatitis, characterized by erythema, scaling, vesicles and hyperkeratosis, that particularly involves the palms and finger-tips [20]. Friction can be caused by many activities, such as repetitive handling of tools, working in kneeling position, contact to rough textile fabrics, paper, dust or wood materials [21, 22].

In wet work professions, meteorological factors (dry and cold weather) can contribute to the pathogenesis of irritant hand dermatitis [19, 23].

Endogenous Factors

Alterations in the skin barrier seem to increase the risk of getting ICD. Particularly, patients with atopic dermatitis (AD) are more susceptible of developing ICD [24–26]. Interestingly, it has been shown that loss-of-function mutations in the filaggrin gene (FLG) are a strong predisposing

Table 3.1 Substances which commonly cause ICD (modified from [4, 10, 33, 45])

Categories	Examples
Water	
Soaps and detergents	
Alkalis	Soap, soda, ammonia, potassium and sodium hydroxides, cement, lime, sodium silicate, trisodium phosphate, and various amines
Acids	Sulfuric, hydrochloric, nitric, chromic, and hydrofluoric acids
Metalworking fluids	
Organic solvents	Aliphatics, chlorinated aliphatics, aromatics, ketones
Other petroleum products	
Oxidizing agents	Peroxides, halogens
Reducing agents	Aluminum hybrids, boranes, silanes
Animal products	
Man-made vitreous fibers	Fibers made of glass, ceramic, rock, slag wool
Physical factors	Friction, sharp edges of hard materials, plants, woods
Extreme thermic influences	

factor for ICD [26–28]. The increased odds ratio for getting ICD is highest in individuals having mutations in FLG and atopic dermatitis. However, individuals with mutations in FLG without having atopic dermatitis have also an increased risk of acquiring ICD compared to healthy individuals [25]. Twin studies also indicate that genetic factors other than atopy may play a role in inter-individual variability to ICD [29].

Diagnosis

The diagnosis of ICD may be challenging. Currently there is no specific diagnostic test to confirm ICD. It is usually an exclusion diagnosis after patch testing, based on a temporal relationship to a history of relevant irritant exposure [19, 30]. Irritant exposures should be systematically assessed. The history must be detailed to clearly identify potential irritants and allergens. It includes the daily activities, manipula-

Table 3.2 Sectors of activity and/or professions associated with irritant and allergic contact dermatitis modified from (TE7007049ENC) [3, 10, 16, 45]

Sectors of activity and/or professions	Irritants involved	Allergens involved
1. Cleaning and food handling • Cleaners, domestic help. • Food handlers, cooks, butchers, bakers, pastry makers, grocers, cheese-makers.	• Acids (phosphoric, hydrochloric, acetic, citric, vinegar). • Bases/alkalis (sodium hydroxide, potassium hydroxide, ammonium hydroxide, concentrated, Javelle water). • Repeated physical microtrauma (abrasion). • Solvents (acetone), diluted Javelle water, vinegar. • Wet work, soaps, detergents. • Foodstuffs.	• Gloves and rubber articles. • Biocides. • Fragrances and flavoring agents. • Fruit and vegetables (such as onions, garlic, lemons, and lettuce, artichokes). • Spices. • Metals (knife and tools handles).
2. Construction		
Construction workers	• Cement, particularly rapid-hardening or quick-setting cement, very alkaline (pH = 13–14), lime. • Physical agents: Traumas, heat, cold. • Wet work, washing hands with detergents, washing powders or soaps with abrasives, alkalis (pH > 10). • Glass fibers (reinforced, composite plastics).	• Cement (chromate, cobalt). • Gloves and rubber articles. • Additives in shale oils. • Plastics (glues, sealants): Epoxy resin systems, phenol- or urea-formaldehyde resins), polyurethanes. • Wood preservatives. • Teak. • Epoxy resin, rubber strip seals, jointing materials.
Painters	• Paint removers. • Wet work, detergents. • Acids, alkalis (bases). • Solvents and thinners.	• Rubber gloves. • Biocides (in water-based paints and glues. • Plastic resins and additives (paints, varnishes, glues): Epoxy resin systems, phenol- or urea-formaldehyde resins, polyester resins, polyurethanes. • Turpentine, colophonium. • Dyes.
Wood workers (carpenters, cabinet makers)	• Physical agents: Thorn, traumas, wood dust. • Detergents. • Paints and glues. • Wood preservatives.	• Rubber gloves. • Biocides. • Exotic woods (teak, rosewood…), colophonium, turpentine. • Plastic resins and additives: Epoxy resin systems, acrylates and methacrylates, formaldehyde, polyurethane.
3. Hairdressing, cosmetology Hairdressers, beauticians, manicurists	• Wet work, soaps, detergents, shampoos. • Perms (base: ammonium thioglycolate and acid). • Bleach (hydrogen peroxide). • Hair dyes. • Glues (acrylates).	• Hair dyes, decoloring agents (persulphates), perms (thioglycolates). • Acrylates and methacrylates. • Rubber gloves. • Biocides. • Fragrances. • Cosmetic excipients. • Modified rosin (depilatory waxes).

(continued)

Table 3.2 (continued)

Sectors of activity and/or professions	Irritants involved	Allergens involved
4. Heatlhcare workers	• Wet work, soaps, detergents. • Antiseptics and disinfectants.	• Rubber gloves. • Biocides/disinfectants. • Drugs. • Acrylates and methacrylates. • Cosmetic excipients.
5. Metal industry Metalworkers, solderers, brazers, welders	• `Physical agents: Trauma, sharp particles of various metallic oxide, various fibers, insulating materials. • Motor fuels. • Abrasives. • Battery electrolytes (sulfuric acid). • Glues with cyanoacrylates. • Degreasing agents (TRI, gasoline, bases). • Dewaxing agents. • Protection removers (alkalis: pH > 12). • Cleaning products. • Acids and alkalis. • Cooling lubricants (especially water-soluble).	• Rubber additives. • Metals. • Biocides. • Cutting oils: Biocides, emulsifiers, fragrances, antioxidants, colophonium. • Plastic resins and additives (glues) acrylates and methacrylates, epoxy resin systems.
6. Chemical industry Plastic manufacturers, plastic-processes operators. Applicators of glues and adhesives.	• Glass fibers (reinforced, composite plastics). • (meth)acrylates • Epoxy systems.	• Rubber gloves. • Biocides (paints and glues). • Plastic resins and additives (paints, varnishes, glues): Epoxy resin systems, phenol- or urea-formaldehyde resins, polyester resins, polyurethanes. • Turpentine, colophonium. • Dyes.
Pharmaceutical industry	• Wet work. • Chemicals. • Drugs.	
7. Agriculture and professions with plants or animal exposure	• Wet work, soaps, detergents. • Disinfectants. • Fertilizers, pesticides. • Trauma: Thorns, cereal beards, wood, calcium oxalate (crystals, raphides or microscopic airborne needles). • Flowers. • Processionary caterpillars from oak, pine. • Sea products: Jellyfish, coral.	• Rubber (boots, gloves). • Plants and lichens: (Asteraceae, tulips, Alstroemeria…). • Local remedies for veterinary use. • Wood preservatives. • Pesticides. • Turpentine.

tions at work, such as the types of soaps and (abrasive) hand cleaning products used, products handled at work, specific types of gloves used, exposure to dust, as well as the hobbies [19]. Important indicators for ICD are significant exposures to known irritants and a related temporal course of the disease. Lack of itching and slow aggravation after resuming work are typical. However, in occupational settings, ICD and ACD can be both involved. Therefore, careful patch testing is often required to exclude ACD.

Occupational Allergic Contact Dermatitis

Allergic contact dermatitis is a common and potentially disabling disease. The clinical definition of the disease is based on the history of the patient, clinical examination, positive and relevant patch tests, and a detailed, often repeated exposure assessment. It also frequently complicates irritant contact dermatitis in occupational cases.

In contrast to ICD, allergic contact dermatitis (ACD) is highly dependent on an allergen-specific activation of the adaptive immune response (type IV hypersensitivity Reaction) [31, 32]. The response can be divided into two phases: the sensitization phase and the elicitation phase. It involves "allergen-specific" T cells as mediators of the inflammatory skin reaction. Therefore, previous contact is needed to induce allergy. It is specific to one chemical and its close relatives. When a sensitized individual is re-exposed to the culprit contact sensitizer in sufficient concentrations, ACD occurs at the site of skin exposure. Sensitization can persist all the life.

Clinical Features

Allergic contact dermatitis can mimic or be associated with other types of eczematous eruption. As other eczematous dermatoses, it is characterized in variable degrees by pruritus, erythema, vesiculation, exudation, fissuring, excoriations, papulation, scaling, hyperkeratosis, lichenification, and dryness.

The dermatitis in occupational cases is usually localized on the hands and most prominent on those parts which have the most intense contact with the occupational irritant(s) and/or allergen [33]. In many occupations eczematous lesions are also present on the worker's lower arms, neck, and face. This may be due to dusts (wood, stone) or vapors of fluids and gases and either by airborne exposure or (accidental) transfer by contaminated hands or soiled clothes. If the degree of sensitization is high, dermatitis may develop in "ectopic areas" by transfer of small amounts from the fingers – also by gloved fingers.

Acute Allergic Contact Dermatitis

In acute allergic contact dermatitis, the main signs are erythema, weeping and crusting, blistering usually with vesicles (but, in severe cases with large blisters), redness, papules, swelling and scaling (Figs. 3.3, 3.4, and 3.5). Usually the border is ill-defined.

Chronic Allergic Contact Dermatitis

In case of continued or repeated exposure to the allergen, and/or association with irritant exposure, chronic contact may develop. Skin is less vesicular, exudative and more scaly, pigmented and thickened, with fissures, lichenification, and hyperkeratosis (Figs. 3.5 and 3.6). At this stage, it

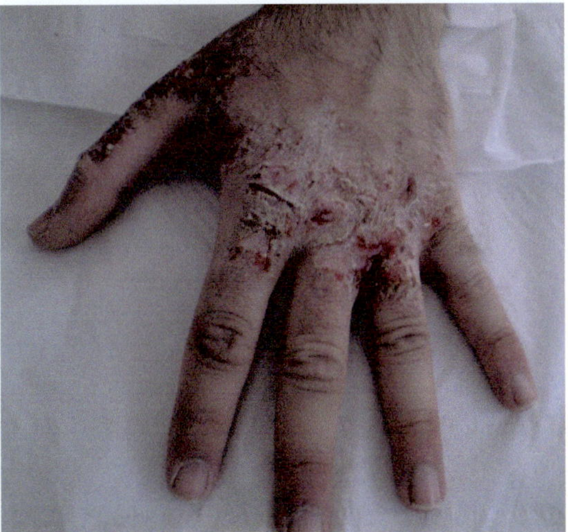

Fig. 3.3 Chronic ICD in a metalworker to cooling fluids

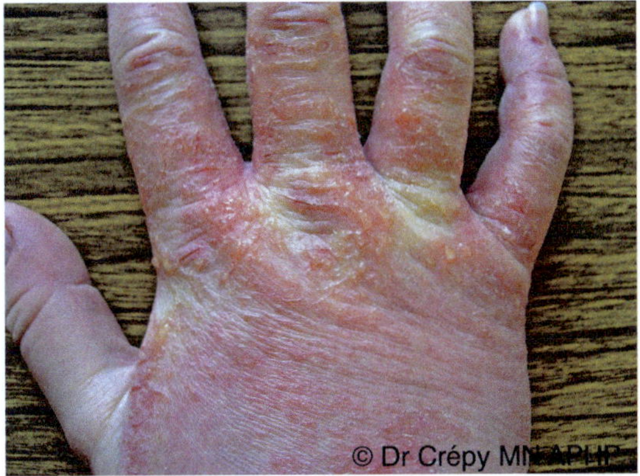

Fig. 3.4 First photo: Positive patch tests to hair dyes in a hairdresser Second photo: Acute ACD in a nurse to thiuram-dithiocarbamates and diphenylguanidine in rubber gloves

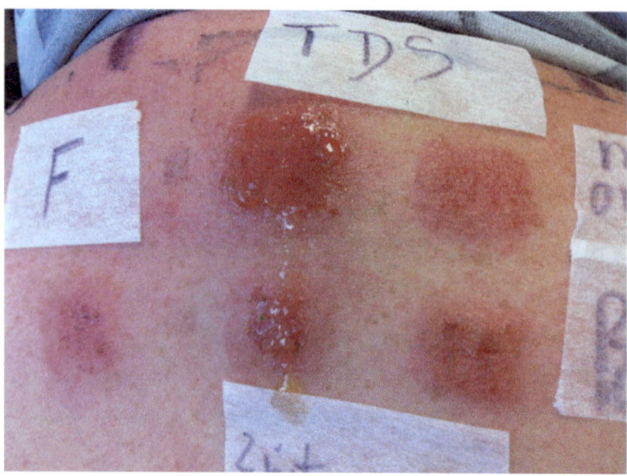

Fig. 3.4 (continued)

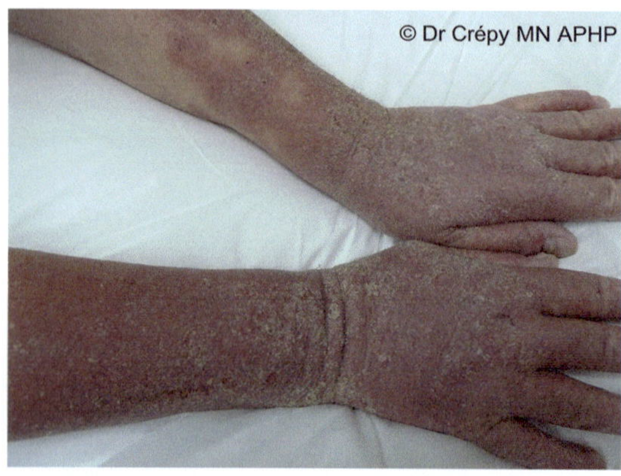

Fig. 3.5 Chronic ACD in a hospital cleaner to accelerators of rubber gloves and tricresyl phosphate of vinyl gloves

is very difficult to distinguish between allergic and irritant contact dermatitis. The main differences between irritant and allergic contact dermatitis are listed in Table 3.3.

Specific Patterns According to Localization

Hand Eczema

A classification of hand eczema (HE) recommended in guidelines from the ESCD is based on a combination of etiology and morphological signs, with the following subgroups [1]:

- Etiological subtypes: Irritant Contact Dermatitis; Allergic Contact Dermatitis; Protein Contact Dermatitis/Contact Urticaria; Atopic Hand Eczema.

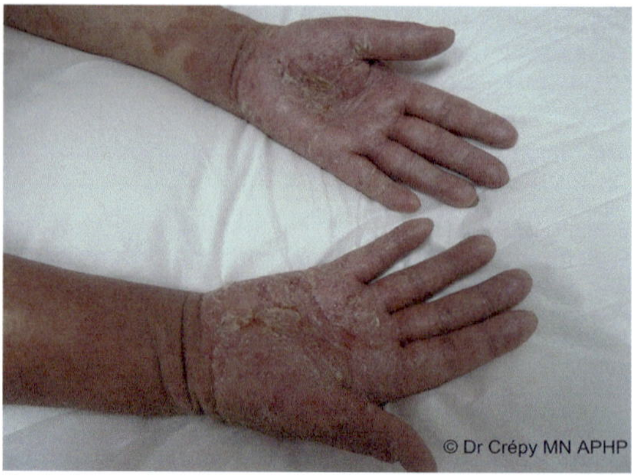

Fig. 3.6 Chronic ACD in a hospital cleaner to accelerators of rubber gloves and tricresyl phosphate of vinyl gloves (the same patient as Fig 3.5)

- Clinical subtypes: Hyperkeratotic palmar HE; Acute recurrent vesicular HE; Nummular HE; Pulpitis (fingertip eczema) (Fig. 3.7).
- Mixed forms: More than one etiological and clinical subtype may be present.

The morphology of HE does not reflect the etiology of the disease [34].

Airborne Allergic Contact Dermatitis

Contact with some allergens may be airborne such as vapors, gasses (volatile allergens), droplets, or dust particles. The most common sites of airborne allergic contact dermatitis are the parts of the body that are directly exposed to the air: the face, neck, upper part of the chest, hands, wrists, and forearms. In the face, the upper eyelids are particularly susceptible to airborne allergens, because the skin is thin in this area, and allergens penetrate more easily. The main causes are occupational exposure to plastic (epoxy and (meth)acrylate resins), biocides (in paints for instance), drugs, plants (Compositae plant extracts, etc.), natural resins and woods, rubber and glue components [35].

Photoallergic Contact Dermatitis

It is the result of an interaction in the skin between a photohapten (an exogenous low molecular weight compound much like a contact allergen) and UV or visible light [13]. It presents

Table 3.3 The main differences between irritant and allergic contact dermatitis [6, 10]

	Irritant contact dermatitis	Allergic contact dermatitis
Physiopathology	Innate immune system: Non-allergic inflammatory reaction of the skin to an external irritant	Innate and adaptive immune system (sensitization phase) specific type IV hypersensitivity Reaction to an allergen
Number of people affected	A majority of exposed people	Few people
Onset	– Rapid for strong irritants – late for weak irritants	24–72 h in clinically sensitized individuals
Subjective symptoms	Burning, painful	Itchy
Distribution of eczema	Localized to area in contact	Spreads to other parts of the body
Patch tests	Negative	Positive and relevant
Histopathological criteria	Necrosis of epidermal cells	Spongiosis, exocytosis

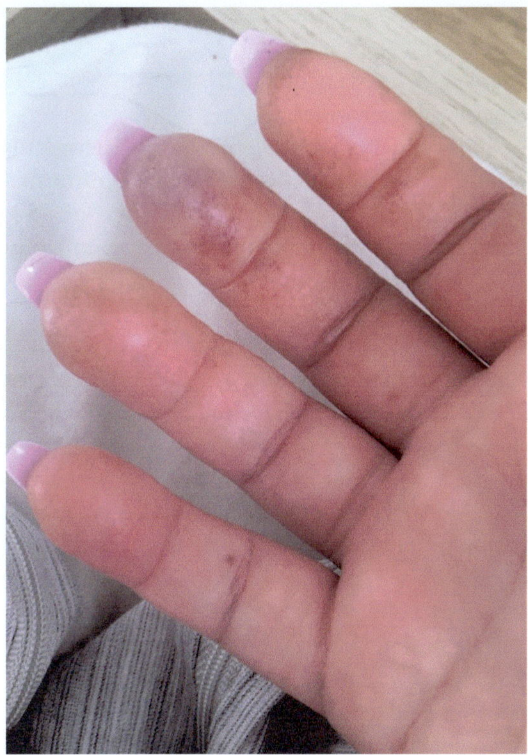

Fig. 3.7 Pulpitis to methacrylates in a beautician

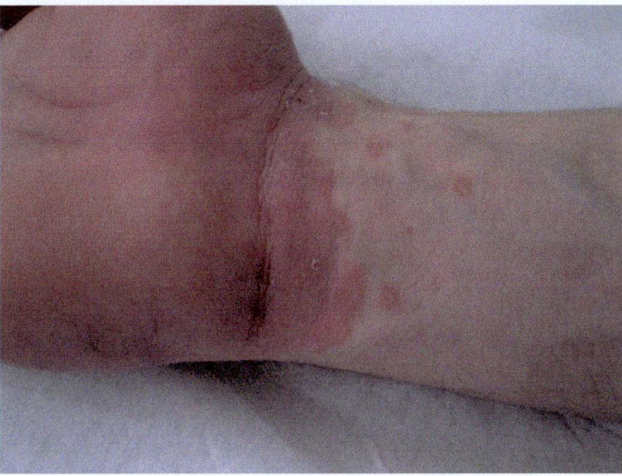

Fig. 3.8 Erythema-multiforme-like ACD to Pao ferro in a cabinetmaker

as a dermatitis which predominantly affects sunlight-exposed skin.

Non-Eczematous Reactions

Contact reactions may present as non-eczematous dermatitis: erythema-multiforme-like eruptions, lichenoid eruption, lymphomatoid contact dermatitis.

Erythema-multiforme-like eruptions show eczema on the primary contact site as usually the first clinical sign. Within a few days, papular and plaque lesions appear on the primary contact site, spreading to adjacent skin and occasionally distant sites [36]. The eruptions persist longer than the primary eczematous lesions and tend to persist after the disappearance of the initial dermatitis. In all cases, a positive patch test to the contact allergen can be elicited. The patch-test reaction is always eczematous and often severe. Allergens of wood (mainly pao ferro) (Fig. 3.8) and plants have been the most frequently reported occupational causes [36, 37].

Lichenoid Reactions

The clinical presentation is an eruption of itchy, violaceous, dusky papules on the skin exposed to the allergen. The main incriminated allergens have been color developers [38].

Lymphomatoid Contact Dermatitis

This type of allergic contact dermatitis is very rare [39]. It is characterized by clinical and histological features suggestive of cutaneous T-cell lymphoma, but remains responsive to anti-inflammatory topical treatment and allergen avoidance. Patch testing, skin biopsies, and molecular studies are helpful in making the correct diagnosis. In 2007, lymphomatoid contact dermatitis received significant attention from the European dermatological and regulatory communities because of the initially widespread outbreak of a severe dermatitis, termed "toxic sofa" dermatitis primarily presenting on the hips, legs, and buttocks [39]. The identified culprit was the contact allergen dimethyl fumarate, a mold inhibitor contained in sachets in the leather furniture. The main incriminated allergens are rubber chemicals, dyes, metals, phosphorus sesquisulfide, and preservatives [39].

Histopathological Features

The histopathological picture of allergic contact dermatitis is a typical example of a spongiotic dermatitis [40] (Fig. 3.9).

In the epidermis, spongiosis is an almost constant sign, resulting from the accumulation of fluid around individual keratinocytes (exoserosis) and the consequent stretching of intercellular desmosome complexes (or "prickles"). A more plentiful accumulation of fluid results in the rupture of the desmosomes and the formation of vesicles. Thus, in allergic contact dermatitis, spongiotic vesiculation can be defined as an intraepidermal cavity with ragged walls and surrounding spongiosis. There is migration of inflammatory cells into the epidermis (exocytosis), mainly lymphocytes.

At the electron microscopic level, dissolution of interdesmosomal areas, or "microacantholysis," can be demonstrated; remaining desmosomes show tension and alignment of tonofilament bundles.

In the dermis: a dense lymphocytic infiltrate is usually present in upper dermis. Dermal edema is prominent with deposits of acid mucopolysaccharides.

Interestingly, when allergic contact dermatitis lesions are not eczematous (erythema multiforme-like, lichenoid or lymphomatoid), the positive patch test is always morphologically eczematous, sometimes with additional features [40].

Causative Factors

The most frequently and consistently reported agents in cases of occupational allergic occupational contact dermatitis include rubber additives, biocides, allergens of plastics (epoxy resin systems and acrylates and methacrylates), metals (cobalt, chromates, nickel), allergens of cosmetics and fragrances, plants, dyes [10, 41]. They are listed in Table 3.4.

The allergens in the European baseline series associated with a markedly increased risk of occupational contact dermatitis include rubber additives (thiurams, mercapto compounds, and IPPD,) epoxy resin, and biocides (isothiazolinone and formaldehyde) [42].

Diagnosis

The diagnosis of occupational allergic contact dermatitis is based on medical history, clinical examination, and performance of skin tests. If necessary, the diagnostic spectrum may be further extended by histopathology examination and microbiology tests [1, 43].

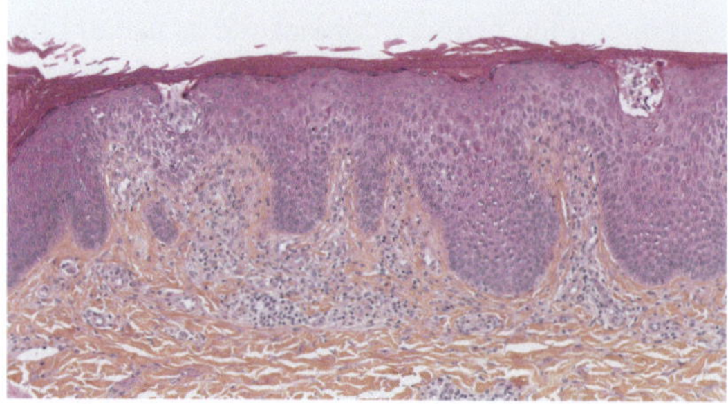

Fig. 3.9 "Skin biopsy showing features of acute spongiotic dermatitis: association of diffuse epidermal spongiosis, spongiotic vesicles containing Langerhans cells and lymphocytes and dermal superficial perivascular lymphocytic inflammatory infiltrate. Hematoxylin Eosin Saffron (×140)." Courtesy of Dr. P Sohier

Table 3.4 Substances which commonly cause ACD (modified from [10, 33, 45]: Rubber, metals, plastics, tensioactifs, dyes, hair dyes, rosin, plants, huile de coupe, fragrances

Products/categories	Examples of allergens
Biocides	Isothiazolinones, formaldehyde releasers
Metals	Chromium, nickel, cobalt
Plastics	Epoxy resin systems (diglycidyl ether derivatives and hardeners) Acrylates and methacrylates, urea- and phenol-formaldehyde, polyurethanes, polyester resins
Rubber	Thiurams, dithiocarbamates, mercaptobenzothiazoles, antioxidants (N-isopropyl-N′-phenyl-p-phenylenediamine derivatives)
Fragrances	Oxidized limonene and various fragrances (linalool…)
Plants and woods	Sesquiterpene lactones
Dyes	p-phenylenediamines and derivatives
Rosin	
Emulsifiers, surfactants excipients	Cocamide DEA, glucosides

Table 3.5 Differential diagnosis of irritant and allergic contact dermatitis

All other types of eczema: – Atopic dermatitis.   – Dyshidrotic eczema.   – Asteatotic eczema.   – Seborrheic dermatitis.   – Nummular (discoid) eczema.   – Stasis dermatitis.
Psoriasis
Mycosis
Scabies
Lichen simplex chronicus
Cutaneous T-cell lymphomas, parapsoriasis en plaque
Lupus erythematosus

A careful history is therefore very important in the diagnosis work-up of patients with occupational contact dermatitis. This should detail both occupational and domestic exposures including the analysis of ingredient labels of products and safety data sheets, the use and type of protective equipment, as well as products used for skin care, personal hygiene, and medical and alternative therapy [1].

The temporal relationship between work activities and onset of dermatitis and healing/improvement away from work are important diagnostic clues.

The gold standard for diagnosing allergic contact dermatitis is the epicutaneous or patch test [44]. The clinical relevance of positive skin test reactions should be assessed, based on past and present exposures and contact eczema locations.

Differential Diagnosis

Allergic contact dermatitis has to be distinguished from other types of eczema (mainly irritant contact dermatitis and atopic dermatitis) and other skin conditions that look like it. They are listed in Table 3.5.

Conclusion

Occupational contact dermatitis is the most frequent type of occupational skin diseases. This disabling skin condition strongly impacts the quality of life and occupational performance of affected individuals. The correct etiological diagnosis is a prerequisite for successful treatment and prevention.

References

1. Thyssen JP, Schuttelaar MLA, Alfonso JH, et al. Guidelines for diagnosis, prevention and treatment of hand eczema. Contact Dermatitis. 2022;86:357.
2. Smith HR, Basketter DA, McFadden JP. Irritant dermatitis, irritancy and its role in allergic contact dermatitis. Clin Exp Dermatol. 2002;27(2):138–46.
3. Vannina S, Marie-Noëlle C. Irritant contact dermatitis: why it happens, who suffers it and how to manage. Curr Treat Options Allergy. 2020;7(1):124–34.
4. Brans R, John SM, Frosch PJ. Clinical aspects of irritant contact dermatitis. In: Johansen D, et al., editors. Contact dermatitis. Switzerland: Springer Nature; 2019.
5. Higgins CL, Palmer AM, Cahill JL, Nixon RL. Occupational skin disease among Australian healthcare workers: a retrospective analysis from an occupational dermatology clinic, 1993–2014. Contact Dermatitis. 2016;75(4):213–22.
6. Belsito DV. Occupational contact dermatitis: etiology, prevalence, and resultant impairment/disability. J Am Acad Dermatol. 2005;53(2):303–13.
7. Cherry N, Meyer JD, Adisesh A, et al. Surveillance of occupational skin disease: EPIDERM and OPRA. Br J Dermatol. 2000;142(6):1128–34.
8. Diepgen TL, Coenraads PJ. The epidemiology of occupational contact dermatitis. Int Arch Occup Environ Health. 1999;72(8):496–506.

9. Jacobsen G, Rasmussen K, Bregnhøj A, et al. Causes of irritant contact dermatitis after occupational skin exposure: a systematic review. Int Arch Occup Environ Health. 2022;95:35.

10. Crépy MN, Nosbaum A, Bensefa-Colas L. Dermatoses professionnelles. EMC Elsevier masson SAS Pathologie professionnelle et de l'environnement. 2021;[16-533-A-10].

11. Chiang A, Bruze M, Fregert S, Gruvberger B. Chemical skin burns. In: John SM, et al., editors. Kanerva's occupational dermatology. Cham: Springer; 2018.

12. Slodownik D, Lee A, Nixon R. Irritant contact dermatitis: a review. Australas J Dermatol. 2008;49(1):1–9; quiz 10-1

13. Crépy M-N. Photosensibilisation, cancers cutanés et exposition professionnelle aux ultraviolets. Fiche d'allergologie-dermatologie professionnelle TA 69. Doc Méd Trav. 2004;97:109–19.

14. Frings VG, Böer-Auer A, Breuer K. Histomorphology and immunophenotype of eczematous skin lesions revisited-skin biopsies are not reliable in differentiating allergic contact dermatitis, irritant contact dermatitis, and atopic dermatitis. Am J Dermatopathol. 2018;40(1):7–16.

15. Willis CM. The histopathology of irritant contact dermatitis. In: van der Valk PGM, Maibach HI, editors. The irritant contact dermatitis syndrome. Boca Raton: CRC Press; 1996. p. 291–303.

16. Diepgen TL. Occupational skin diseases. J Dtsch Dermatol Ges. 2012;10(5):297–313; quiz 314-5

17. Bundesanstalt für Arbeitsschutz und Arbeitsmedizin 2008. Risks resulting from skin contact: determination, evaluation, measures. TRGS401 [Internet]. Disponible sur: www.baua.de/en/Topics-from-A-to-Z/Hazardous-Substances/TRGS/pdf/TRGS-401.pdf?__blob=publicationFile&v=4

18. Hamnerius N, Svedman C, Bergendorff O, et al. Wet work exposure and hand eczema among healthcare workers: a cross-sectional study. Br J Dermatol. 2018;178(2):452–61.

19. Uter W, Bauer A, Bensefa-Colas L, et al. Extended documentation for hand dermatitis patients: pilot study on irritant exposures. Contact Dermatitis. 2018;79(3):168–74.

20. McMullen E, Gawkrodger DJ. Physical friction is under-recognized as an irritant that can cause or contribute to contact dermatitis. Br J Dermatol. 2006;154(1):154–6.

21. Berndt U, Hinnen U, Iliev D, Elsner P. Hand eczema in metalworker trainees—an analysis of risk factors. Contact Dermatitis. 2000;43(6):327–32.

22. Morris-Jones R, Robertson SJ, Ross JS, et al. Dermatitis caused by physical irritants. Br J Dermatol. 2002;147(2):270–5.

23. Uter W, Gefeller O, Schwanitz HJ. An epidemiological study of the influence of season (cold and dry air) on the occurrence of irritant skin changes of the hands. Br J Dermatol. 1998;138(2):266–72.

24. Löffler H, Effendy I. Skin susceptibility of atopic individuals. Contact Dermatitis. 1999;40(5):239–42.

25. Visser MJ, Landeck L, Campbell LE, et al. Impact of loss-of-function mutations in the filaggrin gene and atopic dermatitis on the development of occupational irritant contact dermatitis. Br J Dermatol. 2012;168:326.

26. Visser MJ, Verberk MM, Campbell LE, et al. Filaggrin loss-of-function mutations and atopic dermatitis as risk factors for hand eczema in apprentice nurses: part II of a prospective cohort study. Contact Dermatitis. 2014;70(3):139–50.

27. Scharschmidt TC, Man M-Q, Hatano YC, et al. Filaggrin deficiency confers a paracellular barrier abnormality that reduces inflammatory thresholds to irritants and haptens. J Allergy Clin Immunol. 2009;124(3):496–506, 506.e1–6.

28. de Jongh CM, Khrenova L, Verberk MM, et al. Loss-of-function polymorphisms in the filaggrin gene are associated with an increased susceptibility to chronic irritant contact dermatitis: a case-control study. Br J Dermatol. 2008;159(3):621–7.

29. Lerbaek A, Kyvik KO, Mortensen J, et al. Heritability of hand eczema is not explained by comorbidity with atopic dermatitis. J Invest Dermatol. 2007;127(7):1632–40.

30. Friis UF, Menné T, Schwensen JF, et al. Occupational irritant contact dermatitis diagnosed by analysis of contact irritants and allergens in the work environment. Contact Dermatitis. 2014;71(6):364–70.

31. Martin SF, Esser PR, Weber FC, et al. Mechanisms of chemical-induced innate immunity in allergic contact dermatitis. Allergy. 2011;66(9):1152–63.

32. Nosbaum A, Nicolas J-F, Vocanson M, et al. Dermatite de contact allergique et irritative. Physiopathologie et diagnostic immunologique. Arch Mal Prof. 2010;71:394–7.

33. Frosch PJ, Mahler V, Weisshaar E, Uter W. Occupational contact dermatitis: general aspects. In: Johansen JD, et al., editors. Contact dermatitis. Switzerland: Springer Nature; 2019.

34. Agner T, Elsner P. Hand eczema: epidemiology, prognosis and prevention. J Eur Acad Dermatol Venereol. 2020;34(Suppl 1):4–12.

35. Swinnen I, Goossens A. An update on airborne contact dermatitis: 2007–2011. Contact Dermatitis. 2013;68(4):232–8.

36. Crépy MN. Dermatites de contact chez les professionnels du bois. RST. 2014:FAP 139.

37. Bonny M, Aerts O, Lambert J, et al. Occupational contact allergy caused by pao ferro (santos rosewood): a report of two cases. Contact Dermatitis. 2013;68(2):126–8.

38. Goh CL, Kwok SF, Rajan VS. Cross sensitivity in colour developers. Contact Dermatitis. 1984;10(5):280–5.

39. Knackstedt TJ, Zug KA. T cell lymphomatoid contact dermatitis: a challenging case and review of the literature. Contact Dermatitis. 2015;72(2):65–74.

40. Lachapelle JM, Marot L. Histopathological and immunohistopathological features of irritant and allergic contact dermatitis. In: Johansen JD, et al., editors. Contact dermatitis. Berlin: Springer; 2019.
41. Nicholson PJ, Llewellyn D, English JS. Evidence-based guidelines for the prevention, identification and management of occupational contact dermatitis and urticaria. Contact Dermatitis. 2010;63(4):177–86.
42. Pesonen M, Jolanki R, Larese Filon F, et al. Patch test results of the European baseline series among patients with occupational contact dermatitis across Europe – analyses of the European Surveillance System on Contact Allergy network, 2002–2010. Contact Dermatitis. 2015;72(3):154–63.
43. Alfonso JH, Bauer A, Bensefa-Colas L, et al. Minimum standards on prevention, diagnosis and treatment of occupational and work-related skin diseases in Europe - position paper of the COST Action StanDerm (TD 1206). J Eur Acad Dermatol Venereol. 2017;31(S4):31–43.
44. Johansen JD, Aalto-Korte K, Agner T, et al. European Society of Contact Dermatitis guideline for diagnostic patch testing - recommendations on best practice. Contact Dermatitis. 2015;73(4):195–221.
45. Crépy M-N. Allergènes responsables de dermatites de contact allergiques en milieu de travail: classement par secteur d'activité professionnelle. Doc Méd Trav. 2010;123:319–41.

Occupational Contact Urticaria Syndrome

Ana M. Giménez-Arnau, David Pesqué, and Howard I. Maibach

Introduction and Epidemiology

Contact urticaria syndrome (CUS), which includes contact urticaria (CoU), protein contact dermatitis (PCD), and contact pruritus, is characterized by the development of immediate contact skin reactions (ICSR), mainly consisting of wheals and/or eczema [1].

The CUS comprises a heterogeneous group of immediate contact inflammatory reactions that appear within minutes after the contact with the eliciting substances (chemicals or proteins). These reactions may be due to an immunological—normally IgE-mediated mechanism—or a non-immunological mechanism. CoU refers to the appearance of wheals following the contact with a substance, within 30 minutes after this contact. This reaction clears completely within hours, without residual signs [2]. PCD is considered by many authors as a part of CUS [3]. PCD refers to the appearance of an immediate dermatitis after contact with proteins that can present as an urticarial or eczematous reaction [4].

Despite the epidemiology of ICSR is not well known, it has been suggested that CoU and PCD could be underreported and unrecognized entities [5]. There is convincing data not only about the importance of CUS in occupational settings [6], but also about the association with other allergic occupational diseases such as asthma [7]. The prevalence of occupational CoU is 0.4% and could account for up to 30% of all occupational skin diseases [5]. However, with the exception of natural rubber latex allergy, there are limited data on the prevalence of ICSR. CoU can cause important health consequences and disability at work [8].

A. M. Giménez-Arnau (✉)
Department of Dermatology, Hospital del Mar – Institut Mar d'Investigacions Mèdiques, Universitat Autònoma de Barcelona (UAB), Barcelona, Spain

Department of Dermatology, Hospital del Mar – Institut Mar d'Investigacions Mèdiques, Universitat Pompeu Fabra (UPF), Barcelona, Spain

D. Pesqué
Department of Dermatology, Hospital del Mar – Institut Mar d'Investigacions Mèdiques, Universitat Autònoma de Barcelona (UAB), Barcelona, Spain

H. I. Maibach
Department of Dermatology, University of California San Francisco, San Francisco, CA, USA

Contact Urticaria

Clinical Features

CoU mainly occurs within minutes after skin or mucosal contact with eliciting agent and disappears within minutes or hours (<24 h). It consists in erythema and swelling, sometimes angioedema, associated with itching and/or pain, on the site of the contact with the eliciting agent. Spreading of urticarial lesions, generalized urticaria, or extracutaneous symptoms are possible.

© The Author(s), under exclusive license to Springer Nature Switzerland AG 2023
A. M. Giménez-Arnau, H. I. Maibach (eds.), *Handbook of Occupational Dermatoses*, Updates in Clinical Dermatology, https://doi.org/10.1007/978-3-031-22727-1_4

The symptoms progression of CUS, described in four stages, are summarized in Table 4.1 below.

Pathophysiology

CoU is traditionally divided into immunological and non-immunological urticaria.

Immunological CoU is a type I mediated hypersensitivity reaction which occurs in patients with specific IgE against a specific agent. Indeed, immunological CoU needs sensitization and will thus appear after repeated contact with the culprit agent. Concomitant history of allergic disorders like asthma, eczema, or hay fever is a risk factor [5]. In such cases, skin testing is positive in the affected individuals and negative in controls. There are two different groups of allergens that may cause CoU. The former group includes high molecular weight proteins (10,000 kD or more), whereas the second includes hapten chemicals of low molecular weight (less than 10 kD) [5]. A classification on the agents leading to CoU has been proposed and can be found in Table 4.2. In addition, the determination of specific IgE for this group of agents is feasible. The main exam-

ple of immunological CoU is natural rubber latex, for which 13 different allergenic proteins have been described, named Heb b1 to b13. Figure 4.1 depicts positive skin testing to the leaves and petals of a Lilium specimen in a patient with suspicion of CoU.

Non-immunological CoU elicits the case of contact urticaria without prior sensitization. Therefore, it can appear after the first contact with the agent. It is usually considered more common than immunologic CoU and less severe as it is not accompanied by systemic manifestations [5]. Among the substances that can induce non-immunological CoU, cinnamaldehyde, benzoic acid, sorbic acid, and nicotinic acid esters are to be enhanced [2]. Histamine is not believed to play a key role due to the therapeutic inefficacy of antihistamines. Contrarily to immunological CoU, skin testing will be positive in both affected individuals and controls.

Table 4.1 Clinical stages of CUS

Stage	Symptoms
1	– Localized urticaria – Localized eczema/dermatitis – Non-specific symptoms (burning, itching)
2	– Generalized urticaria
3	– Systemic upper and lower airway and oropharyngeal manifestations (asthma, rhinitis, angioedema, lip swelling) – Systemic digestive manifestations (nausea, diarrhea) – Other allergic systemic manifestations (conjunctivitis)
4	– Generalized anaphylactic reaction, including anaphylactic shock

Table 4.2 Agents leading to immunological CoU classification

Group I	Proteins of plant origin
Group II	Proteins of animal origin
Group III	Grains
Group IV	Enzymes

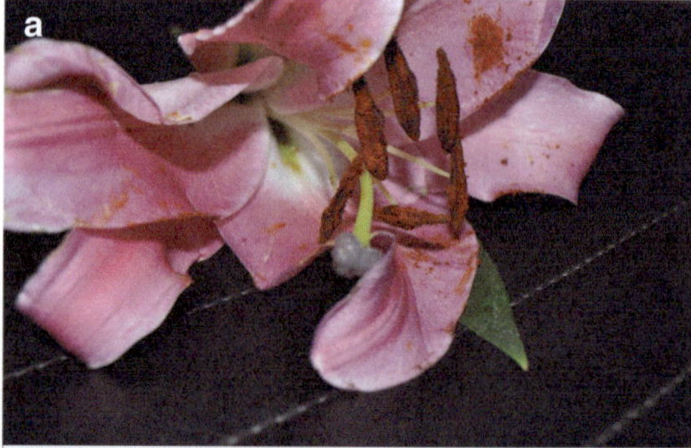

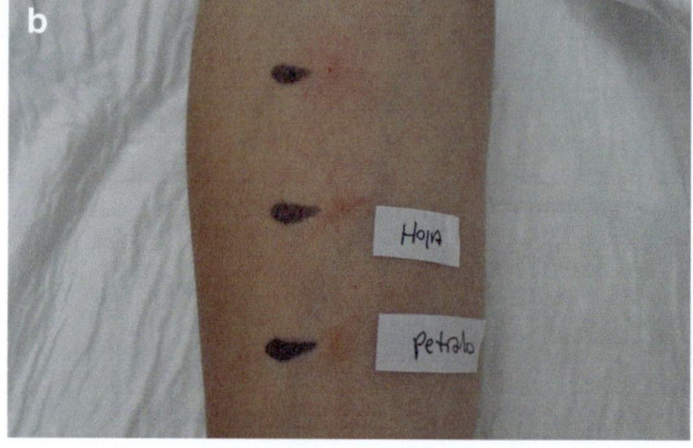

Fig. 4.1 (**a** and **b**) Immediate Contact Skin Reaction, induced by occupational exposure to Lilium "Stargazer" showing CoU demonstrated by prick by prick with the petals and leaves of the plant. The potential contact allergen is a Tuliposide

Protein Contact Dermatitis

Clinical Features

PCD affects the hands (especially the fingertips) and sometimes extends to the wrists and arms. Rarely some other locations, like the face, have been reported [9]. Pruritus, erythema, wheals, or angioedema are characteristic of the acute phase, which occurs within minutes, followed by vesicular lesions in the subacute phase. Examination after the acute crisis shows chronic or cured hand dermatitis, chronic paronychia, or even fingertip dermatitis [10]. In the chronic phase excoriations and finally lichenification can be found (Fig. 4.2).

Various foods such as fruits, vegetables, meats, and seafood or non-food proteins have been reported as responsible for PCD [10].

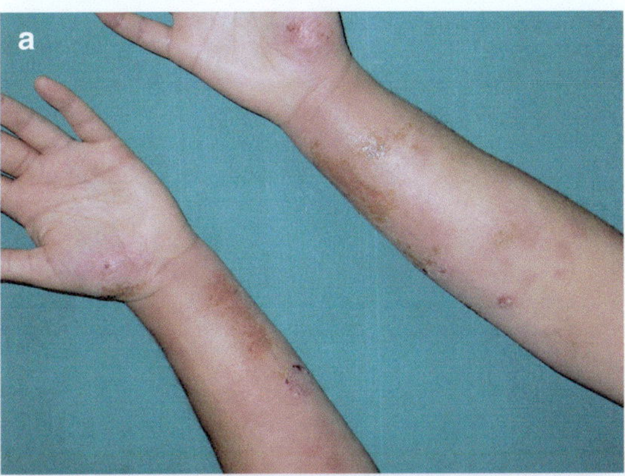

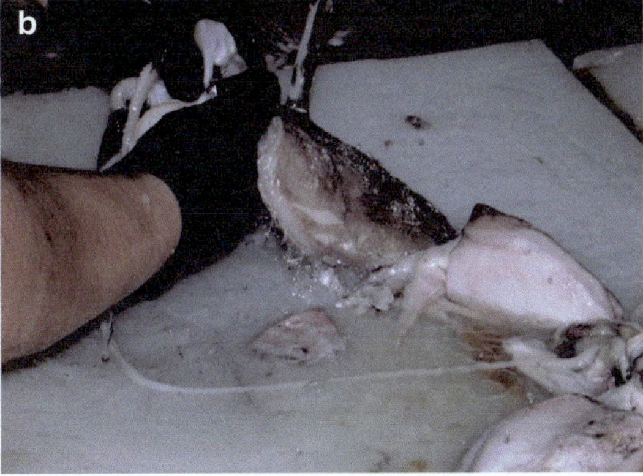

Fig. 4.2 (**a** and **b**) Occupational Protein Contact Dermatitis due to cuttlefish in an occupational setting due to manufacturing of fish for freezing

Pathophysiology

The pathogenesis of PCD remains seen as a thorny issue, but most authors claim the co-occurrence of type I and IV reactions against proteins, normally with a molecular weight of 10,000 to several hundred thousand or low molecular weight molecules that act as haptens, as it has been described for CoU [11]. In fact, some of these proteins can induce both CoU and PCD. The diagnosis of PCD lies in prick tests and/or scratch tests, as patch tests are rarely positive; specific IgE may be useful if available [11]. Although initially the diagnosis of PCD was restricted to those patients with positive scratch but negative patch test result, further studies expanded PCD to cases showing an additional type IV contact allergy to proteins. Furthermore, isolated reports of non-occupational PCD cases showing both positive prick-by-prick and patch tests have been reported [12, 13].

Diagnosis

Diagnosis of ICSR is based on full medical history and skin testing with suspected substances. In vitro techniques can be used only for a few allergens. For instance, natural rubber latex allergy can be studied with the use of basophil histamine release, RAST, enzyme-linked immunosorbent assay (ELISA), and IgE immunoblots of peptides present in natural rubber [14].

The investigation of these skin reactions with in vivo procedures has to be performed with caution. A sequential order has been proposed for the evaluation with skin testing procedures. If a positive reaction is evidenced, further studies are discouraged. Positive and negative controls are recommended. The proposed order can be seen in Table 4.3 [15].

The initial cutaneous provocation test for ICSR is the open test, which entails the application of the suspected substance gently rubbed on a normal-looking or slightly affected area of the skin, either on the upper back or the extensor side

Table 4.3 Diagnosis scheme for ICSR

1. Open application on unaffected skin.
2. Open application on affected skin.
3. Occlusive application on unaffected skin.
4. Occlusive application on affected skin.
5. Intraepidermal administration (prick test, scratch test, scratch chamber test).
6. Intradermal injection.

of the upper arm. The substances should be applied to skin sites suggested by the patient's history. A positive result is defined as edema and/or erythema typical of CoU, or tiny intraepidermal spongiotic vesicles typical of acute eczema. An immunological and non-immunological contact reaction usually appears within 15–20 min. Immunological CoU can also show a delayed onset, although this is rare.

When the open test results are negative, these tests can be repeated with occlusion of the suspected products. If these results are negative, prick testing of the suspected allergen or prick by prick with a part of the suspected product is often the method of choice for immediate contact reactions (Fig. 4.3). Scratch test and chamber scratch test (contact with a small aluminum chamber for 15 min) are less standardized than the prick test, but are useful when a non-standard allergen must be studied. When testing with poorly or non-standardized substances, control tests should be assessed on at least 20 people to avoid false positive interpretations [1].

It is important to enhance that some authors have proposed prick testing as a screening method for immediate-type allergy/hypersensitivity. To prevent systemic reactions, prick testing technique is commenced by using very low concentrations. A benefit of this approach is that prick testing permits to screen a large number of substances [16].

Many cases found in daily practice involve a differential diagnosis approach that may include other tests such as patch testing or photopatch testing [17].

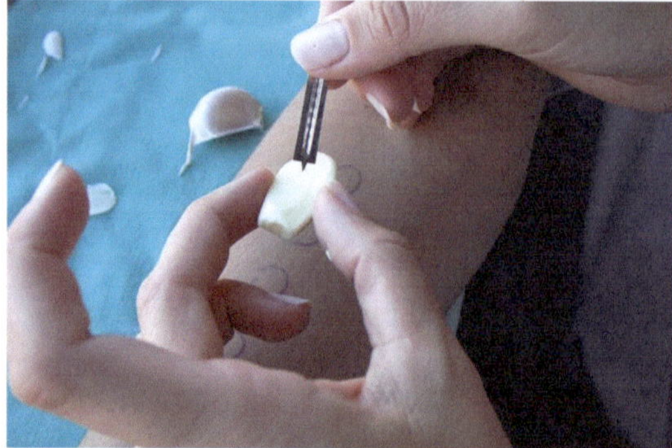
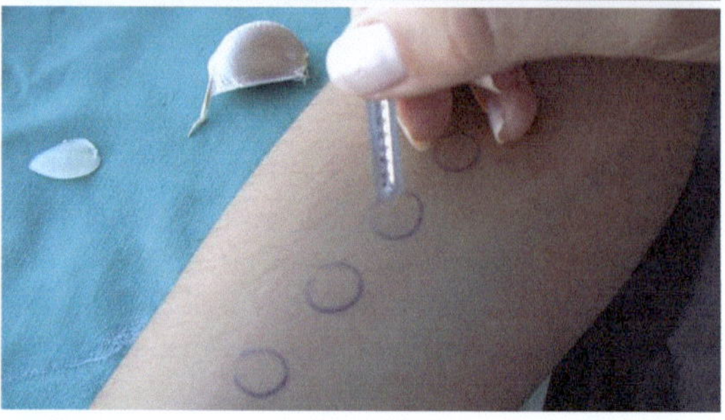

Fig. 4.3 Immediate Contact Skin Reaction due to garlic, induced by occupational exposure in a cook, that was studied with a prick-by-prick test. The allergen commonly tested for delayed contact dermatitis to garlic for patch testing is diallyl sulfide

Occupational Relevance

Despite CoU and PCD are infrequent, these conditions are mostly seen in occupational settings [18]. Finnish registers depict CoU as the second most common cause of occupational allergic contact dermatoses. The three most commonly responsible agents reported in this register were cow dander, flour and grains, and natural rubber latex [19]. In two German cohorts, the most frequent elicitors of CoU were cosmetics and rubber latex, respectively [18]. An Australian retrospective study highlighted that nearly 10% of the occupational skin disease corresponded to CoU. The three most common occupations involved were health workers, food handlers, and hairdressers due to natural rubber latex, foodstuffs, and ammonium persulfate, respectively [20]. A French study evidenced a decrease in terms of occupational CoU due to rubber natural latex, but did not evidence this decrease for other causes [8].

Atopic dermatitis or jobs that are a risk factor for irritant dermatitis (wet working, glove wearers, etc.) eases the disruption of the cutaneous barrier and thus facilitates allergic sensitization. These groups have an increased risk for both CoU and PCD.

Workers in the food industries, agriculture, farming, floriculture, health care, plastics, pharmaceutical and other laboratories, as well as hunters, veterinarians, biologists, or hairdressers are among those most frequently suffering CoU or PCD [1]. The prevalence of CoU in health care workers in Europe varies from 5 to 10%, whereas in the general population it lies between 1 and 3% ([2]; Fig. 4.4).

Healthcare workers have traditionally presented occupational skin diseases associated with natural rubber latex gloves.

The reactions vary from mild erythema, with itching at the site of contact, to severe anaphylactic reactions occasionally leading to death [21]. The proteins of natural rubber latex are emitted from gloves and other latex objects into the air, and the

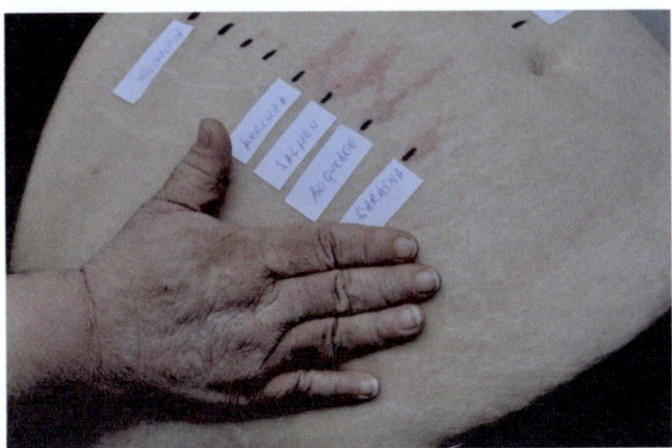

Fig. 4.4 Chronic hand eczema due to occupational fish exposure in a fishmonger seller. Initial exposure started with itch and hives and chronic exposure became eczematous with lichenified and fissured skin. Prick-by-prick testing revealed different positivities to different types of fish, including salmon

starch and other powders used in latex gloves may act as carriers of latex proteins. Healthcare workers with latex allergy produce IgE specific for a 20 kDa latex peptide (prohevein). A 17 kDa recombinant h antigen (Hev b5) is allergenic for over 90% of the latex allergic healthcare workers but just over half of the spina bifida patients allergic to latex [22]. The introduction of unpowdered latex gloves enables workers to avoid the air contamination, and lower later release of these gloves prevents new cases of sensitization [23]. A declining trend in the evolution of CoU has been described in different studies [8, 21]. In addition, healthcare personnel work also entails working with many different sensitizers (drugs, disinfectants, etc.). The use of gloves does not always prevent from being in contact with the aforementioned substances. Drugs that can lead to skin manifestations of the CUS are antibiotics, antineoplastics, and neuroleptics, among others. Some important disinfectants and biocides known to cause CoU are ethyl alcohol and chlorhexidine.

Industry workers deal with highly reacting sensitizing chemicals, like epoxy resins, acrylates, metals, and metallic salts, among others. The contact with these chemicals has led to immunological and non-immunological CoU, airborne CoU, and more generalized clinical presentations with respiratory symptoms. In the pharmaceutical industry, occupational CoU has also been reported from latex and drugs.

Hairdressing workers are exposed to bleaching agents (ammonium persulfate and other types of persulfates), hair dyes and protein hydrolysates (collagen or keratin) which can lead to occupational CoU.

Laboratory workers are veterinarians who are in contact with animals and have a high risk of allergy to such animals (20–30%). Veterinarians are frequently in contact with animal proteins (saliva, blood, and animal hair). Obstetric procedures give the higher risk of CoU and PCD that is likely enhanced by the repeated hand washing and occlusion due to gloves [24]. Rats (the most frequently responsible for skin symptoms), mouses, guinea pigs, rabbits, hamsters, and monkeys have been reported to cause CoU, PCD, or extracutaneous symptoms like conjunctivitis, rhinitis, asthma, or even anaphylaxis [25].

Workers in food industry are exposed to food and food additives. In addition, they may work under wet conditions. In this industry, work involves working with proteinaceous substances that are cause of CoU and PCD. Bakers may be most frequently affected by CoU or PCD [26], principally due to wheat proteins. Suspected allergens are peroxidase, purple acid phosphatase (Matsuo 2010), and the additive alpha-amylase [27]. Cow dander is the first cause of CoU in Finland [19]. In addition, chefs, cooks, and butchers are in contact with animal proteins. Occupational seafood allergy manifests as rhinitis, conjunctivitis, asthma, CoU, and PCD [28]. Among vegetal proteins, numerous fruits, vegetables, plants and plant products, and food additives can induce both CoU and PCD.

Contact with plants also leads to occupational CoU and PCD. This phenomenon is observed in different jobs: farmers, florists, gardeners, workers in the wood industry, horticulturists, etc. Numerous plants have been reported as inducers of CoU and/or PCD. Some induce CoU by an irritant mechanism, while some others lead to immunological CoU. If the best-known urticant plants are the nettles (*Urtica dioica*), the description of other plant wild species, domestic species, pollens, and other environmental factors (fungicides, pesticides, insects) highlights the difficulty of establishing the culprit agent.

In addition, the type of workplace can also ease the appearance of inducible chronic urticaria in patients suffering from this condition. Some clear examples of this can be seen in several occupations: jackhammers and the worsening of vibratory urticaria, heat urticaria in cooks or cold urticaria in workers who deal with frozen products [29].

Responsible Agents of Occupational ICSR (Table 4.4)

Table 4.4 Relevants agents classified according to their occupational origin

Industrial and chemical products	– Benzonitrile – Phthalic anhydride – Xylene – Dibutyl phthalate
Cosmetic products	– Ammonium persulfate – Basic Blue 99 – Balsam of Perú – *Lawsonia inermis* – Protein hydrolysate – Paraphenylenediamine – Ammonium thioglycolate
Pharmaceutical products	
– Antibiotic	– Cefotiam – Penicillin – Amoxicillin – Piperacillin – Streptomycin – Sulbactam – Azithromycin
– Fungicides	– Albendazole – Chlorothalonil
– Antineoplastic drugs	– Cisplatin
– Antiparasitic drugs	– Pentamidine
– Neuroleptics	– Levomepromazine – Donepezil
Biocides	– Chloramine – Chlorhexidine – Chlorocresol – Ethanol – Formaldehyde – Phenylmercuric acetate – Sodium benzoate
Metals and metallic salts	– Aluminum – Chromium – Iridium – Nickel – Platinum – Rhodium – Zinc
Animal and vegetal products**	
– Meat	– Beef – Chicken – Pork – Horse – Calf – Frog – Roe deer

Table 4.4 (continued)

– Seafood	– Crab
	– Cuttlefish
	– Large prawns
	– Lobster
	– Mussel
	– Oysters
– Fish	– Cod
	– Haddock
	– Herring
	– Mackerel
	– Monkfish
	– Perch
	– Plaice
	– Red mullet
	– Salmon
	– Sea bream
	– Sea perch
	– Sole
	– Squid
	– Trout
	– Tuna
– Other animal products	– Blood
	– Cheese
	– Dander and hair
	– Eggs
	– Liver
	– Milk
	– Mites
	– Saliva
	– Serum
	– Silk
	– Spider mites
	– Skin
	– Urine
– Vegetables	– Artichoke
	– Asparagus
	– Beans
	– Cabbage
	– Carrot
	– Castor bean
	– Celery
	– Chicory
	– Chive
	– Coffee
	– Cucumber
	– Endive
	– Garlic
	– Leek
	– Lettuce
	– Mustard
	– Onion
	– Olives
	– Pepper
	– Potato
	– Soybean
	– Tomato

Table 4.4 (continued)

– Fruits	– Apple
	– Lemon
	– Lime
	– Strawberry
	– Watermelon
– Mushrooms	– Shiitake
– Nuts and seeds	– Almonds
	– Hazelnuts
	– Nuts
	– Sesame
– Grains	– Corn starch
	– Barley
	– Rice
	– Wheat
– Food additives	– Beer
	– Caraway
	– Coriander
	– Curry
	– Paprika
– Enzymes	– Alpha–amylase
	– Cellulase
	– Papain
	– Phytase
	– Protease
	– Xylanase
– Flavorings	– Benzaldehyde
	– Cinnamic aldehyde
Plants and derivatives**	– *Ammi majus*
	– *Cannabis sativa*
	– Chamomile
	– *Chrysanthemum sp.*
	– Cinchona
	– Colophony
	– Cornstarch
	– *Dianthus sp.*
	– *Ficus sp.*
	– *Lilium sp.*
	– *Limonium sp.*
	– *Mentha sp.*
	– Meranti wood dust
	– Obeche
	– Pollens
	– *Schlumbergera sp.*
	– Tobacco
	– Tropical woods
	– *Tulipa sp.*
	– *Verbena sp.*
	– *Yucca sp.*

"**" implies that agents in these categories can cause both CoU and PCD

Treatment and Prognostic

Discovering the responsible agent is required to promote the correct avoidance of the eliciting trigger. Avoidance of further exposure improves occupational CoU. Primary and secondary prevention are highly recommended. Considering their good safety profile, second-generation antihistamines must be considered the preferred first-line symptomatic treatment of most of CoU. Before considering alternative treatment, higher doses of antihistamines should be used. When dermatitis is present, topical immunomodulation is conducted using topical steroids. Severe cases of CUS require a short course of oral steroids [2].

Occupational CoU seems to have a better prognosis than occupational dermatitis, even if previous studies show that workers may still lose their job. A Danish study on occupational CoU indicated a risk of prolonged sick leave [30]. In addition, job change may occur during the first years after recognition of occupational CoU and more often among patients with positive skin testing reactions, or with a severe condition [31].

Nicholson et al. guidelines advise that employers have to remove or reduce the exposure to agent causing occupational CoU, promote the use of afterwork creams, refer workers with occupational CoU to specialists, and provide appropriate gloves and cotton liners when it is not possible to remove risk of occupational CoU [32]. In addition, health practitioners need to advise atopic workers to maximize safety measures, have a detailed study of history on the job and materials used at work when a worker is affected by CoU or PCD and confirm it with skin testing.

Conclusions

ICSR pose an important challenge, as its occupational relevance has been seriously considered in only a few countries. Skin clinical manifestations of ICSR can be expressed as urticaria and/or dermatitis. The identification of occupational CoU require a high level of clinical suspicion, detailed occupational history, physical examination and complementary tests, such as prick testing. Cosmetics, plants, vegetables, and foods continue to be the most common agents responsible for new cases of immediate contact skin reactions. However, further studies are required to further understand the impact of these reactions in the occupational setting. Avoiding the trigger factor seems to be the best treatment. After symptoms control, a global approach is required to treat immediate contact skin reactions. This includes appropriate and early diagnosis, the report of the occupational condition, and the development of preventive measures.

References

1. Gimenez-Arnau A, Maurer M, De La Cuadra J, Maibach H. Immediate contact skin reactions, an update of Contact Urticaria, Contact Urticaria Syndrome and Protein Contact Dermatitis—"A Never Ending Story". Eur J Dermatol. 2010;20:552–62.
2. Gimenez-Arnau AM, Maibach H. Contact Urticaria. Immunol Allergy Clin N Am. 2021;41:467–80.
3. Ale SI, Maibach HI. Occupational contact urticaria. In: Kanerva L, Maibach HI, Wahlberg J, editors. Occupational dermatology. Berlin/Heidelberg: Saunders; 2000. p. 200–16.
4. Hjorth N, Roed-Petersen J. Occupational protein contact dermatitis in food handlers. Contact Dermatitis. 1976;2:28–42.
5. Vethachalam S, Persaud Y. Contact urticaria. In: StatPearls [Internet]. Treasure Island, FL: StatPearls Publishing; 2021; 2021 Jan. Available from: https://www.ncbi.nlm.nih.gov/booksNBK549890/
6. Kanerva L, Jolanki R, Toikkanen J. Frequencies of occupational allergic diseases and gender differences in Finland. Int Arch Occup Environ Health. 1994;66:111–6.
7. Helaskoski E, Suojalehto H, Kuuliala O, Aalto-Korte K. Occupational contact urticaria and protein contact dermatitis: causes and concomitant airway diseases. Contact Dermatitis. 2017;77:390–6.
8. Bensefa-Colas L, Telle-Lamberton M, Faye S, Bourrain JL, Crépy MN, Lasfargues G, et al. Occupational contact urticaria: lessons from the French National Network for Occupational Disease Vigilance and Prevention (RNV3P). Br J Dermatol. 2015;173:1453–61.
9. Pesqué D, Canal-Garcia E, Rozas-Muñoz E, Pujol RM, Giménez-Arnau AM. Non-occupational protein contact dermatitis induced by mango fruit. Contact Dermatitis. 2021;84:458–60.

10. Amaro C, Goossens A. Immunological occupational contact urticaria and contact dermatitis from proteins: a review. Contact Dermatitis. 2008;58:67–75.
11. Walter A, Seegräber M, Wollenberg A. Food-related contact dermatitis, contact Urticaria, and atopy patch test with food. Clin Rev Allergy Immunol. 2019;56:19–31.
12. Perez-Carral C, Garcia-Abujeta JL, Vidal C. Non-occupational protein contact dermatitis due to crayfish. Contact Dermatitis. 2001 Jan;44:50–1.
13. Paulsen E, Christensen LP, Andersen KE. Tomato contact dermatitis. Contact Dermatitis. 2012;67:321–7.
14. Palosuo T, Mäkinen-Kiljunen S, Alenius H, Reunala T, Yip E, Turjanmaa K. Measurement of natural rubber latex allergen levels in medical gloves by allergen-specific IgE-ELISA inhibition, RAST inhibition, and skin prick test. Allergy. 1998;53:59–67.
15. Li BS, Ale IS, Maibach HI. Contact urticaria syndrome: occupational aspects. In: John SM, Johansen JD, Rustemeyer T, Elsner P, Maibach HI, editors. Kanerva's occupational dermatology. Cham: Springer; 2020. p. 2595–628.
16. Aalto-Korte K, Kuuliala O, Helaskoski E. Skin tests and specific IgE determinations in the diagnosis of contact urticaria and respiratory disease caused by low-molecular-weight chemicals. In: Giménez-arnau AM, Maibach H, editors. Contact urticaria syndrome. Boca Raton: CRC Press; 2015. p. 129–34.
17. Nishiwaki K, Matsumoto Y, Kishida K, Kaku M, Tsuboi R, Okubo Y. A case of contact dermatitis and contact urticaria syndrome due to multiple allergens observed in a professional baseball player. Allergol Int. 2018;67:417–8.
18. Süß H, Dölle-Bierke S, Geier J, Kreft B, Oppel E, Pföhler C, et al. Contact urticaria: frequency, elicitors and cofactors in three cohorts (Information Network of Departments of Dermatology; Network of Anaphylaxis; and Department of Dermatology, University Hospital Erlangen, Germany). Contact Dermatitis. 2019;81:341–53.
19. Pesonen M, Koskela K, Aalto-Korte K. Contact urticaria and protein contact dermatitis in the Finnish Register of Occupational Diseases in a period of 12 years. Contact Dermatitis. 2020;83:1–7.
20. Williams JD, Lee AY, Matheson MC, Frowen KE, Noonan AM, Nixon RL. Occupational contact urticaria: Australian data. Br J Dermatol. 2008;159:125–31.
21. Chowdhury MM. Occupational contact urticaria: a diagnosis not to be missed. Br J Dermatol. 2015;173:1364–5.
22. Alenius H, Kalkkinen N, Lukka M, Turjanmaa K, Reunala T, Mäkinen-Kiljunen S, et al. Purification and partial amino acid sequencing of a 27-kD natural rubber allergen recognized by latex-allergic children with spina bifida. Int Arch Allergy Immunol. 1995;106:258–62.
23. Filon FL, Radman G. Latex allergy: a follow up study of 1040 healthcare workers. Occup Environ Med. 2006;63:121–5.
24. Bulcke DM, Devos SA. Hand and forearm dermatoses among veterinarians. J Eur Acad Dermatol Venereol. 2007;21:360–3.
25. Hesford JD, Platts-Mills TA, Edlich RF. Anaphylaxis after laboratory rat bite: an occupational hazard. J Emerg Med. 1995;13:765–8.
26. Kanerva L, Toikkanen J, Jolanki R, et al. Statistical data on occupational contact urticaria. Contact Dermatitis. 1996;35:229–33.
27. Morren MA, Janssens V, Dooms-Gossens A, Van Hoeyveld E, Cornelis A, De Wolf-Peeters C, et al. Alpha-amylase, a flour additive: an important cause of protein contact dermatitis in bakers. J Am Acad Dermatol. 1993;29:723–8.
28. Jeebhay MF, Robins TG, Lehrer SB, Lopata AL. Occupational seafood allergy: a review. Occup Environ Med. 2001;58:553–62.
29. Miranda-Romero A, Navarro L, Pérez-Oliva N, González-López A, García-Muñoz M. Occupational heat contact urticaria. Contact Dermatitis. 1998;38:358–9.
30. Cvetkovski RS, Zachariae R, Jensen H, Olsen J, Johansen JD, Agner T. Prognosis of occupational hand eczema: a follow-up study. Arch Dermatol. 2006;142:305–11.
31. Carøe TK, Ebbehøj NE, Bonde JP, Agner T. Occupational hand eczema and/or contact urticaria: factors associated with change of profession or not remaining in the workforce. Contact Dermatitis. 2018;78:55–63.
32. Nicholson PJ, Llewellyn D, English JS, Guidelines Development Group. Evidence-based guidelines for the prevention, identification and management of occupational contact dermatitis and urticaria. Contact Dermatitis. 2010;63:177–86.

Cara Symanzik [iD] and Swen Malte John [iD]

Introduction

Occupational skin cancers account for a considerable share of all reported occupational diseases [1, 2]. Over the previous few decades, the number of people diagnosed with skin cancer has steadily increased [3, 4]. Consequently, skin cancers have become a major public health concern in fair skinned populations globally; the most important external risk factor for developing skin cancer is exposure to ultraviolet radiation (UVR) [5]. Recently, one specific high-risk population has come into the scientific focus: outdoor workers [2, 6, 7]. In terms of the number of employees exposed and incidence, solar UVR is the most important occupational carcinogenic exposure [8–10], as solar UVR is the leading cause of non-melanoma skin cancer (NMSC), more precisely referred to as keratinocyte carcinoma (KC), which manifests as actinic keratosis (AK, intra-epidermal SCC), invasive cutaneous squamous cell carcinoma (SCC), and/or basal cell carcinoma (BCC) [11–13].

Despite the reality that millions of workers globally are subjected to the occupational carcinogenic exposure represented by solar UVR for a huge proportion of their working time, this work-related risk factor is still not formally recognized by occupational safety and health (OSH) directives and regulations in many regions of the world [11, 14, 15]. Furthermore, no specific occupational exposure limit values are generally accepted, however the International Commission on Non-Ionizing Radiation Protection (ICNIRP) has suggested an occupational UVR exposure limit equivalent to 1.0–1.3 Standard Erythema Doses (SED) per day; 1 SED equals 100 J/m^2 of the biologically weighted erythema action spectrum [15, 16].

There is a deficiency of acknowledgment of cases, a lack of evidence on the effectiveness of health surveillance programs and screenings for high-risk groups of outdoor workers, a lack of indemnification for cases of cancer, and a lack of political understanding and acceptance of this growing work-related health issue, among the negative consequences of this under-recognition of health hazards associated with solar UVR [17–19]. This chapter focuses on evidence for causation of occupational skin cancer induced by solar UVR and strategies for prevention.

C. Symanzik · S. M. John (✉)
Institute for Interdisciplinary Dermatological Prevention and Rehabilitation (iDerm) and Department of Dermatology, Environmental Medicine and Health Theory at Osnabrück University, Osnabrück, Germany

© The Author(s), under exclusive license to Springer Nature Switzerland AG 2023
A. M. Giménez-Arnau, H. I. Maibach (eds.), *Handbook of Occupational Dermatoses*, Updates in Clinical Dermatology, https://doi.org/10.1007/978-3-031-22727-1_5

Outdoor Workers as High-Risk Group for Skin Cancer by Solar Ultraviolet Radiation (UVR)

Because they spend the most of their working hours outside, outdoor workers are exposed to high amounts of solar UVR [20] and are as a result significantly more likely to acquire KC than the average population; risk is increased at least twofold, with SCC being the cancer most directly related to *cumulative* UVR exposure [11, 21–23]. Examples for occupations with a high share of outdoor work are, for instance, construction workers, gardeners, fishers, and farmers. Table 5.1 lists further vocations with direct and indirect occupational exposures to solar UVR.

Table 5.1 Extract of vocations (sorted alphabetically) with direct and indirect occupational exposures to solar ultraviolet radiation (UVR) according to the Australian and New Zealand Standard Classification of Occupations (ANZSCO)

Direct occupational solar UVR exposure	Indirect occupational solar UVR exposure
Agricultural workers	Aircraft maintenance engineers
Animal trainers	Building and construction managers
Bricklayers	Bulldozer operators
Builders	Caravan and camping ground stuff
Construction workers	Childcare workers
Drillers	Defense force staff
Earthmoving laborers	Door-to-door salespeople
Farm hands	Firefighters
Gardeners	Forklift operators
Jockeys	Motor mechanics
Leaflet or newspaper deliverers	Outdoor ushers and ticket people
Lifeguards	Panel beaters
Miners	Plumbers and assistants
Outdoor billboard and sign writers	Police officers
Outdoor car park attendants	Primary and secondary school teachers
Painters and decorators	Professional drivers
Roof tilers and slaters	Railway assistance
Sports people, coaches, and support persons	Street vendors
Sugarcane workers	Supermarket trolley collectors
Traffic controllers	Tree surgeons
Vegetable, fruit, and nut growers	Zoo workers

UVR ultraviolet radiation

Malignant Melanoma (MM)

Malignant melanoma (MM) is linked to UVR exposure, however, especially intermittent UVR exposure and, in particular, exposure during younger years as well as genetic traits seem to be predisposing [24]. In fact, the correlation between (*cumulative*) occupational solar UVR exposure and MM is viewed as not convincing, even though some recent studies suggested a possible link between chronic occupational sun damage and specific MM subtypes, such as lentigo maligna melanoma (LMM) [12, 17].

Non-melanoma Skin Cancer (NMSC)

NMSC is on the rise at a global scale, and particularly in outdoor workers. The massive actinic damage they often suffer frequently leads to a life-long chronicity with numerous freshly developing lesions, necessitating continuous therapy [2]. Outdoor workers are subjected to solar UVR doses that are at least 2–3 times greater than those of indoor employees and are frequently exposed to daily solar UVR doses that are regularly 5 times higher than the ICNIRP exposure limits [15, 16, 20, 25–30]. Epidemiologic studies reveal a particularly high frequency of both BCC and SCC among outdoor workers after years of cumulative sunlight exposure, demonstrating a strong link between occupational solar UVR exposure and the incidence of NMSC [21, 22, 31, 32]. Because of the extended latency period between exposure and (chronic) sickness of up to 20 years, for the patient the disease often remains "invisible," much like the causal UVR. Over 80% of cases occur in persons aged 60 and elder [33], exceptions may be outdoor workers under immuno-suppression, who tend to develop especially AK/SCC rather early. Due to demographic change, the prevalence of occupational NMSC is expected to continually rise, putting an even greater strain on health care requirements and insurance systems across the world [2]. NMSC is, however, one of the rare cancers that is curable, easily detectable, and—most importantly—fully preventable [2].

The use of objective dosimetric measures has aided in the characterization of at-risk groups among outdoor workers [2, 26, 28–30]. It was discovered that it is not the industrial sector as a whole that is troublesome, but rather the occupation and duties associated with this activity within the industrial sector—these are the deciding factors in determining the quantity of solar UVR exposure encountered at work [2, 29, 30]. As a corollary, the German statutory social accident insurance has implemented a mathematical model known as "Wittlich's algorithm" to assess individual occupational lifetime solar UVR exposure based on the obtained dosimetric data, which is now being used to improve prevention measures, healthcare services, and compensation for affected workers [29]. The underlying concept of Wittlich's algorithm being, if the job adds 40% UVR exposure to the individual's lifetime UVR exposure, that then the risk for developing AK/SCC doubles, thus the occupational influences are considered relevant and occurring skin cancer in occupationally exposed body areas therefore is acknowledged as an occupational disease and open for compensation. Considering that the large dosimetric measuring campaign conducted by Wittlich et al. in Germany in over thousand outdoor workers for three complete April to October periods have revealed unexpectedly high occupational exposures of up to 600 SED per summer period [30], outdoor workers usually satisfy the above condition if they work for longer than 10 years in a high-risk profession full-time.

The dangers of solar UVR exposure in the workplace are mostly overlooked, and the obvious future problems are contrasted with the existing position in terms of legal recognition, patient treatment, and compensation [2]. While prevention is critical in reducing cancer risks for outdoor workers, improved protection through legally enforceable laws and regulations is as important [2]. Table 5.2 summarizes recommendations to prospectively address the unmet needs

Table 5.2 Fields of activity concerning non-melanoma skin cancer (NMSC) patients' unmet needs according to the global Call to Action, launched on 26 April 2019 at the 1st Multi-Stakeholder Summit on Occupational Skin Cancer, held in Paris at the occasion of the 15th European Association of Dermato-Oncology (EADO) Congress (24–27 April 2019) [2]

Number	Recommendation
1	Policymakers should enhance the legal framework to better safeguard outdoor workers and provide access to frequent screenings and, as a result, early treatment. NMSC should be recognized as an occupational disease in the European Union within the next legislative period.
2	Doctors, other health professionals, and politicians should collaborate to ensure that NMSC registration is harmonized across the European Union.
3	Employers should utilize technologies to track levels of UVR exposure in the workplace. They must also develop cost-effective methods for sun-safe behavior and assure that outdoor workers receive regular skin cancer screenings.
4	Occupational NMSC (including actinic keratosis) should be considerably better reported by doctors and other health professionals.
5	Patient advocacy organizations, doctors, and other healthcare professionals, as well as employers, should work together to increase skin cancer prevention and sun-safe work conditions, as well as to answer the unmet needs of retired outdoor workers experiencing NMSC.

NMSC non-melanoma skin cancer, *UVR* ultraviolet radiation

of NMSC patients. In this context, health professionals are of utmost importance [2], dermatologists will play a progressively important role in improving patient care and outcomes in dermato-oncology in the future, particularly in light of novel diagnostic methods and treatments for early and advanced skin cancer, as well as the increasingly diverse skills, knowledge, and expertise required to manage this heterogeneous spectrum of diseases [4]. Regarding occupational causation, it is pivotal, however, that cases are reported to the respective authorities. Versatile multi-purpose notification forms for reporting suspected cases to respective authorities were recently published open access [34].

Unfortunately, to date, even in the few countries where NMSC is acknowledgeable as an occupational disease, affected workers mostly are not awarded the benefits of legal recognition, because underreporting is massive: the responsible physician or dermatologist does not notify, as the correlation between the disease and the occupation is not yet routinely made [2]. In Denmark, only 36 cases of skin cancer had been recognized since its inclusion in the list of occupational diseases in 2000 until 2013 [35]. In Italy, where UVR-induced NMSC is also on the national occupational diseases list, the situation is no different: averagely, only 34 cases were reported annually between 2002 and 2017 [17]; a similarly dramatic underreporting applies to other countries [19]. In 2015, in Germany, the picture changed, when some forms of NMSC (SCC, multiple AK) were officially included in the national decree of occupational diseases. Within the first 12 months of its introduction, >7700 occupational skin cancer cases were notified. In 2019, the number of notifications amounted to 9931, making skin cancer the third most frequently notified occupational disease and the second most frequently legally acknowledged illness. It is worth noticing that a financial incentive has been instituted which encourages physicians to report—which undoubtedly has been essential to the high notification figures. Further, patients with acknowledged occupational skin cancer are provided with priority medical care and, in more severe cases, substantial compensation. The unexpectedly high UVR exposures in outdoor workers, revealed by the recent measurement campaigns in this country [30], and consistently in many other countries [15, 20, 25–28], together with the drastically increasing number of skin cancer notifications have enabled a breakthrough in health and safety legislation in Germany. For the first time, as of 12 July 2019, employers are specifically required to conduct a special UVR exposure risk assessment, provide personal protective equipment (including sunscreens), and offer UVR-exposed employees a consultation by an occupational physician every three years [36].

The recent German example shows that only if there are notifications there is an inclination for politicians to take action. For that reason, the 11th revision of the World Health Organization (WHO) International Classification of Diseases (ICD), adopted 25 May 2019, can be considered an important milestone to tackle underreporting and obtain improved and objective disease data at global level. NMSC, incl. AK can now for the first time be coded for as occupational, and BCC and SCC are now separate entities [37]. Thus, when ICD 11 will come into force by 1 January 2022, it will likely reveal the true epidemiological magnitude of work-related UVR-induced skin cancer and may provide pivotal new global public health data for cancer prevention in outdoor workers [2]. Loney et al. have recently demonstrated the current lack of data on skin cancer in occupationally UVR-exposed workers in large parts of the globe [11]. Given the pressing nature of the growing numbers of NMSC cases linked to occupational UVR exposure, the WHO and the International Labour Organization (ILO) are currently assessing—within the United Nations (UN) Sustainable Development Goals 2030 framework—the global disease burden of NMSC. Both UN agencies have classified it among the ten most relevant occupational risk factors and health outcomes that have never been included in previous global estimation strategies but are very likely to account for a considerable disease burden [6, 7].

Prevention

Sun protection belongs to the field of occupational safety. In general, a considerable decrease in occupationally acquired UVR doses in outdoor workers is required to avoid skin cancers caused by UVR exposure. The quantity of UVR exposure and the specific activities to be done in the sun, as well as the employees' UVR protective practices, are important factors determining *cumulative* sun exposure in outdoor workers. Recommendations generally follow the so-called TOP principle and include technical, organizational, and person-related measures, which is explained in Table 5.3. Further, preventative efforts can be subdivided into primary, secondary, and tertiary preventative measures.

Table 5.3 Measures according to the TOP principle (technical, organizational, and person-related) for the reduction of the occupational ultraviolet radiation (UVR) exposure in ascending order, i.e., the next step of measures should only be instigated if the previous stage has been exhausted to the full extent

Measure	Explanation	Example
T	Technical	Checking technical measures that can be used to avoid exposure to sunlight. All forms of shading, such as sun sails or weather protection tents, are suitable for this.
O	Organizational	Avoidance of outdoor work when the sun is shining intensely. Even shifting working hours away from the midday heat can be an important aspect in terms of occupational safety. In Europe, this is particularly the case between April and September from around 11 a.m. to 4 p.m. relocation of working hours in the early mornings, having breaks in the shade and—if feasible—performance of individual work task in the shade is recommended.
P	Person-related	If precedent measures are not sufficient, personal protection for employees should be ensured including appropriate clothing (long sleeves and long trousers), protective brimmed headgear, and suitable sunglasses. Protective clothing with UVR protection factor (UPF) is desirable, however, even ordinary cotton T-shirts seem to offer reasonable protection against solar UVR ("better a T-shirt than no shirt"). Sunscreens should only be used where protection by other means is not possible.

UVR, ultraviolet radiation

Primary Prevention

As defined by the International Agency for Research on Cancer (IARC), any preventive activity aimed at lowering the occurrence of cancer in humans is classified as primary prevention [38], whereby the collective level and the individual level are further subclassified [39]. Primary prevention should not be limited to the corporate level; it may also be part of a broader strategy that includes governmental and institutional preventative measures and policies, as well as the adoption of certain norms, standards, and preventive initiatives [19, 39]. The implementation of an effective risk assessment procedure, which must be evaluated and updated on a regular basis, is the first step in primary prevention in the workplace. Based on the results of the risk assessment, appropriate steps can be implemented, including, but not restricted to, technical measures [39]. The supply of informational materials (e.g., brochures) and the implementation of specialized health-pedagogical training programs (e.g., sun-safety trainings and skin cancer prevention trainings) are key strategies in terms of collective prevention. Particularly those efforts including health-education can improve employees' understanding and perception of the occupational solar UVR risk and are regarded essential in the prevention of skin cancer in outdoor workers [14, 39, 40]. Individual prevention involves providing outdoor workers with proper Personal Protective Equipment (PPE), which comprises i) sunglasses with wide, solar UVR filtering lenses, ii) UVR filtering clothing (i.e., long-sleeved shirts and pants), and iii) headgears (i.e., broad-brimmed helmets or hats with sun shields as well as ear and neck guards) [38, 39]. A further protective strategy—which does not belong to PPE—is the use of sunscreens, which must filter UV-A and UV-B rays, have a Sun Protection Factor (SPF) of at least 30 but preferably 50+, and need to be water/sweat-resistant as well as easily applicable so that they can be frequently re-applied throughout the day [38, 39, 41, 42]. Essential new methods for assessing secondary performance attributes of sunscreens in order to specifically design them for this purpose and thus increase acceptance in professional outdoor work have recently been developed [42].

Secondary Prevention

Secondary prevention, according to the IARC, comprises strategies that can lead to the early identification of precancerous states or malignancies in an early phase—screening and early diagnosis are the two fundamentals of secondary prevention [38]. Occupational health surveillance (HS) of employees who are exposed to relevant levels of solar UVR and hence at greater risk of harmful effects is the most substantial approach of secondary prevention in the workplace. Workers with conditions that may determine a particular vulnerability to the hazard (e.g., fair skin photo-types I & II; workers under immuno-suppression or hydrochlorothiazide) should be given special consideration. Periodic health checks of the workforce by certified occupational health specialists are commonly incorporated in HS; additional medical professionals, such as dermatologists, are involved in supplemental health management on an individual basis [14, 17, 19].

Tertiary Prevention

Measures of intervention at a stage when harmful effects have already manifested are referred to as tertiary prevention. Medical and occupational rehabilitation of employees with UVR-related skin malignancies after treatments are examples of tertiary preventive measures, which seek to provide a safe return to work, recovery from the condition, and a good quality of life as well as compensation [16, 19].

Challenges in Prevention

Irregular and lacking recognition of the occupational risk of developing occupational skin cancer in outdoor workers, as evidenced by the wide range of studies reporting high levels of individual solar UVR exposure at work and inadequate adoption of sun-protective activities and routines by outdoor workers, substantially impedes adequate implementation of effective preventive interventions in this occupational group [14, 40, 43]. Table 5.4 depicts priorities in dermato-

Table 5.4 Priorities in dermato-oncology according to a position paper of the European Association of Dermato Oncology (EADO), European Academy of Dermatology and Venereology (EADV) and Task Forces, European Dermatology Forum (EDF), International Dermoscopy Society (IDS), European Board of Dermato-Venereology at the European Union of Medical Specialists (EBDV–UEMS) and European Organization for Research and Treatment of Cancer (EORTC) Cutaneous Lymphoma Task Force. Primary prevention (i.e., actions to reduce solar UVR exposure in the general and high-risk populations), secondary prevention (i.e., early detection of thick, aggressive tumors, and tumors that develop in individuals at high risk for adverse outcomes), and tertiary prevention alongside expansion and improvement of skin cancer registry (i.e., monitoring the current state, measuring the efficacy of preventive strategies, and planning of appropriate interventions) are all necessary to effectively address occupational skin cancer caused by solar UVR [4]

Classification	Concrete actions
Primary prevention	• Conception and implementation of health educational measures, such as specialized health-pedagogical training programs. • Collaboration with authorities and scientific communities to organize campaigns and other actions. • Integration of legislators to change statutes with regard to solar UVR exposure.
Secondary prevention	• Conception and implementation of health educational measures, such as promotion of self-examinations and to seek physician skin examinations or educating non-healthcare professionals (e.g., hairdressers) in recognizing skin cancer. • Collaboration with authorities and scientific communities to organize campaigns and other actions. • Establishing standards and determining the optimum population to screen. • Creating a system for healthcare professionals to receive updated and ongoing training.
Tertiary prevention	• Creating patient management algorithms that are standardized. • For more complex matters, encouraging the creation of interdisciplinary cancer boards. • Collaborating with providers to enhance patient access to new therapies. • Strengthening patient access to randomized controlled trials.

UVR ultraviolet radiation

oncology which should be focused on the future in order to facilitate better prevention of occupational skin cancer by solar UVR.

Interventions to enhance outdoor workers' sun protection behavior have already been identified as being urgently needed. A recent investigation examined the risk perceptions and attitudes of outdoor workers toward sun protection measures and demonstrated that these factors might impact practical sun protection behavior at work [44]. Another contemporary study found that the unique needs of outdoor workers are seldomly considered, despite the fact that several occupational groups have shown an inclination to enhance their sun protection behavior [45]. Prevailing evidence supports the notion that, on the one hand, structures are deemed necessary to enable the implementation of technical and organizational sun-protective measures, and that, on the other hand, educational interventions and clear instructions designed for specific needs and attitudes of outdoor workers are mandatory to strengthen UVR protection behavior and mitigate widespread errors in sun protection [2, 42, 45].

References

1. Diepgen TL. New developments in occupational dermatology. J Dtsch Dermatol Ges. 2016;14(9):875–89. https://doi.org/10.1111/ddg.13128.
2. John SM, Garbe C, French LE, Takala J, Yared W, Cardone A, et al. Improved protection of outdoor workers from solar ultraviolet radiation: position statement. J Eur Acad Dermatol Venereol. 2021;35(6):1278–84. https://doi.org/10.1111/jdv.17011.
3. Park YJ, Kwon GH, Kim JO, Kim NK, Ryu WS, Lee KS. A retrospective study of changes in skin cancer characteristics over 11 years. Arch Craniofac Surg. 2020;21(2):87–91. https://doi.org/10.7181/acfs.2020.00024.
4. Garbe C, Peris K, Soura E, Forsea AM, Hauschild A, Arenbergerova M, et al. The evolving field of Dermato-oncology and the role of dermatologists: position paper of the EADO, EADV and task forces, EDF, IDS, EBDV-UEMS and EORTC cutaneous lymphoma task force. J Eur Acad Dermatol Venereol. 2020;34(10):2183–97. https://doi.org/10.1111/jdv.16849.
5. Trakatelli M, Barkitzi K, Apap C, Majewski S, De Vries E. Skin cancer risk in outdoor workers: a European multicenter case-control study. J Eur Acad Dermatol Venereol. 2016;30(Suppl 3):5–11. https://doi.org/10.1111/jdv.13603.
6. Paulo MS, Adam B, Akagwu C, Akparibo I, Al-Rifai RH, Bazrafshan S, et al. WHO/ILO work-related burden of disease and injury: protocol for systematic reviews of occupational exposure to solar ultraviolet radiation and of the effect of occupational exposure to solar ultraviolet radiation on melanoma and non-melanoma skin cancer. Environ Int. 2019;126:804–15. https://doi.org/10.1016/j.envint.2018.09.039.
7. Boniol M, Hosseini B, Ivanov I, Náfrádi B, Neira M, Olsson A, et al. The effect of occupational exposure to solar ultraviolet radiation on malignant skin melanoma and nonmelanoma skin cancer: a systematic review and meta-analysis from the WHO/ILO joint estimates of the work-related burden of disease and injury. Geneva: World Health Organization; 2021.
8. Peters CE, Ge CB, Hall AL, Davies HW, Demers PA. CAREX Canada: an enhanced model for assessing occupational carcinogen exposure. Occup Environ Med. 2015;72(1):64–71. https://doi.org/10.1136/oemed-2014-102286.
9. McKenzie JF, El-Zaemey S, Carey RN. Prevalence of exposure to multiple occupational carcinogens among exposed workers in Australia. Occup Environ Med. 2020; https://doi.org/10.1136/oemed-2020-106629.
10. Kauppinen T, Toikkanen J, Pedersen D, Young R, Ahrens W, Boffetta P, et al. Occupational exposure to carcinogens in the European Union. Occup Environ Med. 2000;57(1):10–8. https://doi.org/10.1136/oem.57.1.10.
11. Loney T, Paulo MS, Modenese A, Gobba F, Tenkate T, Whiteman DC, et al. Global evidence on occupational sun exposure and keratinocyte cancers: a systematic review. Br J Dermatol. 2021;184(2):208–18. https://doi.org/10.1111/bjd.19152.
12. Armstrong BK, Kricker A. The epidemiology of UV induced skin cancer. J Photochem Photobiol B. 2001;63(1–3):8–18. https://doi.org/10.1016/s1011-1344(01)00198-1.
13. Fitzmaurice C, Abate D, Abbasi N, Abbastabar H, Abd-Allah F, Abdel-Rahman O, et al. Global, Regional, and National Cancer Incidence, mortality, years of life lost, years lived with disability, and disability-adjusted life-years for 29 cancer groups, 1990 to 2017: a systematic analysis for the global burden of disease study. JAMA Oncol. 2019;5(12):1749–68. https://doi.org/10.1001/jamaoncol.2019.2996.
14. Modenese A, Korpinen L, Gobba F. Solar radiation exposure and outdoor work: an underestimated occupational risk. Int J Environ Res Public Health. 2018;15:10. https://doi.org/10.3390/ijerph15102063.
15. Peters CE, Pasko E, Strahlendorf P, Holness DL, Tenkate T. Solar ultraviolet radiation exposure among outdoor workers in three Canadian Provinces. Ann Work Expo Health. 2019;63(6):679–88. https://doi.org/10.1093/annweh/wxz044.
16. International Commission on Non-Ionizing Radiation Protection. ICNIRP statement—protection of workers against ultraviolet radiation. Health

Phys. 2010;99(1):66–87. https://doi.org/10.1097/HP.0b013e3181d85908.

17. Gobba F, Modenese A, John SM. Skin cancer in outdoor workers exposed to solar radiation: a largely underreported occupational disease in Italy. J Eur Acad Dermatol Venereol. 2019;33(11):2068–74. https://doi.org/10.1111/jdv.15768.

18. John SM, Trakatelli M, Ulrich C. Non-melanoma skin cancer by solar UV: the neglected occupational threat. J Eur Acad Dermatol Venereol. 2016;30(Suppl 3):3–4. https://doi.org/10.1111/jdv.13602.

19. Ulrich C, Salavastru C, Agner T, Bauer A, Brans R, Crepy MN, et al. The European Status Quo in legal recognition and patient-care services of occupational skin cancer. J Eur Acad Dermatol Venereol. 2016;30(Suppl 3):46–51. https://doi.org/10.1111/jdv.13609.

20. Wittlich M, John SM, Tiplica GS, Sălăvăstru CM, Butacu AI, Modenese A, et al. Personal solar ultraviolet radiation dosimetry in an occupational setting across Europe. J Eur Acad Dermatol Venereol. 2020;34(8):1835–41. https://doi.org/10.1111/jdv.16303.

21. Schmitt J, Haufe E, Trautmann F, Schulze HJ, Elsner P, Drexler H, et al. Is ultraviolet exposure acquired at work the most important risk factor for cutaneous squamous cell carcinoma? Results of the population-based case-control study FB-181. Br J Dermatol. 2018;178(2):462–72. https://doi.org/10.1111/bjd.15906.

22. Schmitt J, Haufe E, Trautmann F, Schulze HJ, Elsner P, Drexler H, et al. Occupational UV-exposure is a major risk factor for basal cell carcinoma: results of the population-based case-control study FB-181. J Occup Environ Med. 2018;60(1):36–43. https://doi.org/10.1097/jom.0000000000001217.

23. Bauer A, Haufe E, Heinrich L, Seidler A, Schulze HJ, Elsner P, et al. Basal cell carcinoma risk and solar UV exposure in occupationally relevant anatomic sites: do histological subtype, tumor localization and Fitzpatrick phototype play a role? A population-based case-control study. J Occup Med Toxicol. 2020;15:28. https://doi.org/10.1186/s12995-020-00279-8.

24. Watson M, Holman DM, Maguire-Eisen M. Ultraviolet radiation exposure and its impact on skin cancer risk. Semin Oncol Nurs. 2016;32(3):241–54. https://doi.org/10.1016/j.soncn.2016.05.005.

25. Kovačić J, Wittlich M, John SM, Macan J. Personal ultraviolet radiation dosimetry and its relationship with environmental data: a longitudinal pilot study in Croatian construction workers. J Photochem Photobiol B. 2020;207:111866. https://doi.org/10.1016/j.jphotobiol.2020.111866.

26. Modenese A, Gobba F, Paolucci V, John SM, Sartorelli P, Wittlich M. Occupational solar UV exposure in construction workers in Italy: results of a one-month monitoring with personal dosimeters. 2020 IEEE International Conference on Environment and Electrical Engineering and 2020 IEEE Industrial and Commercial Power Systems Europe (EEEIC/I&CPS Europe) 2020. p. 1–5.

27. Modenese A, Gobba F, Paolucci V, John SM, Sartorelli P, Wittlich M. A one-month monitoring of exposure to solar UV radiation of a group of construction workers in Tuscany. Energies. 2020;13(22):6035.

28. Moldovan HR, Wittlich M, John SM, Brans R, Tiplica GS, Salavastru C, et al. Exposure to solar UV radiation in outdoor construction workers using personal dosimetry. Environ Res. 2020;181:108967. https://doi.org/10.1016/j.envres.2019.108967.

29. Wittlich M, Westerhausen S, Kleinespel P, Rifer G, Stöppelmann W. An approximation of occupational lifetime UVR exposure: algorithm for retrospective assessment and current measurements. J Eur Acad Dermatol Venereol. 2016;30(Suppl 3):27–33. https://doi.org/10.1111/jdv.13607.

30. Wittlich M, Westerhausen S, Strehl B, Schmitz M, Stöppelmann W, Versteeg H: Exposition von Beschäftigten gegenüber solarer UV-Strahlung—Ergebnisse des Projekts mit Genesis-UV. https://publikationen.dguv.de/widgets/pdf/download/article/3993 (2020). Accessed 31 December 2021.

31. Schmitt J, Seidler A, Diepgen TL, Bauer A. Occupational ultraviolet light exposure increases the risk for the development of cutaneous squamous cell carcinoma: a systematic review and meta-analysis. Br J Dermatol. 2011;164(2):291–307. https://doi.org/10.1111/j.1365-2133.2010.10118.x.

32. Bauer A, Diepgen TL, Schmitt J. Is occupational solar ultraviolet irradiation a relevant risk factor for basal cell carcinoma? A systematic review and meta-analysis of the epidemiological literature. Br J Dermatol. 2011;165(3):612–25. https://doi.org/10.1111/j.1365-2133.2011.10425.x.

33. Breitbart EW, Choudhury K, Anders MP, Volkmer B, Greinert R, Katalinic A, et al. Benefits and risks of skin cancer screening. Oncol Res Treat. 2014;37(Suppl 3):38–47. https://doi.org/10.1159/000364887.

34. Skudlik C, Tiplica GS, Salavastru C, John SM. Instructions for use of the OSD notification forms. J Eur Acad Dermatol Venereol. 2017;31(Suppl 4):44–6. https://doi.org/10.1111/jdv.14320.

35. Carøe TK, Ebbehøj NE, Wulf HC, Agner T. Recognized occupational skin cancer in Denmark—data from the last ten years. Acta Derm Venereol. 2013;93(3):369–71. https://doi.org/10.2340/00015555-1484.

36. Federal Ministry of Justice and for Consumer Protection: German "Ordinance on Preventive Occupational Health Care (ArbMedVV)". http://www.gesetze-im-internet.de/englisch_arbmedvv/index.html, 2019. Accessed 31 December 2021.

37. World Health Organization: WHO Website. Classifications. ICD. https://www.who.int/classifications/icd/en/, 2021. Accessed 31 December 2021.

38. International Agency for Research on Cancer of the World Health Organization: IARC Handbooks of Cancer Prevention—Preamble for Primary

Prevention.   https://handbooks.iarc.fr/docs/HB-Preamble-Primary-Prevention.pdf, 2019. Accessed 21 October 2021.

39. Alfonso JH, Bauer A, Bensefa-Colas L, Boman A, Bubas M, Constandt L, et al. Minimum standards on prevention, diagnosis and treatment of occupational and work-related skin diseases in Europe—position paper of the COST Action StanDerm (TD 1206). J Eur Acad Dermatol Venereol. 2017;31(Suppl 4):31–43. https://doi.org/10.1111/jdv.14319.

40. Reinau D, Weiss M, Meier CR, Diepgen TL, Surber C. Outdoor workers' sun-related knowledge, attitudes and protective behaviours: a systematic review of cross-sectional and interventional studies. Br J Dermatol. 2013;168(5):928–40. https://doi.org/10.1111/bjd.12160.

41. Tenkate T, Strahlendorf P. Sun safety at work: a management systems approach to occupational sun safety. Toronto: Ryerson University; 2020.

42. Rocholl M, Weinert P, Bielfeldt S, Laing S, Wilhelm KP, Ulrich C, et al. New methods for assessing secondary performance attributes of sunscreens suitable for professional outdoor work. J Occup Med Toxicol. 2021;16(1):25. https://doi.org/10.1186/s12995-021-00314-2.

43. Schmalwieser AW, Casale GR, Colosimo A, Schmalwieser SS, Siani AM. Review on occupational personal solar UV exposure measurements. Atmos. 2021;12(2):142. https://doi.org/10.3390/atmos12020142.

44. Rocholl M, Ludewig M, John SM, Bitzer EM, Wilke A. Outdoor workers' perceptions of skin cancer risk and attitudes to sun-protective measures: a qualitative study. J Occup Health. 2020;62(1):e12083. https://doi.org/10.1002/1348-9585.12083.

45. Ludewig M, Rocholl M, John SM, Wilke A. Secondary prevention of UV-induced skin cancer: development and pilot testing of an educational patient counseling approach for individual sun protection as standard procedure of patient care. Int Arch Occup Environ Health. 2020;93(6):765–77. https://doi.org/10.1007/s00420-020-01532-7.

Occupational Skin Infections

Orianna Yilsy Marcantonio Santa Cruz
and Gemma Martin-Ezquerra

Among the exposures to hazards at work, biologic agents are of extreme importance. Biologic hazards range from bacteria, fungi, viri, to skin parasites. They can lead to severe cutaneous infections, and its prompt diagnosis is mandatory to avoid delay in treatment that can lead to significant morbidity. Most of them are preventable, and measures have to be applied to reduce its risk. It is essential to know the commonest skin infections related to work activities.

The European schedule of occupational diseases dedicates a section to occupational skin diseases [1], and includes a reference (reference number 4) to "Infectious and parasitic diseases; with the subreference number 401 to "Infectious or parasitic diseases transmitted to man by animals or remains of animals" and number 407 to "Other infectious diseases caused by work in disease prevention, health care, domiciliary assistance and other comparable activities for which a risk of infection has been proven". The ILO list [2] also includes a section for them (1.3.9. "Diseases caused by other biological agents at work not mentioned in the preceding items where a direct link is established scientifically, or determined by methods appropriate to national conditions and practice, between the exposure to these biological agents arising from work activities and the disease(s) contracted by the worker." Most of the diseases described in this chapter can be classified herein.

Almost all dermatologic infections can be caused by occupational exposure. Professions at risk include health care workers, animal handlers and veterinaries, agriculture workers, and food process workers. Some specific infections will be discussed in this chapter:

- Bacterial occupational skin infections: **erysipeloid, fish tank granuloma, tuberculosis.**
- Viral occupational skin infections: **milker's nodule.**
- Fungal occupational skin infections.
- Parasitic occupational infestations, such as **scabies.**

Baker-Rosenbach's Erysipeloid

Erysipelothrix rhusiopathiae is a facultative, non-spore forming, non-acid fast, small, Gram-positive bacillus [3]. The organism was first established as a human pathogen late in the nineteenth century. Three clinical presentations of erysipeloid are known: the localized cutaneous form ("true" erysipeloid), the generalized variety, and a septicemia form often associated with endocarditis [3].

O. Y. M. S. Cruz · G. Martin-Ezquerra (✉)
Department of Dermatology, Hospital del Mar,
Barcelona, Barcelona, Spain

© The Author(s), under exclusive license to Springer Nature Switzerland AG 2023

A. M. Giménez-Arnau, H. I. Maibach (eds.), *Handbook of Occupational Dermatoses*, Updates in
Clinical Dermatology, https://doi.org/10.1007/978-3-031-22727-1_6

It is a pathogen or a commensal in a wide variety of wild and domestic animals, birds, and fish. Swine erysipela caused by *E. rhusiopathiae* is a disease of high prevalence and economic importance. Humans acquire the infection with exposure to infected animals, their products or wastes, or soil. The disease is most common among farmers, butchers, cooks, housewives, and fishermen. Reflection of the occupational attributes of the disease is some of the names used to describe this infection, including whale finger, seal finger, speck finger, blubber finger, fish poisoning, fish handler's disease, and pork finger [4].

The disease manifests in a similar way in animals and humans. Erysipeloid is the most common form of human infection. After an incubation period ranging from 2 to 7 days, the disease appears at the site of inoculation (usually hand or fingers) as a well-defined, slightly elevated, bright red-violaceous zone, with a peripheral edge that spreads as the center fades; ulceration can also be present. The pain is often severe and may be described as a burning or as itching sensation. Systemic symptoms can occur in some cases: fever, joint aches, lymphadenitis, and lymphadenopathy. Arthritis of an adjacent joint may be seen. The disease is self-limiting and usually resolves in 3–4 weeks without therapy [4]. Occasionally the organism can escape the immunologic system and disseminate producing generalized and septicemic forms. The rare cases of severe sepsis reported in the literature are more frequently secondary to ingestion of undercooked pork. Endocarditis is often associated with it, involving a life-threatening prognosis.

The infection could be underdiagnosed due to the resemblance it bears to other infections, and problems encountered in isolation and identification. When not suspected the diagnosis of erysipeloid can be difficult.

High-dose penicillin G (12–20 million units per day) for a period of time of at least 2 weeks is the treatment of choice for *E. rhusiopathiae*. Cephalosporins and Clindamycin can be an alternative in case of penicillin allergy [5]. Prevention with veterinary surveillance of the germ reservoirs, animal vaccination, and above all compliance with the rules of hygiene by those at risk remain the best solution to avoid this infection.

Tuberculosis Verrucosa (Tuberculosis Verrucosa Cutis)

Cutaneous tuberculosis (TB) consists of only 1–2% of all extrapulmonary TB infections. The clinical manifestations may vary depending on the immune status of the host and previous sensitization to the pathogen [6].

Tuberculosis verrucosa cutis is a paucibacillary subtype of cutaneous TB caused by a reexposure (reinoculation) to *M. tuberculosis* or *Bacillus Calmette-Guérin* in previously sensitized individuals with moderate to high immunity. It can be acquired in occupational settings, such as may occur to dentists treating the mouth of a patient with pulmonary TB or to butchers handling contaminated meat (in the latter case it is usually due to infection by *M. bovis*). The lesions commonly occur at sites prone to trauma such as hands, feet, or buttocks [6, 7].

Clinically, it appears as painless, hyperkeratotic, verrucous, violaceous plaque with irregular borders, the lesions initially are chronic and persistent but slowly tend to resolve, leaving residual scar changes. Regional adenopathies or associated systemic symptoms are rarely seen. Only exceptionally underlying bone lesions (solitary or multiple) have been described. Other entities that present in form of verrucous lesions should be included in the differential diagnosis, such as paracoccidioidomycosis, leishmaniasis, sporotrichosis, chromomycosis, lobomycosis, atypical mycobacteriosis, hypertrophic lichen planus, verrucous carcinoma, iododerma, bromoderma, verruca vulgaris, keratoacanthoma centrifugum, and pyoderma vegetans.

Histopathological studies demonstrate pseudocarcinomatous hyperplasia with poorly defined noncaseating, tuberculous granulomas. Owing to its paucibacillary nature, bacillus is rarely identified by tissue Ziehl-Neelsen staining, making it difficult to diagnose without tissue culture or PCR. The visualization of the mycobacterium and/or their isolation from culture is the exception rather than the rule. The treatment of cutaneous TB is generally similar to that of pulmonary TB Lesions. The good response to specific anti-TB treatment itself can act as a diagnostic tool [6, 7].

Fish Tank Granuloma (*Mycobacterium marinum*)

Mycobacterium marinum is an acid-fast, non-tuberculous mycobacterium. In the past, these non-tuberculosis mycobacteria were thought to be unusual, so they were referred to as "atypical." But actually, they are widely known as environmental mycobacteria. *M. marinum* is the most common form of atypical cutaneous mycobacteriosis in our environment, it was originally reported after its discovery on saltwater fish in the Philadelphia Aquarium in 1926, and was recognized as a human pathogen after the first skin infection was reported in 1951 [8].

M. marinum is usually found on plants, in soil, and on fish in household aquariums, and in fresh and saltwater, worldwide. It is a known pathogen of fresh and saltwater fish, causing the so-called "fish tuberculosis" and occasionally can cause opportunistic infections in humans [9].

The infection usually starts when skin lesions (after trauma, lacerations in an aquatic environment or injury when cleaning an aquarium) come into contact with contaminated water (in fish tanks or swimming pools for instance) with an incubation period of 2 weeks (can vary between 1 and 8 weeks) [9]. Typically it begins with a papulonodular lesion at the inoculation site that slowly grows and frequently ulcerates or abscesses, adopting a warty appearance (Fig. 6.1). The lesions are usually located on the back of the fingers of the hand (aquarium granuloma), or on the knees (swimming pool granuloma), although there are cases described of any location. Subsequently, in a significant percentage of cases (5–70%), a string of purplish painless nodules develops along the lymphatic drainage pathway, producing the typical sporotrichoid appearance. The injuries sustained resolve spontaneously leaving residual hyperpigmentation or atrophic scars [8, 10].

M. marinum cannot divide at a temperature above 30 °C and the infection, therefore, remains much localized to the skin. Infection only occasionally involves deeper structures, like the joints and tendons leading to synovitis and arthritis. Disseminated infections are extremely rare and exclusive of immunocompromised individuals, with a poor prognosis [10].

The diagnosis of *M. marinum* infection can be challenging. The clinical characteristic with an epidemiological history of injury or contact with an aquatic environment, altogether, with the histopathological image showing epithelioid granulomas with multinucleated giant cells, and the visualization of acid-fast bacilli allow suspicion of the diagnosis. Testing for acid-fast bacilli is unreliable and confirmation only can be made by culturing or PCR. The tuberculin skin test is often

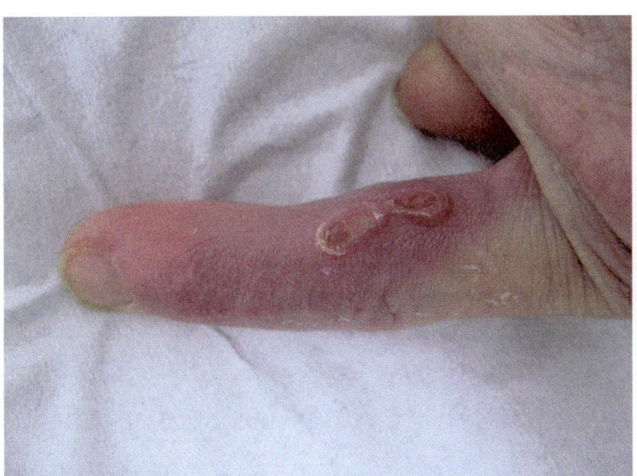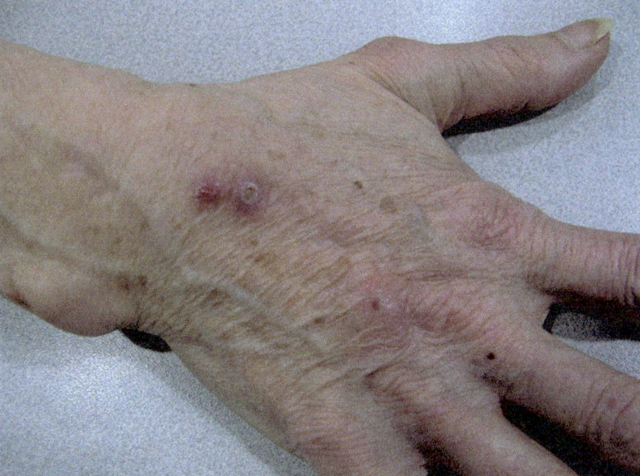

Fig. 6.1 Nodules on the fingers and dorsum of the hand secondary to *M. marinum* infection

positive due to cross-reactivity with others mycobacteria.

The differential diagnosis should be established with other granulomatous lesions in lymphocutaneous distribution such as sporotrichosis and cat scratch disease.

Untreated infection tends to resolve spontaneously after years of evolution. Small lesions can be treated surgically. *M. marinum* is sensitive to rifampin and ethambutol and is resistant to pyrazinamide, isoniazid, and streptomycin. The best treatment regimen is still under debate. Rifampicin, minocycline, clarithromycin, and ciprofloxacin are the drugs most commonly prescribed. Duration of the different regimens is variable (between 3 and 9 months) [8].

The Milker's Nodule

The milker's nodule, also called pseudocowpox, is a cosmopolitan zoonosis mainly found in agro-livestock areas resulting from the infection with paravaccinia. Paravaccinia is a double-stranded DNA virus member of the Parapoxvirus genus and Poxvirus family. In affected cattle, it produces the so-called bovine stomatitis, with erosive lesions or crusty ulcers on the udders and alopecia. Humans usually acquire it by inoculation through contact with their udders, muzzles, or by handling their meat. Visible lesions on the cattle may be absent, but transmission may still occur. Since the virus is viable in a dried state, indirect fomite infection is possible. It is considered an occupational disease, found in farmers, milkers, slaughterers, butchers, cooks, and veterinarians. Those infected often report not wearing personal protective equipment when interacting with bovine and ovine [11, 12].

The incubation period ranges from 5 to 15 days; some of 2–5 nodules then develop, commonly on areas where skin contact was made with the infected animal, such as the hands and forearms. It typically evolves through 6 clinical stages—erythematous maculopapular, targetoid, oozing papulopustular, dry crusted nodular, papillomatous, and regressing. Each stage lasts approximately 1 week. Lesions are typically asymptomatic or not very painful, of relatively rapid appearance and usually do not compromise the general condition. Multiple lesions have rarely been described [11]. The initial lesion, at first, may go unnoticed, but then the nodule becomes larger and usually ulcerates. The surrounding skin often shows lymphangitis. In most cases, after 1–2 months, the nodule will resolve without scaring. However, the lesions may last for months and it tends to recur in immunocompromised individuals. Uncommonly, the patients may present with fever, lymphadenopathy, lymphangitis, erythema multiforme, and secondary bacterial overgrowth of the lesions [11, 12].

The diagnosis is based on epidemiological, clinical, and histopathological criteria. Histological findings might vary according to the stage of presentation. Earlier stages, namely maculopapular and target stages, are characterized by viral cytopathic effects, including cytoplasmic inclusion bodies and epidermal reticular degeneration along with predominantly neutrophilic inflammatory infiltration. Throughout epidermal necrosis and massive infiltration of mononuclear cells are observed in acute weeping stage. In later stages, acanthosis and vasodilation with chronic inflammatory cell infiltrate are predominant in the dermis and subcutis [13].

Orfis, a similar zoonosis caused by a different virus from the same Parapoxvirus genus with nearly identical clinical and histopathologic features is the main differential diagnosis. It is commonly transmitted to humans through direct contact with infected sheep and goats. The similarities, both clinically and histologically between orf and milker's nodules, have led to the joint term "farmyard pox" when describing both viruses. Current PCR assays are unable to distinguish between pseudocowpox and orf with only subtle differences in tissue culturing. Thus, the clinical history of suspected infection sources and exposures is key to an accurate diagnosis. Other differential diagnoses include anthrax, atypical mycobacteriosis, sporotrichosis, tularemia, loxoscelism, piogenic granuloma, and cowpox [11].

As the majority of cases of milker's nodules resolve spontaneously an expectant behavior with supportive measures and counselling is recommended to avoid overtreatment. For small lesions, treatment include Idoxuridine, imiquimod topical creams, cryosurgical ablation or surgical excision. In cases of large lesions or immunocompromised hosts, intralesional alfa-interferon or cidofovir cream have been described [13].

Scabies

Scabies is an infectious disease caused by the infestation with the parasite *Sarcoptes scabiei var. hominis*. The infestation occurs by skin-to-skin contact or contact with fomites. *S. scabiei* mites burrow into the human epidermis in which the female parasite lays eggs. Adult parasites will appear in 2 weeks.

Affected individuals can acquire the infection both in the community, typically spreading to all household members. However, occupational scabies has to be suspected in those individuals at risk, especially workers in nursing homes, health care workers, and workers in social services and prisons. Occupational history has to be always recorded when facing patients with scabies.

Clinical manifestations include abrupt incoercible pruritus, exacerbated at night, and typically unresponsive to antihistamines. It can affect any part of the body and usually spares the head in adults.

Skin examination shows a crusted exanthema, sometimes with small erythematous papules, which is unspecific. Careful examination can reveal specific scabies signs that include the burrow, which is considered pathognomonic, as a thin, brown-gray line of 0.5–1 cm or vesicles at the start of a burrow [14] (Fig. 6.2). They are typically located on the interdigital spaces or on the volar wrists. Scabies nodules are round brownish nodules or papules, more commonly on folds or genitalia. In children, papulopustular acral eruptions have to be included in the differential diagnosis of scabies. In immunosuppressed and elderly patients pruritus can be absent. Crusted scabies affects particularly those groups and it is characterized by large thick scaly plaques, mainly in the extensor surfaces (Fig. 6.3). It is highly con-

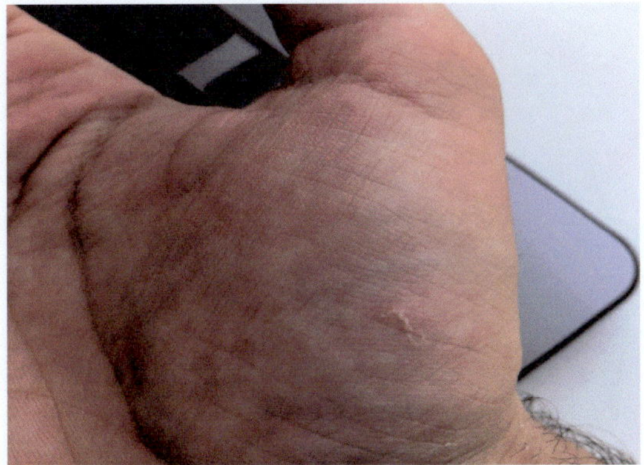

Fig. 6.2 Burrow in scabies

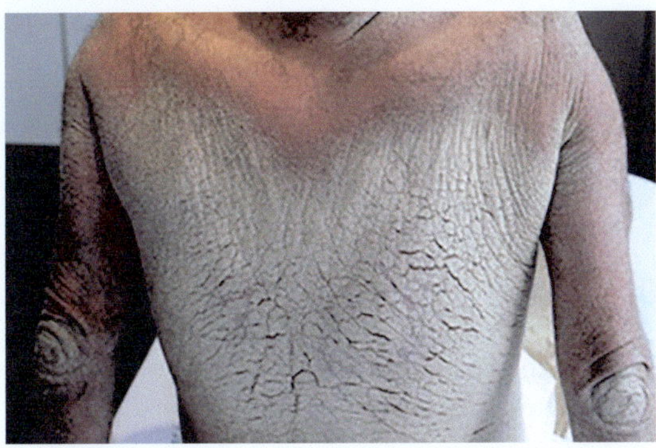

Fig. 6.3 Scaly plaques in an immunosuppressed patient with crusted scabies

tagious and it is commonly the source of infections in occupational settings.

Diagnosis can be challenging at firsts symptoms. Clinical suspicion can be made in patients with professions at risk or with intrafamiliar pruritus. Examination can reveal the eruption with specific signs. Confirmation can be performed with dermoscopy which can demonstrate the parasite on the burrow (delta-wing jet sign) and Müller test, that visualizes the parasite, feces, or eggs under the microscope (Fig. 6.4).

Treatment of individuals can be made following guidelines with permethrin 5%, as first-line treatment, 10–25% benzyl benzoate, 2–10% precipitated sulfur, 10% crotamiton, 0.5% malathion, and 1% lindane [15]. Oral ivermectin is available in most countries as an alternative to topical treatments due to its efficacy and simplicity. It is especially useful in outbreaks in big

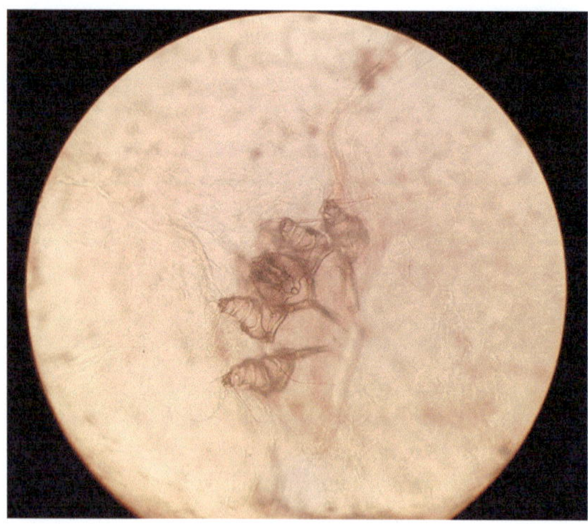

Fig. 6.4 Mite visualized under an optic microscope after scraping the burrow

facilities where a high number of residents and workers have to be simultaneously treated.

Treatment of close contacts is highly advisable to avoid recurrences. Fomites have to be treated, and recommendations include washing at high temperatures all clothes and linen.

In cases of occupational infestations, it is crucial to investigate the source of the infection, detect other individuals infected (among both residents and workers), decide to early treat simultaneously all contacts to avoid transmission, and close follow-up to detect new cases. Special circuits to manage fomites should be implemented during the outbreak. Attack rates in health care facilities have been calculated to be between 26% and 32% of workers with direct contact with the index patient, and up to 5% to 9% of the household members of these workers being infected as well [16].

References

1. EUR-Lex - 32003H0670 - EN - EUR-Lex [Internet]. [citado 14 de noviembre de 2021]. Disponible en: https://eur-lex.europa.eu/legal-content/EN/ALL/?uri=CELEX%3A32003H0670

2. ILO List of Occupational Diseases (revised 2010) [Internet]. 2010 [citado 14 de noviembre de 2021]. Disponible en: https://www.ilo.org/global/topics/safety-and-health-at-work/resources-library/publications/WCMS_125137/lang%2D%2Den/index.htm

3. Brooke CJ, Riley TV. Erysipelothrix rhusiopathiae: bacteriology, epidemiology and clinical manifestations of an occupational pathogen. J Med Microbiol. 1999;48(9):789–99.

4. Reboli AC, Farrar WE. Erysipelothrix rhusiopathiae: an occupational pathogen. Clin Microbiol Rev. 1989;2(4):354–9.

5. Barnett JH, Estes SA, Wirman JA, Morris RE, Staneck JL. Erysipeloid. J Am Acad Dermatol. 1983;9(1):116–23.

6. Dias MFRG, Bernardes Filho F, Quaresma MV, do Nascimento LV, Nery JADC, Azulay DR. Update on cutaneous tuberculosis. An Bras Dermatol. 2014;89(6):925–38.

7. Bravo FG, Gotuzzo E. Cutaneous tuberculosis. Clin Dermatol. 2007;25(2):173–80.

8. Aubry A, Chosidow O, Caumes E, Robert J, Cambau E. Sixty-three cases of Mycobacterium marinum infection: clinical features, treatment, and antibiotic susceptibility of causative isolates. Arch Intern Med. 2002;162(15):1746–52.

9. Kiesch N. Aquariums and mycobacterioses. Rev Med Brux. 2000;21(4):A255–6.

10. Wolinsky E. Mycobacterial diseases other than tuberculosis. Clin Infect Dis. 1992;15(1):1–10.

11. Adriano AR, Quiroz CD, Acosta ML, Jeunon T, Bonini F. Milker's nodule—Case report. An Bras Dermatol. 2015;90(3):407–10.

12. Werchniak AE, Herfort OP, Farrell TJ, Connolly KS, Baughman RD. Milker's nodule in a healthy young woman. J Am Acad Dermatol. 2003;49(5):910–1.

13. Groves RW, Wilson-Jones E, MacDonald DM. Human orf and milkers' nodule: a clinicopathologic study. J Am Acad Dermatol. 1991;25(4):706–11.

14. Salavastru CM, Chosidow O, Boffa MJ, Janier M, Tiplica GS. European guideline for the management of scabies. J Eur Acad Dermatol Venereol. 2017;31(8):1248–53.

15. Thomas C, Coates SJ, Engelman D, Chosidow O, Chang AY. Ectoparasites: Scabies. J Am Acad Dermatol. 2020;82(3):533–48.

16. Buehlmann M, Beltraminelli H, Strub C, Bircher A, Jordan X, Battegay M, et al. Scabies outbreak in an intensive care unit with 1,659 exposed individuals—key factors for controlling the outbreak. Infect Control Hosp Epidemiol. 2009;30(4):354–60.

Identification of Occupational Dermatoses. The Role of the Occupational Physician and the Dermatologist

Vera Mahler

Occupational Dermatoses

Occupational dermatoses range among the four most frequently notified occupational diseases and have significant economic and social repercussions (Fig. 7.1). In this chapter, "occupational dermatosis" and "occupational skin disease" are used synonymously. Though occupational dermatoses are subject to mandatory reporting in most countries, they are often underdiagnosed [1–3].

Definitions

"Work-related (skin) disease" and "occupational (skin) disease" are differently defined. Work-related diseases are generally defined as diseases, which have multiple causes, including factors of the work environment [1]. Work-related diseases are defined as diseases with solid scientific evidence concerning a possible occupational origin, which may, however, not fulfil all given legal criteria for recognition of an

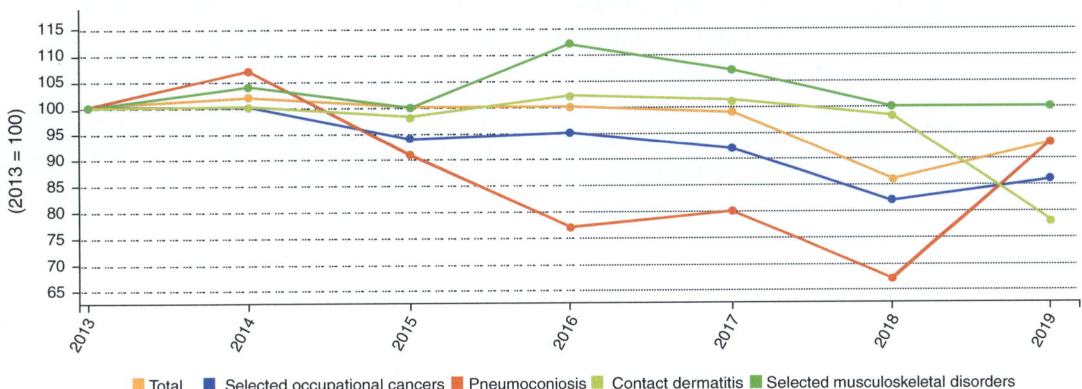

Fig. 7.1 Development of occupational diseases—total and groups (European Union* 2013–2019). *Note: excluding Germany, Greece and Portugal. Based on the median value of available data for other EU Member States. Source: Eurostat (online data code: hsw_occ_ina)

V. Mahler (✉)
Division of Allergology, Paul-Ehrlich-Institut,
Langen, Germany

© The Author(s), under exclusive license to Springer Nature Switzerland AG 2023
A. M. Giménez-Arnau, H. I. Maibach (eds.), *Handbook of Occupational Dermatoses*, Updates in Clinical Dermatology, https://doi.org/10.1007/978-3-031-22727-1_7

occupational disease [1]. Therefore, when making the diagnosis of an occupational or work-related (skin) disease, it is necessary to establish a causal link between exposure to a risk factor and development of the disease, since definitions for both conditions are based on the notion of occupational risk. Work-related skin diseases are caused or worsened by a professional activity [2]. To be recognized as "occupational skin diseases" they need to fulfil additional legal criteria, which differ from country to country [2]. Most European countries have an ILO/EU recommendation-based official list of occupational diseases; only a few have an "open" list of occupational diseases [1, 4].

The European schedule of occupational diseases lists diseases that have been scientifically recognized as occupational in origin [4]. As a result, they qualify for compensation and are the subject of compulsory preventive measures to reduce their prevalence [5]. European Member States determine for themselves the criteria for recognizing occupational diseases and are free to implement more comprehensive and detailed national laws and regulations. Occupational diseases caused by physical, chemical, or biological factors are recognized in all EU Member States [5]. Especially with regard to physical exposures (e.g., heat and cold), a distinction has to be made as to whether the noxious work-related exposures occurred once (traumatically within a single work shift) or repetitively (in several work shifts): In the former case an occupational accident is recognized, in the case of repetitive effects an occupational skin disease has to be assessed. Differences concerning the recognition procedure and recompensation between work accidents and occupational skin diseases apply.

The official recognition of occupational skin diseases is in most countries based on the recognition of a so-called "occupational risk" and the application of three key criteria [5]:

- There has to be a causal relationship between the disease and exposure to a harmful situation or agent.
- This exposure is linked to the work place.

- The disease occurs among specific groups with a frequency exceeding the average morbidity of the rest of the population.

EU countries recognize the risks of dermal exposure leading to skin diseases and have transposed the requirements of all relevant Directives into their legislation [5]. However, it remains unclear how far individual countries have translated this recognition into national law [5].

Existing definitions for occupational skin diseases differ between countries, and the point in time when an occupational dermatosis is being notified varies from first suspicion to when a person had to quit the job [2]. Consequently, the figures for work-related skin diseases and occupational skin diseases, respectively, incorporated in national statistics vary dramatically from one country to the other, since the steering of the notification process is not comparable [2].

Concerning occupational dermatoses, a survey conducted among occupational dermatologists and occupational health experts has shed light on the situation in 28 countries, including the recognition of UV light-induced skin cancer as an occupational disease [2]. However, recognition or rejection as an occupational disease may change over time in a country, e.g.,:

- Due to fundamental changes in legislation (regarding general recognition criteria) (e.g., 2021 in Germany [6]).
- Increasing scientific knowledge regarding a work-related disease (e.g., on doubling of basal cell carcinoma risk in outdoor workers [7]).
- The emergence of a novel work-related disease (e.g., COVID-19 [8]).

In view of the prevalence of skin diseases throughout the European Union, skin diseases and their prevention are recognized as an important issue [5]. Effective prevention of skin diseases requires a combination of technical, organizational, and medical measures to eliminate or minimize the skin's exposure to risk factors [5]. The occupational dermatologist and the occupational physician play important roles at the interface between technical, organizational, legal, and medical requirements for the successful prevention and early treatment of occupational skin diseases. This chapter summarizes relevant aspects of the identification of occupational dermatoses from a European perspective.

Spectrum of Occupational Skin Diseases

Exposure to chemical, physical, and biological risk factors can lead to different occupational skin diseases, though several individual (genetic) factors influence the outcome too [9]. Most frequent occupational dermatoses are allergic (ICD-code L23) and irritant contact dermatitis (L24) predominantly located at the hands (Fig. 7.2a–c), and less frequently arms and face [10–13]. They belong to the core (short) list of the European occupational diseases statistics (EODS) of the most reported ICD codes [14]—together with selected occupational cancers (Malignant neo-plasm of bronchus (C34); Mesothelioma (C45)), Pneumoconiosis (J61 due to asbestos and other mineral fibers and J62 due to dust containing silica), and selected musculoskeletal disorders (G56 Mononeuropathies of upper limb; I73 Other peripheral vascular diseases; M51 Other intervertebral disc disorders; M65 Synovitis and tenosynovitis; M70 Soft tissue disorders related to use, overuse and pressure; M75 Shoulder lesions; M77 Other enthesopathies) (Fig. 7.1). This short list represents around 70% of the total number of occupational diseases reported in the EODS database (2013–2019) by 24 participating EU Member States (Germany, Greece, and Portugal not included).

Between 2013 and 2019, the total index for the number of people recognized as having occupational diseases declined overall by 7% [14]. Both allergic and irritant contact dermatitis recorded a lower level in 2019 than in 2013, down by 21% for the allergy-based variant and by 1% for the irritant-based variant [14].

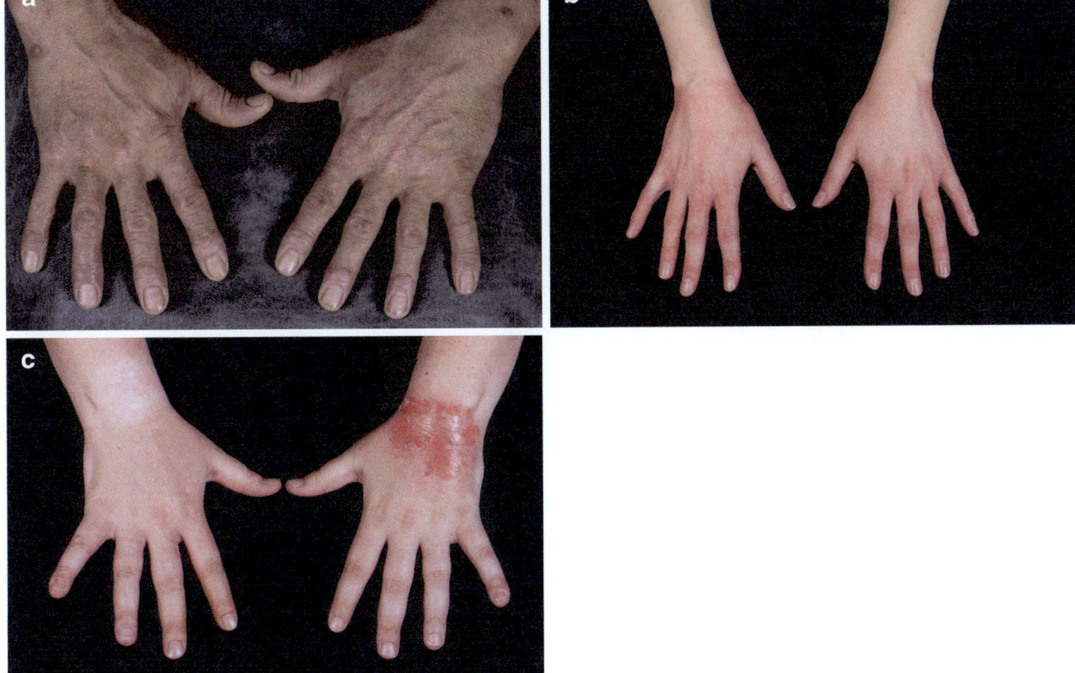

Fig. 7.2 (**a**) chronic irritant contact dermatitis in a metal worker; (**b**) allergic contact dermatitis to nitril gloves in a dental assistant; (**c**) artifact in a warehouse worker pre-sented for medical assessment under the diagnosis of occupational contact dermatitis to colophony

Table 7.1 gives an overview of frequent and less frequent work-related diseases, which may be recognized as occupational dermatoses depending on the occupational exposure and respective legal framework. Concurrent non-occupational exposures have to be considered [9, 15, 16]. The table is not exhaustive but is intended to raise awareness of less common occupational dermatoses beyond the predominant manifestations of contact dermatitis. In addition to dermatoses primarily caused by occupational exposures, endogenous inflammatory dermatoses can be aggravated by specific occupational exposures: e.g., atopic eczema (mostly by irritants, less frequently by heat or cold), psoriasis (mostly by mechanical, but also other physical triggers), progressive systemic scleroderma (by cold, rapid temperature changes, or vibration), dermatomyositis (UV, cold, rapid temperature changes, or vibration), cutaneous lupus erythematodes (mostly UV-light, but also cold, heat, rapid temperature changes, and mechanical triggers). The manner of dealing with work-related aggravation of a congenital skin disease with regard to recognition as an occupational disease varies in different countries (the situation in 28 European countries has been summarized in [2].

The most important thing in identifying occupational dermatoses is to even think about the possibility that occupational influences may play a role in the disease manifestation that a patient presents with. The occupational dermatologist and the occupational physician must be aware of the pathology and possible occupational induction or exacerbation of these diseases, and accordingly, identify relevant exposures in an exploratory manner.

As with any occupational disease, a certain degree of causal relationship between the skin disease and the occupation must be verified during

Table 7.1 Work-related skin diseases caused by exposure to hazards at work (modified from [9, 15, 16])

Chemical hazards	Examples (for agents and *occupational exposures*)	Work-related or occupational dermatosis	Principles of prevention of occupational dermatoses
Irritants	For example, • Wet work and detergents (*healthcare, food processing*) • Organic solvents (*used in many industries, e.g., in the production of dyes, polymers, plastics, textiles, printing inks, pharmaceuticals. Paints, varnishes, laquers, adhesives glues, and degreasing agents*) • Acids (*used in many industries, e.g., aerated beverages, car batteries, manufacture of paints, dyes, synthetic fibers, fertilizers, electrolytes, detergents, polymers, plastics, explosives*) • Alkalies (*used in many industries, e.g., manufacture of paper, metal industries, food industries, cleaning agents in industrial processes, water treatment, crude oil treatment*)	Irritant contact dermatitis Also, post-traumatic irritant contact dermatitis at the site of previous physical damage (burns, chemical burns)	Rule out allergic contact dermatitis (patch test). Reduce irritant exposure by technical and organizational measures. Exchange agent if possible against less irritating substance (e.g., in healthcare: Reduce frequent handwashing by disinfection instead); Review the skin protection concept including personal protection gear, skin cleansing, skin protection, and care products
Phototoxic agents	e.g. • Furocoumarins (psoralens) in plants (*gardeners, florist, manufacturer of cosmetic*) • Tar derivatives (*road construction and building insulation workers*) • Pharmaceuticals (*drug manufacturing based on phototoxic pharmaceutical plant materials*)	Phototoxic contact dermatitis	Rule out (photo)allergic contact dermatitis (patch test). Reduce exposure by technical and organizational measures. Review the skin protection concept including personal protection gear, skin cleansing, skin protection, and care products

Table 7.1 (continued)

Chemical hazards	Examples (for agents and *occupational exposures*)	Work-related or occupational dermatosis	Principles of prevention of occupational dermatoses
Sensitizing agents: (i) Haptens or (ii) proteins	For example, *occupational fields with contact to (i) haptens* • Metals—chromium, nickel, cobalt, mercury • p-phenylenediamine (PPD) • Rubber additives • Natural resins • Artificial resins • Biocides • Preservatives • Animal feeds • Plants • Pharmaceuticals To (ii) proteins: • Animal proteins • Plant proteins, grains • Enzymes For example, *as aerogen (iii) occupational exposure:* • Wood dust • Textile fibers • Cement • Glass fibers • Other chemical compounds in the air (epoxy resins, acrylates) • Dusts from plant materials (e.g., from the Compositae/Asteraceae family) • Pollens	(i) Allergic contact dermatitis (ii) Protein contact dermatitis (iii) Airborne allergic contact dermatitis (or rarely airborne protein contact dermatitis)	Identifying the culprit is essential. (i) if an occupational origin is suspected the baseline series should be supplemented by occupational series of a given sector/occupation and/or substances used at work (based on the safety data sheets) (ii) If proteinaceous substances might be a potential elicitor, skin prick test with these and in vitro IgE-test should be done additionally: Stringent avoidance measures (e.g., by ban of substance from the work environment or—if ban is not possible—personal protection gear) have to be implemented after identification of the culprit allergen(s)
Photosensitizing agents	e.g. • Fragrances (*cleaning, chemical industry*) • Optical brighteners (e.g., *in laundries, washing powder manufacturing*) • Sun screens • Pharmaceuticals (*pharmaceutical industries*)	Photoallergic contact dermatitis	As above in sensitizing agents. Additionally, a photo patch test is necessary to identify the culprit
Urticariatogenic substances: (i) High molecular (ii) Low molecular (iii) Direct urticariatogens	(i) Proteins (e.g., latex (*glove-wearing sectors, e.g., healthcare, food processing, catering, and cleaning*); fish, meats, eggs (food processing); plants (crops and ornamental plants, wood) (ii) For example, bisphenol-A, chromium, and cobalt (iii) For example, stinging-nettle, fragrances, balsam of Peru, preservatives, additives, fruits, vegetables, and dyes	(i)/(ii) Immunologic contact urticarial syndrome (iii) Non-immunogenic contact urticaria	Identifying the culprit is essential. Skin prick test with these substances and in vitro IgE-test should be done additionally. Stringent avoidance measures including total elimination of the allergen due to the risk of more serious complications are necessary; if technical and organizational measures do not succeed change of job might be necessary to avoid/prevent exposure

(continued)

Table 7.1 (continued)

Chemical hazards	Examples (for agents and *occupational exposures*)	Work-related or occupational dermatosis	Principles of prevention of occupational dermatoses
Acnegenic agents	• Industrial oils and greases (via *direct skin*, e.g., *in contact car mechanics*, and *maintenance workers*) • Tar derivatives (via *direct skin*, e.g., *construction, paving, roofing, wood-preserving industries*) • Halogen-containing compounds (*contamination* via *skin, gastrointestinal system or lung; e.g., occupational exposure to polychlorinated naphthalenes, polychlorinated phenoxy phenols, 3 4-dichloroaniline and similar herbicides, iodides, and bromides*) • Certain pharmaceuticals	Oil acne Tar acne Halogen acne	Personal and work hygiene is of utmost importance. Frequent change and centralized washing of dirty work wear are necessary
Skin cancers due to chemical exposure	• Pitch, tar, soot, anthracene and compounds thereof • Mineral and other oils • Raw paraffin • Carbazole and compounds thereof • Arsenic	Basal cell Squamous cell carcinomas Bowen carcinoma Keratotic papilloma Keratoacanthoma Arsenic hyperkeratosis	Prevention of occupational skin cancers due to chemical exposure consists of: Proper occupational safety and health organization and instructions; clothing. Medical surveillance with early detection and treatment of skin lesions
Physical hazards	Examples (for agents and *occupational exposures*)	Work-related or occupational dermatosis	Principles of prevention of occupational dermatoses
Mechanical	(i) Recurrent rubbing or increased pressure can thicken the inflamed skin (e.g., *in shoulders of sack carriers, fingertips of guitarists and violinists, knuckles of masseurs*, and *hands of blacksmiths*) (ii) Vibrations (*such as working*, e.g., *with a jackhammer*) can trigger vibrational urticaria Repetitive use (for months to years) of hand-held tools that generate vibration in the frequency range of 20–1000 Hz can lead to vasospasm and sensitivity disorders in the area of the hands (preferably digitus II–V of the operating hand). (*occupations operating high-speed tools (drills, milling cutters, saws, chisels, grinding and polishing machines, riveting hammers, and tapping machines), e.g., in forestry, civil engineering, metalworking industry, and shipbuilding*)	(i) Lichenification; callosities (these conditions are mostly of esthetic nature and reversible) (ii) Vibratory urticaria/ angioedema Vibration-induced vasospastic syndrome	Reduction of mechanical stress by technical measures, however, prevention is usually impossible

Table 7.1 (continued)

Physical hazards	Examples (for agents and *occupational exposures*)	Work-related or occupational dermatosis	Principles of prevention of occupational dermatoses
Radiation: (i) Ionizing (ii) Non-ionizing (e.g. UV-light)	(i) • Medical imaging and therapy • Industrial quality inspection • Sterilization of medicines and foods (ii) • Natural UV-radiation (*outdoor workers*) • Artificial UV-radiation (*welding, UV lamps and lasers used in medicine, industry, trade and at home*)	(i) Acute radiodermatitis; Chronic radiodermatitis (due to increased occupational safety standards both are very rare nowadays); epithelial skin tumors, further tumor development depending on the dose and exposure (ii) Acute: Various levels of sunburn; Chronic: Photoaging; actinic keratosis; keratoacanthoma; Bowen carcinoma; squamous cell cancer; basal cell carcinoma (concerning melanoma: It is not verified whether occupational exposures are involved in the development of melanoma: The findings are contradictory)	(i) Prevention is mainly technical (enclosure of system, segregation, proper maintenance) accompanied by strict protocols, shielding devices and personal protective equipment (ii) Prevention of occupational skin cancers due to radiation consists of: Proper occupational safety and health organization and instructions Shields, hats and (UV-absorbent) clothing, sun screens Medical surveillance with early detection and treatment of precancerous skin lesions
Temperature: (i) Heat (ii) Cold	(i) Sweat stagnation can cause miliaria; in skin folds intertrigo may develop. Localized heat may cause heat contact urticaria. Intense heat can cause burns or scalds (*the metallurgy sector, bakeries, kitchens, summer outdoor jobs (agriculture, construction), and deep mining*) (ii) The effects of cold on the skin may range from progressive vasoconstriction (narrowing of blood vessels and Raynaud-like symptoms (blanching attacks of fingers) to chilblains and frostbites. Cold storage and winter outdoor (e.g., maintenance and construction) jobs are examples of such exposure. Localized colds may also cause cold contact urticaria	(i) Miliaria (~crystallina, rubra, profunda) Intertrigo Heat contact urticaria Burns and scalds of different degrees (ii) Raynaud-like symptoms; chilblains (perniones) Frostbites of different degrees Cold contact urticaria	Technical and organizational measures: The prevention is based on insulation, appropriate clothing, and work organization (rotation of workers and specified recovery areas for breaks and shelter)

(continued)

Table 7.1 (continued)

Biological hazards	Examples (for agents and *occupational exposures*)	Work-related or occupational dermatosis	Principles of prevention of occupational dermatoses
Bacteria	Several infectious agents may be contracted from various sources during work, including animals at work (occupational zoonoses) For example, **Infection** of (i) *Streptococcus* and *Staphylococcus* bacteria which generate pus (*health and welfare occupations*[a]) (ii) Erysipelothrix rhusiopathiae (*animal breeders, veterinarians, butchers, fishermen, cooks*) (iii) *Mycobacterium tuberculosis* hominis (*pathologist, dissectors, and surgeons*) (iv) *M. tuberculosis* bovis (*veterinarians, animal handlers, butchers, farmers*) (v) *M. marinum* (*workers handling fish and water in tanks or pools*) (vi) *Borrelia burgdorferi* (*common occupational skin disease among forestry and horticultural workers*) **Colonization,** which is the presence of microorganisms on the worker without apparent disease, and manifest infection with antibiotic-resistant bacteria (e.g., MRSA) among healthcare workers is an emerging issue with implications for patient safety (however, is mostly not recognized as an occupational disease)	(i) Occupational pyodermas (folliculitis, furuncle, carbuncle, impetigo, ecthyma, paronychia, etc.) (ii) Erysipeloid (iii) Skin tuberculosis (iv) Cutaneous manifestation of bovine tuberculosis (in humans) (v) Fish tank granuloma (atypical mycobacteriosis) (vi) *Erythema chronicum migrans* (ECM)	Prevention is based on the risk assessment of the given workplace that takes into account unintentional exposure to biological agents. The measures follow the hierarchy of control and include proper personal and work hygiene, the use of germicide agents and gloves (and further protective gear depending on the exposure and mode of transmission). In case of zoonoses, the cooperation with the veterinarian is essential
Fungi	(i) Yeasts mainly Candida albicans (*workers in canneries and confectioneries, and healthcare workers are at risk. Wearing rubber gloves and boots (wet work) and handling of sweets can be contributing factors to the development*) (ii) Dermatophytes: *Trichophytia verrucosum* (*farmers, milkers, animal handlers, and veterinarians may acquire it from infected cattle*) *Microsporum canis* (*pet traders and breeders, vets, laboratory workers*); *Microsporum gypseum* (*agriculture workers*)	(i) Onychomycosis; paronychia; interdigital mycosis (ii) Trichophytia profunda Microsporiasis (ringworm)	Prevention is based on the risk assessment of the given workplace that takes into account unintentional exposure to biological agents. The measures follow the hierarchy of control and include proper personal and work hygiene, the use of germicide agents and gloves. In case of zoonoses, the cooperation with the veterinarian is essential

Table 7.1 (continued)

Biological hazards	Examples (for agents and *occupational exposures*)	Work-related or occupational dermatosis	Principles of prevention of occupational dermatoses
Viri	(i) Paravaccinia virus (*milkers and other animal handlers; the source is the udder of the cow, less frequently of sheep or goats*) (ii) Zoonotic Orthoxpoxviruses (e.g., Orthopoxvirus simiae) (*veterinarians, animal handlers, zoo workers*) (iii) Parapox virus, which is common in sheep and goats (*shepherds, goatherds, veterinarians*) (iv) Human-to-human transmitted viruses (e.g., Varizella-Zoster-Virus) under special occupational exposure conditions (*health and welfare occupations*)	(i) Milker's nodules (Nodus mulgentium) (ii) Zoonotic orthopoxvirus infections (e.g., monkey pox) (iii) Orf (Ecthyma contagiosum) (iv) Virus-related dermatoses (e.g., chickenpox)	Prevention is based on the risk assessment of the given workplace that takes into account unintentional exposure to biological agents. The measures follow the hierarchy of control and include proper personal and work hygiene, the use of germicide agents and gloves (and further protective gear depending on the exposure and mode of transmission). In case of zoonoses, cooperation with the veterinarian is essential
Skin parasites	Although frequently unrecognized, parasitic skin diseases may have an occupational origin. For example, (i) Scarcoptes scabiei infection (*health and welfare occupations*) (ii) Arthropod bites from animal parasites or granary mites (Pyemotes mites) (*common in agricultural workers and grain storage workers*)	(i) Scabies (ii) Pyemotes dermatitis	Prevention is based on the risk assessment of the given workplace that takes into account unintentional exposure to biological agents. The measures follow the hierarchy of control and include proper personal and work hygiene, the use of germicide agents and gloves (and further protective gear depending on the exposure and mode of transmission). In case of zoonoses, the cooperation with the veterinarian is essential

[a] *Streptoccus suis* has been described as an emerging infectious disease (mainly in China, Australia, and Europe) presenting in *pig breeders, butchers veterinarians* as zoonosis. Primary risk factors are occupational exposure and eating contaminated undercooked food. Due to the predominantly systemic disease manifestation, it is only briefly mentioned here: Clinical characteristics of this infection include meningitis, sepsis, endocarditis, arthritis, hearing loss, and skin lesions (mostly petechial or hemorrhagic) in approximately 10%. Toxic shock syndrome also was reported as a distinct severe clinical feature at high rates in a few outbreaks in Asia [16]

the investigation. Accordingly, there are two requisites: (i) making the right and specific medical diagnosis and (ii) verifying that the skin disease is related to the occupation [5]. For the latter, it is essential to be familiar with the work activity, the hazards at work, the occupational safety and health instructions and skin protection program at the workplace [5]. In addition, it is necessary for the occupational dermatologist and the occupational physician to keep up to date regarding new developments (new diseases and their treatment, as well as new legal developments. For example, the recognition of COVID-19 as an occupational disease or accident at work is already a reality in 25 Member States. France, for example, introduced a government decree in September 2020, which allows for the automatic recognition of healthcare and similar workers and professionals in cases leading to severe respiratory infection. In addition, France allows for compensation in such cases. In Denmark, cases of COVID-19 can be recognized and compensated as both, occupational disease and accident at work in all professions, following an assessment of relevant authorities [8].

Work-related skin diseases due to different exposures (chemical, physical, biological) are displayed in more detail on the internet pages of EU-OSHA, the European Union information agency for occupational safety and health ([9]. http://oshwiki.eu/index.php?title=Work-related_

skin_diseases&oldid=247465 (last visited July 31, 2022). To enable the sharing of occupational safety and health (OSH) knowledge, information, and best practices, in order to support all stakeholders in ensuring safety and health at the workplace, EU-OSHA has developed OSHwiki, which aims to be an authoritative source of information that is easily updated, edited or translated and reaches beyond the OSH community. It holds additional valuable updated information that appears useful for the occupational dermatologist and the occupational physician.

Legal Framework

Article 153 of the Treaty on the Functioning of the European Union [Consolidated version of the Treaty on the Functioning of the European Union [17] gives the EU the authority to adopt legislation (directives) in the field of safety and health at work, in order to support and complement the activities of Member States.

Directive 89/391/EEC, the so-called occupational safety and health (OSH) "Framework Directive" [Council Directive 89/391/EEC], lays down the main principles to encourage improvements in the safety and health of workers at work. It guarantees minimum safety and health requirements throughout the European Union while the Member States are allowed to maintain or establish more stringent measures. The directive was amended three times by legal acts, in 2003, 2007, and 2008.

The Framework Directive is accompanied by further directives focusing on specific aspects of safety and health at work [18–49] (summarized in Table 7.2). As of 2018, 20 individual directives were adopted [19–31, 34–38]. Together they form the fundamentals of European safety and health legislation. Further linked policy documents, guidance documents, publications, and other Commission services in the context of OSH can be found on the internet pages of the European Commission on Employment [50].

Table 7.2 The occupational safety and health (OSH) "Framework Directive" (Directive 89/392/EEC) and further directives focusing on specific aspects of safety and health at work guarantee minimum safety and health requirements throughout the European Union while Member States may maintain or establish more stringent measures

Work environment		References
Abbreviation	**Legislation**	
89/391/EEC	Council directive on the introduction of measures to encourage improvements in the safety and health of workers at work	[18]
89/654/EEC	First individual directive: Council directive concerning the minimum safety and health requirements for the workplace	[19]
2009/104/EC	Second individual directive: Directive of the European Parliament and of the Council concerning the minimum safety and health requirements for the use of work equipment by workers at work	[20]
89/656/EEC	Third individual directive: Council directive concerning the minimum health and safety requirements for the use by workers of personal protective equipment at the workplace	[21]
90/269/EEC	Forth individual directive: Council directive on the minimum health and safety requirements for the manual handling of loads where there is a risk, particularly of back injury to workers	[22]
90/270/EEC	Fifth individual directive: Council directive on the minimum safety and health requirements for work with display screen equipment	[23]
2004/37/EC	Sixth individual directive: Directive of the European Parliament and of the Council on the protection of workers from the risks related to exposure to carcinogens or mutagens at work	[24]
2000/54/EC	Seventh individual directive: Directive of the European Parliament and of the Council on the protection of workers from risks related to exposure to biological agents at work	[25]
92/57/EEC	Eighth individual directive: Council directive on the minimum safety and health requirements at temporary or mobile constructions sites	[26]
92/58/EEC	Ninth individual directive: Council directive on the minimum requirements for the provision of safety and/or health signs at work	[27]

Table 7.2 (continued)

92/85/EEC	Tenth individual directive: Council directive on the introduction of measures to encourage improvements in the safety and health at work of pregnant workers and workers who have recently given birth or are breastfeeding	[28]
92/91/EEC	Eleventh individual directive: Council Directive concerning the minimum requirements for improving the safety and health protection of workers in the mineral-extracting industries through drilling	[29]
92/104/EEC	Twelfth individual directive: Council Directive on the minimum requirements for improving the safety and health protection of workers in surface and underground mineral-extracting industries	[30]
93/103/EC	Thirteenth individual directive: Council Directive concerning the minimum safety and health requirements for work on board fishing vessels	[31]
92/29/EEC	Council Directive on the minimum safety and health requirements for improved medical treatment on board vessels.	[32]
Hazardous substances and exposures		
Abbreviation	**Legislation**	
98/24/EC	Fourteenth individual directive: Council Directive on the protection of the health and safety of workers from the risks related to chemical agents at work	[33]
1999/92/EC	Fifteenth individual directive: Directive of the European Parliament and of the Council on minimum requirements for improving the safety and health protection of workers potentially at risk from explosive atmospheres	[34]
2002/44/EC	Sixteenth individual directive: Directive of the European Parliament and of the Council on the minimum health and safety requirements regarding the exposure of workers to the risks arising from physical agents (vibration)	[35]
2003/10/EC	Seventeenth individual directive: Directive of the European Parliament and of the Council on the minimum health and safety requirements regarding the exposure of workers to the risks arising from physical agents (noise)	[36]
2006/25/EC	Nineteenth individual directive: Directive of the European Parliament and of the Council on the minimum health and safety requirements regarding the exposure of workers to risks arising from physical agents (artificial optical radiation)	[37]
2013/35/EU	Twentieth[a] individual directive: Directive of the European Parliament and of the Council on the minimum health and safety requirements regarding the exposure of workers to the risks arising from physical agents (electromagnetic fields)	[38]
2010/32/EU	Council Directive implementing the Framework Agreement on prevention from sharp injuries in the hospital and healthcare sector concluded by HOSPEEM and EPSU (Text with EEA relevance)	[39]
2009/148/EC	Directive of the European Parliament and of the Council on the protection of workers from the risks related to exposure to asbestos at work	[40]
91/322/EEC	Commission Directive on establishing indicative limit values by implementing Council Directive 80/1107/EEC on the protection of workers from the risks related to exposure to chemical, physical and biological agents at work	[41]
2000/39/EC	Commission Directive establishing a first list of indicative occupational exposure limit values in implementation of Council Directive 98/24/EC on the protection of the health and safety of workers from the risks related to chemical agents at work (Text with EEA relevance).	[42]
2006/15/EC	Commission Directive establishing a second list of indicative occupational exposure limit values in implementation of Council Directive 98/24/EC and amending Directives 91/322/EEC and 2000/39/EC (Text with EEA relevance)	[43]
2009/161/EU	Commission Directive establishing a third list of indicative occupational exposure limit values in implementation of Council Directive 98/24/EC and amending Commission Directive 2000/39/EC (Text with EEA relevance)	[44]
2017/164/EU	Commission Directive establishing a fourth list of indicative occupational exposure limit values pursuant to Council Directive 98/24/EC, and amending Commission Directives 91/322/EEC, 2000/39/EC and 2009/161/EU (Text with EEA relevance)	[45]
2019/1831/EU	Commission Directive (EU) 2019/1831 of 24 October 2019 establishing a fifth list of indicative occupational exposure limit values pursuant to Council Directive 98/24/EC and amending Commission Directive 2000/39/EC (Text with EEA relevance)	[46]

Table 7.2 (continued)

Occupational safety and health (OSH)		
Abbreviation	Legislation	
91/383/EEC	Council directive supplementing the measures to encourage improvements in the safety and health at work of workers with a fixed-duration employment relationship or a temporary employment relationship	[47]
2003/88/EC	Directive of the European Parliament and of the Council concerning certain aspects of the organization of working time	[48]
94/33/EC	Council directive on the protection of young people at work	[49]

[a]Replaces eighteenth individual directive (2004/40/EC) which is no longer in force

The Commission Recommendation 2003/670/EC [4] concerning the European schedule of occupational diseases comprises in Annex I the European schedule of occupational diseases ($n = 108$). The diseases mentioned in this schedule must be linked directly to the occupation. Annex II contains an additional list of diseases suspected of being occupational in origin which should be subject to notification and which may be considered at a later stage for inclusion in Annex I to the European schedule.

Occupational disease statistics are based on administrative data collected nationally by various organizations, usually the national statistical offices. Regulation (EC) No 1338/2008 [51] outlines the domain-specific requirements of the data collection.

The occupational physician—in cooperation with the company management—has a major task in the practical implementation of and compliance with the legal provisions and limit values on site at the workplace to keep employees healthy. If, despite the implemented preventive measures, work-related skin symptoms occur, early occupational dermatological intervention with appropriate measures of secondary and tertiary prevention is sensible and necessary to restore and maintain symptom-free work ability. The occupational dermatologist is required to initiate individual diagnostic and therapeutic measures at an early stage. Good cooperation between occupational physicians and occupational dermatologists is essential in early intervention in identifying the first signs of work-related skin symptoms and substitution of identified irritant or allergenic agents in the workplace and adaptation of personal protective equipment. The above legal framework guarantees minimum safety and health requirements throughout the European Union while Member States may maintain or establish more stringent measures.

If work-related skin diseases are detected at an early stage, the occurrence of a serious skin disease can often be prevented by rapid treatment and, above all, by effective individual preventive measures, and insured persons can continue to perform their occupational activities [52]. For this reason, for example, in Germany already in 1972 the statutory social accident insurance contractually agreed on an early reporting procedure with the medical profession, the so-called "dermatologist procedure" (§§ 41 ff. contract doctors/accident insurance carrier). Doctors have to inform the respective social accident insurance in charge upon the mere possibility of a work-related cause of illness, in order to give them the opportunity for tailored early intervention [52].

Qualification

In Europe, each Member State is responsible to organize the training of medical doctors. For this purpose, national training programs, specific training centers, and national assessments of medical competence have been set up in order to ensure that medical doctors are appropriately trained and able to provide the highest quality of care to the citizens [53].

The European Union of Medical Specialists (UEMS) is a nongovernmental organization representing national associations of medical specialists at the European Level. With a current membership from 41 countries, it is the representative organization of the National

Associations of Medical Specialists in the European Union and its associated countries. Its structure consists of a Council responsible for and working through 43 Specialist Sections and their European Boards, addressing training in their respective specialty [53].

It is the UEMS' conviction that the quality of care is widely directly linked to the quality of training provided to healthcare professionals. Therefore, the UEMS committed itself to contributing to the improvement of medical training at the European level through the development of European Standards in the different medical disciplines.

By its agreed documents, UEMS sets standards for high-quality healthcare practice that are transmitted to the Authorities and Institutions of the EU and the National Medical Associations stimulating and encouraging them to implement its recommendations. The UEMS adopted its Charter on Post Graduate Training aiming at providing recommendations at the European level for good medical training. Made up of six chapters, this Charter set the basis for the European approach in the field of Post Graduate Training. With five chapters being common to all specialties, this Charter provided a sixth chapter, known as "Chap. 6" ("Training Requirements for the Specialty of X"), that each Specialist Section was to complete according to the specific needs of their discipline. This document aims to provide the basic Training Requirements for each specialty and should be regularly updated by UEMS Specialist Sections and European Boards to reflect scientific and medical progress. In doing so, the UEMS Specialist Sections and European Boards did not aim to supersede the National Authorities' competence in defining the content of postgraduate training in their own State but rather to complement these and ensure that high-quality training is provided across Europe.

In 2005, the European Commission proposed to the European Parliament and Council to have a unique legal framework for the recognition of Professional Qualifications to facilitate and improve the mobility of all workers throughout Europe. This Directive 2005/36/EC [54] established the mechanism of automatic mutual recognition of qualifications for medical doctors according to training requirements within all Member States; this is based on the length of training in the Specialty and the title of qualification. Given the long-standing experience of UEMS Specialist Sections and European Boards on the one hand and the European legal framework enabling Medical Specialists and Trainees to move from one country to another, on the other hand, the UEMS is uniquely in a position to provide specialty-based recommendations.

UEMS European Training Requirements (ETRs) in Dermatology and Venerology [55] and, respectively, Occupational Medicine [56] adopted by UEMS Council are available on the Internet pages of the association [54].

The training of the dermatologist accordingly requires (among further qualifications) [55] theoretical knowledge and practical skills in:

- Occupational and environmental dermatology.
- Allergy, diagnostics, and treatment.
- Reactions to physical agents.
- Dermatologic oncology, diagnostic and treatment procedures.
- Prevalence, prevention, diagnosis and therapy of allergic, pseudoallergic, and environmental diseases including occupational dermatoses in relation to the skin and adjacent mucous membranes, toxicology of topical and systemic agents to the skin organ, as well as prevention, diagnosis, medical and surgical treatments, follow-up of tumors of the skin, are a prerequisite for the dermatologist training.
- The resident obligatorily needs to learn regulations for occupational dermatoses and rehabilitation procedures.

The training of the occupational physician requires (among further qualifications) [56] practical and clinical skills on the:

- Framework for practice (practical application of law as it relates to occupational physicians' practice).
- Fitness for work, rehabilitation, and disability assessment (the ability to assess disability, in

patients with chronic disease or rehabilitation from acute injury or ill health, make appropriate decisions on fitness for work, with appropriate workplace adjustments/restrictions and rehabilitation).

- Hazard recognition, evaluation, and control of risk (the ability to carry out a risk assessment of a workplace and make appropriate recommendations recognizing potential hazards, assessment of residual risks; the skills required to understand the application of occupational hygiene in the workplace including appropriate environmental monitoring).
- Epidemiology and preventive health (an understanding of the requirements of health surveillance including legal instruments, how it is implemented within the workplace; an understanding of the role of workplace-based health promotion and other methods of disease prevention in the workplace).
- Dermatological conditions include occupational and environmental skin injuries and dermatoses, which may interfere or be exacerbated by work. Performance requires an understanding of the role of patch testing, the ability to interpret reports, and their use in developing a management plan and advising on risk.

The need for and benefit of a multidisciplinary approach to the management of occupational dermatoses and occupational skin cancer has been highlighted; besides OSH specialists it should also include the participation of the general practitioner [57, 58].

Practical Approach to Diagnosing, Treatment, and Prevention of Occupational Dermatoses

General Aspects in the Identification of Occupational Dermatoses

The identification and prevention of occupational skin diseases require a comprehensive approach with synchronized activities of the dermatologist, the occupational physician, the occupational hygienist, and the occupational safety and health expert [9].

In all countries, the primary approach in work-related skin diseases and occupational skin diseases is medical and occupational rehabilitation of the patient to avoid job loss [2]. Discontinuation criteria, when occupational rehabilitation measures are declared a failure and the patient is advised to leave for good the workplace where the skin lesions have occurred differ in different countries with regard to legal criteria (summarized in [2]). Despite varying definitions for occupational skin diseases, patients do not differ with regard to their clinical diseases (Table 7.1) and upkeep of working ability and maintenance of the job seem to be common goals in all the surveyed countries [1, 2]. Hence, they should be treated and assessed in the same way, based on scientific evidence-based criteria. Only a few countries in Europe have hitherto established recommendations for the diagnosis and management of occupational skin diseases [1], e.g., laying a focus on the most predominant occupational diseases such as occupational contact dermatitis and occupational contact urticaria [1, 59].

The correct etiological diagnosis is a prerequisite for successful treatment and prevention [1]. The diagnosis of any occupational skin disease (Table 7.1) is based on the patient's history, physical examination, and appropriate diagnostic tests (e.g., allergy testing and skin biopsy) [1]. Only trained and qualified specialists such as dermatologists, occupational physicians, or allergologists should perform skin tests [60]. An exploration and accurate documentation of all work-related factors linked to dermatoses is necessary. Correlation of skin lesions (clinical type, localization, and development) and exposure to physical agents, chemicals, or other potential hazards in the work environment and leisure time have to be taken into consideration by every clinician, knowing that for some agents the latency period to induce skin lesions varies (minutes in contact urticaria, days in allergic contact dermatitis, and years in skin cancer) and that there may be indirect effects, apart from direct skin exposure [1]. Occupational skin cancer may even first manifest years after retirement from the causative workplace.

Although the timing of reporting varies in different countries, in most, reporting is required for a diagnosis suggestive of occupational dermatosis [1, 2].

Workers under flexible employment contracts are more vulnerable than, for instance, employees working under standard contracts; they usually carry out hazardous jobs with increased exposure to more dangerous substances in poorer conditions and often receive less occupational safety and health training, which increases the risk of occupational accidents and illness [61]. Cofactors such as chronic infectious comorbidities and psychological factors/illnesses—including occupational dermatitis artifacts—must be considered as concomitant (occult) challenges when treating occupational dermatoses [62–65].

Occupational skin diseases are managed by different medical and paramedical disciplines, e.g., physicians, specialized nurses, and occupational hygienists who help to assess the occupational relevance and implement preventive measures, however, the minimum standards required for a correct diagnosis in the occupational setting should follow common standards of dermatology and occupational medicine [1].

Principals of Diagnosis of Occupational Contact Dermatitis

The diagnosis of occupational contact dermatitis, the most frequent occupational skin disease (with a reported incidence from 0.6 to 6.7 per 10,000 person-years in register studies and 15.9 to 780.0 per 10,000 person-years in cohort studies [66]), is based on a medical history and physical examination [1].

The physical examination should include the entire skin and not only the sites presented by the patient. Affected anatomical sites should be documented carefully, with emphasis on primary locations, extent, severity, and clinical characteristics [1].

Careful correlation of exposure with localization of skin lesions and their evolution is mandatory. The evolution of dermatitis in relation to the workplace, namely improvement during periods off work, and, conversely, in relation to leisure activities, has to be considered and concisely documented [1]. Photographic documentation provided by the patients and by the attending physician is useful in documenting disease evolution.

Patch testing (and further skin testing as required) is indicated in all cases with work-related relapsing or persisting (>3 months) contact dermatitis [1, 60, 67].

Allergic Contact Dermatitis

The gold standard for diagnosing allergic contact dermatitis is epicutaneous patch testing [60], complemented by prick testing in case of immediate symptoms.

The majority of established occupational allergens are also known as non-occupational allergens and emerging occupational allergens are continually described in the literature [68]. The clinical relevance of positive skin test reactions is assessed based on past and present exposures and contact dermatitis locations; positive reactions without current clinical relevance can be important in terms of pointing to former unknown exposures [1, 60]. If patch tests with strongly suspected working materials are negative, several aspects need reappraisal, namely possible changes in composition of working materials or inappropriately low concentrations of the allergens in the working materials, which have to be diluted for patch testing [1].

A limited number of occupationally relevant allergens cause the majority of sensitizations in the workforce, if standard series allergens are concerned [69, 70]. Allergens in the European baseline series associated with an at least doubled risk of occupational contact dermatitis include thiuram rubber chemical accelerators, epoxy resin, and the antimicrobials methylchloroisothiazolinone/methylisothiazolinone, methyldibromo glutaronitrile, and formaldehyde [69, 70]. Data analysis of national and international contact allergy data bases provides valuable information on sensitization rates and profiles in skin risk occupations to implement targeted prevention strategies. However, to diagnose occupational allergic contact dermatitis additional testing of occupation related patch test series as well as patients' own products is commonly inevitable [70]. The following general considerations should be followed when testing with patient-owned material [60]:

- Obtain an overview of the product composition (by reviewing material safety data sheets, frame formulations, and other available information).
- Consult reference works (e.g., [71]).
- If possible, test individual components of patient's own products separately.
- Check and adjust pH (suitable for testing: pH 4–9).
- The test concentration of an individual contact allergen in a finished product should not exceed the recommended test concentration for that allergen.
- A negative test result does not exclude contact allergy to components contained therein.

Contact allergies can affect any part of the body [11, 12], but preferentially occur on the hands, where they are often an expression of occupational disease [11, 12]. In hand eczema, contact with a contact allergen is a frequent (co)factor in eczema elicitation and maintenance [72]. In addition to the common contact allergens of the standard series, which can be found in hand eczema patients without and with occupational dermatosis, in hand eczema patients with occupational dermatosis most frequently positive reactions were found to the rubber accelerators tetramethylthiuram monosulfide, tetramethylthiuram disulfide, 1,3-diphenylguanidine; p-phenylenediamine and p-toluylenediamine (oxidation hair dyes and indicator test substances for haptens from the para group (aminoaromatic compounds)); iodopropynyl butylcarbamate (preservative in technical and cosmetic products); glutaraldehyde (disinfectant in the industrial sector and for disinfecting medical equipment) and monoethanolamine (basic sub-

stance in the chemical industry and additive in cooling lubricants) [72]. In addition to these common contact allergens, less common contact allergens may also be the relevant trigger of work-related hand eczema in specific cases, which is why an individual assessment is required taking into account the individual work-related exposure [72]. In patients with facial dermatitis in addition to non-occupational (e.g., cosmetic) allergen exposure occupational airborne causation should be considered—most frequently induced by allergen sources detected by sesquiterpene lactone mix, compositae mix, epoxy resin, methylisothiazolinone and/or methychlorolisothiazolinone, and oil of turpentine [13].

Irritant Contact Dermatitis

Differential diagnosis should address irritant contact dermatitis by additionally assessing the exposure to irritants [1]. Irritant contact dermatitis is the most common form of contact dermatitis and the most common occupational skin disease [73]. Concomitant exposure to contact allergens and irritants increases the risk of sensitization, emphasizing the need to identify irritant factors [1, 74]. Wet work is the leading cause of irritant contact dermatitis in general and specifically in healthcare [73, 75, 76]. Wet work has been defined as:

- Exposure of skin to liquid for >2 h/day.
- Use of occlusive gloves for >2 h/day.
- Frequent hand washing >20 times per day [77].

or combinations thereof. The diagnosis of irritant contact dermatitis is often difficult, as there is no confirmatory test, and it is often a default diagnosis after allergic contact dermatitis has been excluded. Early recognition, prevention, and treatment are vital in management, especially in the occupational setting [73]. The highest proportions of occupational irritant contact dermatitis were found in metal workers (machinists), bakers, pastry cooks, and confectionery makers [78]. Among patients diagnosed with irritant CD, 45% were found sensitized with no relevance to the current disease [78]. This is exemplary of the crucial impact of a thorough relevance assessment.

Despite some clinical criteria that may be indicative, irritant contact dermatitis and allergic contact dermatitis are not distinguishable from each other with certainty by clinical or histological examinations [9]. Mixed (hybrid) forms (allergic plus irritant) of contact dermatitis are very frequent [79]. Contact substances may have both irritant and sensitizing properties and individuals may be exposed to multiple substances at work as well as off work; furthermore, irritant exposure harms the barrier function of the skin, which promotes sensitization by enabling increased absorption of allergens [74].

Principals of Diagnosis of Contact Urticaria and Protein Contact Dermatitis

As the most common causative agents for occupational contact urticaria and protein contact dermatitis cow dander, flour, and grain, followed by natural rubber latex and other foods were reported [80]. In food-related occupations, wheat and other flours were followed by fish, other animal-derived food, and plant-derived food as causes [80]. Occupations with the highest incidence of occupational contact urticaria and protein contact dermatitis included bakers, chefs and cooks, farmers and farm workers, veterinarians, gardeners, and hairdressers. The diagnosis of occupational contact urticaria or protein contact dermatitis requires, as diagnostic tool, cutaneous in vivo tests such as the skin prick test or the prick-by-prick test of native material as well as specific serum IgE in immunological contact urticaria; other less commonly performed tests such as open tests, closed chamber, scratch, and scratch-patch tests can be useful when investigating skin reactions following contact with food, work chemicals, cosmetics, medicaments, and clothing items [81–84]. These latter tests are non-standardized and considerably more difficult to interpret, thus requiring specialist expertise [84]. For many allergen sources eliciting occupational contact dermatitis and protein contact dermatitis licensed skin prick test extracts may not be commercially available. The safe and meaningful use of self-prepared skin prick test preparations in the diagnosis of occupational contact urticaria, e.g., caused by chemicals (isocyanates, chloramine-T, persulfates) [85], drugs [86, 87], and foods [88, 89] has been reported. For test concentrations and procedures see [85–89].

Diagnosis of UV-Related Occupational Skin Cancer

In some countries, actinic (solar) keratosis, squamous cell carcinoma (and its precursors), basal cell carcinoma, or melanoma can be recognized as occupational skin diseases [2]. The diagnosis of UV-related skin cancer needs to follow the usual procedures of dermatological diagnosis, including a thorough clinical examination often complemented by dermatoscopy, skin biopsy, and dermatopathology [1]. Also, regular follow-up examinations according to established guidelines for non-occupational skin cancer are necessary [e.g., [90–92]].

Assessment of Occupational Exposure

Certain industries and occupations are associated with higher rates of OCD, and as expected, the industries with direct contact with irritants and allergens are highly represented [68]. The highest risk of occupational contact dermatitis was found in occupations classified as "other personal services workers," which includes hairdressers as a large group. A high risk was also seen in nursing and other health professionals, precision workers in metal and related materials, and blacksmiths, tool makers, and related trades workers with varying shares of allergic contact dermatitis, irritant contact dermatitis, or both [69].

Workplace exposure assessment (WEA) is a prerequisite for making a correct diagnosis of work-related/occupational skin disease and is essential for effective treatment and prevention [1]. In many countries, there is no firm rulebook regarding who performs the WEA, when, and how.

The occupational history and assessment of occupational exposure, exploration of product labels, and Material Safety Data Sheet (MSDS) will help establish the occupational relevance of the cutaneous disease [1]. In more than 80% of cases with occupational allergic contact dermatitis WEA in terms of medical history, assessment of product labels and MSDS has been contributory to a correct diagnosis [1]. The incompleteness of MSDS, however, remains a major challenge occasionally not giving the full information about allergens and irritants in a product [1]. Minimum recommended requirements for WEA as part of the diagnostic process for work-related/occupational skin diseases and a checklist covering the most frequent occupational and non-occupational exposures have been proposed (for details see: [1]. Most important occupational exposures comprise:

- Wet exposure
- Chemicals
- Metals
- Specific work-related exposure
- Skin care and cleaning products
- Protective equipment

The gloves and clothes should be checked for their adequacy to prevent exposure. Frequently, erroneously medical examination gloves are being worn in contact with chemicals to which they are not resistant. Furthermore, gloves are often the cause of irritant or contact allergic skin reactions. Airborne exposure may require further prevention measures, like ventilation, special protective masks, and goggles [9]. During the COVID-19 pandemic, besides an anticipated or observed increase in irritant and allergic hand eczema due to enhanced hygiene measurements [93, 94], in the context with increased wearing of medical protection masks, numerous reports of facial allergic and irritant contact dermatitis, acneiform contact eruptions and further mechanical (mostly pressure induced) unwanted side effects to masks have been published and potentially mitigating measures have been reviewed [95–97]. Findings retrieved in workplace exposure assessment should lead to improvement measures.

Treatment of Work-Related Skin Diseases and Occupational Skin Diseases

Besides potentially necessary modifications in the work environment, the dermatological treatment of work-related skin disease and occupational skin diseases does not, in principle, differ from the same non-work-related dermatosis [1]. In this regard, reference is made to the dermatological scientific literature as well as to national and international guidelines, which both are constantly updated. New topical and systemic therapies have improved the range of treatment options for a number of occupational dermatoses, including skin cancer. The treatment of chronic hand dermatitis, the most common work-related disease, has been recently addressed in an updated ESCD guideline [67].

Principles of Prevention of Work-Related and Occupational Skin Diseases

Primary Prevention

Primary prevention strategies to avoid work-related skin diseases and to decrease occupational skin disease incidence are based on proper risk assessment and thereof derived risk management processes, which need to be reviewed and updated regularly [1]. Occupational risk assessment, a crucial step in the prevention process, is based on hazard identification and measurement of different exposures (chemical, physical, biological) at the workplace and on risk classification to define the most appropriate preventive actions [1]. Strategies focus on human behavioral, technical, and organizational prevention measures as well as on avoidance/limitation of exposure to allergic substances or irritants at the workplace according to legislation and on regular training of the use of personal protective measures, adapted to the needs of the employees [1].

Concerning prevention of skin diseases proper workplace skin protection programs adapted to the actual situation are the best way to prevent occupational skin disease [9]. The measures follow the hierarchy of control like in other occupational safety and health programs. The types of measures can be classified as [98]:

1. **Elimination** of the hazards (i.e., hazards no longer present, e.g., by designing new work processes). This kind of measure would be the one with the highest effectiveness. If that is not possible, minimizing and separating the hazards from the workers is necessary (effectiveness in descending order) by
2. **Technical measures** (the hazard is technically separated from workers, e.g., by encasing, exhaust).
3. **Organizational measures** (the hazard is only organizationally separated from the worker, e.g., only qualified employees are allowed to do specified work).
4. **Personal measures** (e.g., personal protection equipment; hazard is still present and effectiveness of the measure depends on wearing).
5. **Behavioral measures** (adapted behavior is hopefully adopted, e.g., by peer observation).

Legislation requires following the hierarchy in order to always select the most effective type of measure [24, 33].

Concerning prevention of skin diseases due to **chemical exposure** proper workplace skin protection programs adapted to the actual situation are the best way to prevent occupational skin disease [9]. In accordance with the hierarchy of control concept disease, includes the following measures [1, 9, 99]:

- The initial target is to eliminate/minimize skin contact with noxious (irritant, sensitizing, carcinogen) material and wet work.
- Personal protective equipment, e.g., gloves should be chosen according to the (chemical) properties of the risk, taking into consideration the tasks, the work environment, and the worker.
- In order to minimize wet work, the duration of uninterrupted wearing of gloves should be minimized as well.
- National initiatives and sectoral guides may provide useful information for the implementation of a skin protection plan. Practical prevention strategies for work-related/occupational chronic hand dermatitis and skin cancer have been outlined [in [1]]. However, it must be always tailored to the actual situation of the given workplace.
- Information and training of workers on exposures, prevention techniques, proper use of personal protective devices and skin hygiene are of fundamental importance.
- Support to the individual in maintaining healthy skin includes the provision of proper skin cleaning agents and skin rehydration products at the workplace.
- Health surveillance is recommended in order to identify the shortcomings of measures, to identify new work-related risks and workers that need advanced protection.

Concerning the prevention of skin diseases due to **physical exposure**, the following principles apply:

- Cold/heat exposure [100]: Technical and organizational measures are necessary. The prevention is based on insulation, appropriate clothing, and work organization (e.g., rotation of workers and specified recovery areas for breaks and shelter). With increasing climate change and unprecedented heat waves already occurring in temperate climate zones, prevention and management of heat-related occupational diseases is a field of growing importance for the occupational physician and the occupational dermatologist.
- Ionizing radiation [101–103]: Prevention consists mainly of technical measures (e.g., enclosure of the technology, segregation, and proper maintenance) accompanied by strict protocols, shielding devices, and personal protective equipment.
- Non-ionizing UV radiation [104, 105]: Prevention of occupational skin cancers due to radiation consists of proper occupational

safety and health organization and instructions, shields, hats, and (UV absorbent) clothing together with medical surveillance. During medical check-ups, precancerous keratoses can be discovered for early treatment, while workers with verified skin cancers should be removed from continuous exposure.

Concerning prevention of skin diseases due to biological exposure (e.g., bacteria, viruses, fungi, and parasites), the following principles apply [106–108]:

- Prevention is based on the risk assessment of the given workplace that takes into account unintentional exposure to biological agents.
- The measures follow the hierarchy of control and include proper personal and work hygiene, the use of germicide agents and gloves (and further protective gear depending on the exposure and mode of transmission).
- In case of zoonoses, cooperation with the veterinarian is essential.

Secondary Prevention

Secondary prevention measures are implemented to detect and treat early stages of the disease, to prevent relapses or chronicity, to induce behavioral change, train employees to protect their skin properly, and change hazardous workplace situations [1].

In the early detection of first signs of occupational dermatoses, which do not yet prompt the person concerned to consult a dermatologist, the occupational physician plays a particularly important role in the context of employment examinations or regular routine examinations. For successful early intervention, the occupational dermatologist should be involved early [52].

Tertiary Prevention

Tertiary prevention measures offer medical and occupational rehabilitation to employees suffering from established work-related skin diseases, who are at risk of losing their job or even having to give up their job because of the disease [1].

All return-to-work measures, including compensation for work-related skin diseases, aim at promoting the social rehabilitation and quality of life of the workers [1].

Here, the experienced occupational dermatologist plays the main role [109]; cooperation with the occupational physician is beneficial, especially if certain substances need to be removed from the work environment and replaced by others. A multidisciplinary model for tertiary prevention of manifest occupational dermatoses established in Germany for many years has been proven successful in enabling the majority of patients to continue working in their chosen profession [110]. It might serve as a blueprint for the development of strategies for tertiary prevention strategies of occupational dermatoses in further European countries [110].

Emerging and Future Challenges

Working environments are constantly changing alongside the introduction of new technologies, substances, and work processes, together with changes in the labor market, and with new forms of employment and work organization [61, 111]. These changes bring new opportunities as well as new risks for workers and employers, which in turn demand political, organizational, technical, and regulatory initiatives to ensure high levels of safety and health at work [61, 111]. The occupational physician and the dermatologist need to be aware of and prepared for these novel challenges. EU-OSHA has been running a series of foresight projects intended to evaluate the possible effects of new technologies, new ways of working, and societal change on workers' safety and health. The projects aim not only to identify new risks as they emerge but also to anticipate changes that could have an impact on workplace safety and health. Most important drivers [61, 112–114] for the changing world of work are summarized in Table 7.3. Specific attention is paid to increased exposure to chemicals (with specific attention to nanomaterials) and biomaterials, which may be

Table 7.3 Important drivers for the changing world of work and emerging OSH risk areas and exposures (modified from [61, 112])

Important drivers for the changing world of work

1. Globalization and growth of the service sector, resulting in more competition, increased economic pressures, more restructuring and downsizing, more precarious work, increase in job insecurity, increased intensification and increased time pressures at work. The number of workers who work in temporary employment is increasing. The current crisis in Europe has increased the economic pressures on companies and this in turn intensifies the effects on EU-employees.

2. Work changes and technical innovation takes place, leading to an employment shift toward services with no clear separation between working time and leisure time. Despite all kinds of opportunities and productivity gains, this possibly results in a poor work-life balance and, in particular a greater complexity of working tasks that requires lifelong learning to secure employability. Additionally, the service economy with its growing number of offices leads to musculoskeletal disorders from inactivity, static postures and repetitive movements. Furthermore, the service economy is creating more and newer human interfaces, and this is leading to increased psychosocial pressures such as violence and harassment[a]. Finally, technical innovations can also lead to new risks caused by new environmental agents [chemical or physical] or via new exposure characteristics.

3. Europe is aging. This demographic change is also a major driver for labor market development in Europe, and this will have a huge impact on occupational safety and health. For governments, enterprises and citizens alike, it will be of crucial importance to be able to prolong working life in a healthy and productive way. For employees this means that they will have to be able and motivated to work until an older age. For companies and enterprises this means that they have to provide opportunities for life long learning and employment opportunities for these aging workers.

The emerging OSH risk areas affected by these drivers are:

1. Important emerging physical risks are physical inactivity and the combined exposure to a mixture of environmental stressors that multiplicatively increase the risks of musculoskeletal disorders, the leading cause of sickness absence and work disability.

2. Important emerging psychosocial risks are job insecurity, work intensification, high demands at work, and emotional demands, including violence, harassments and bullying. Additionally, work-life balance may also be considered a risk.

3. Important emerging dangerous substances due to technological innovation.

Specific attention is paid to an increased exposure to

1. Chemicals (e.g. nanomaterials[b], man-made fibers, expoxy resin, isocyanates, dermal exposure to workplace-specific chemicals).

2. Biological agents (e.g. pathogens of global epidemic significance, human-to-human transmission, transmission as zoonoses, imported tropical diseases)

[a]Successive European Working Conditions Surveys (EWCS), together with several national surveys (i.e. Germany, Finland, The Netherlands, Sweden) have highlighted a trend toward the increasing incidence of workplace bullying, harassment and violence as the basis for work-related health problems [113, 114]

[b]One nanometer is $\times 10^{-9}$ of one meter

potentially important in terms of skin exposure and disease manifestation.

- Nanomaterials have applications in many industrial sectors (currently the main 4 areas are: (1) materials and manufacturing industry including automotive, construction, and chemical industry, (2) electronics and IT, (3) health and life sciences, and (4) energy and environment). A key issue of engineered nanomaterials (ENM) is the unknown human risks of the applied nanomaterials during their life cycle, especially for workers exposed to ENMs at the workplace [112]. Although there is a considerable lack of knowledge, there are indications that because of their size, ENMs can enter the body via the digestive system, respiratory system, or the skin. Once in the body, ENMs can translocate to organs or tissue distant from the portal of entry may accumulate in the body—particularly in the lungs, the brain, and the liver [61]. The size-related effects of nanomaterials on the immune system and allergic disease remain largely unknown at this point. Current knowledge regarding metal nanomaterials and their potential to induce/exacerbate dermal and respiratory allergy have been recently summarized [115]. It was demonstrated in an animal model in BALB/c mice that topical exposure to TiO_2-engineered nanoparticles increases chemical-induced dermal sensitization [116].

- Man-made mineral fibers are increasingly manufactured for all kinds of purposes, and can be classified as being siliceous or non-siliceous (Table 7.4) [61, 112]. The size of the fibers is acknowledged to be linked to their harmful toxic effects: the longer and thinner the fibers, the more dangerous they are. Fibers with a geometric diameter of less than 3 μm may reach the alveolar zone of the lungs [112]. Specific fiber dimensions hypothesized to have biological activity have been proposed but need to be evaluated in epidemiologic studies [112]. Concerning their properties and areas of use for more detail it is referred to [112], in brief:
  - Aluminum silicate wool (ASW), also more commonly called refractory ceramic fibers (RCFs), are aluminum silicate with a diameter varying between 1 and 3 μm [112].
  - ASW/RCFs are mainly used for high-temperature thermal insulation of industrial furnaces or blast furnaces and casting molds, though it is also used in car manufacturing (catalytic exhausts, etc.) and in aeronautical applications [112].
  - While ASW/RFC are vitreous aluminum silicate fibers, mullite fibers are crystalline aluminum silicate fibers. Mullite

fibers are sometimes used as a substitute for ASW/RCF at high temperatures, above 1000 °C [112].
- There are three types of mineral wools—glass, rock, and slag wools—classified according to the type of material they are made out of [112]. Their average geometric diameters are of the order of 1.7–3.5 μm.
- Mineral wools are used for thermal and acoustic insulation in housing, in the tertiary sector, and in technical installations. Special purpose glass fiber types E and 475 are mainly used in filtering applications, and in the aerospace and aeronautics industry as thermal insulation [112].
- Carbon fibers are used for aeronautical and industry engineering applications; they are also used as part of the composition of sports and leisure items [112].
- Potassium titanate fibers and whiskers are used to reinforce high-temperature composite materials.
- Alumina fibers are mainly used as high-temperature thermal insulation [112].
- Finally, some fibers contain up to 25% additives. However, the presence of additives is very rarely taken into account in experimental studies on man-made mineral fibers [112].

In general, fibrous structure increases inflammatory, cytotoxic, and carcinogenic potential [117–121]. The ILO's International Chemical Safety Card (ICSC) for glass wool (ICSC:0157) [118] indicated that repeated or prolonged contact with skin may cause dermatitis and that tumors have been detected in experimental animals but may not be relevant to humans [118]. ILO's ICSC:0194 for rock wool and ICSC:0195 for slag wool warns that both substances are possibly carcinogenic to humans, and that the carcinogenic potential depends on the length, diameter, chemical composition, and biological persistence of the fiber [119–121]. Exposure during the production of these fibers is usually low. However, workers handling fiber-based products—especially during laying, maintenance, or removal operations—may be highly

Table 7.4 Types of man-made fibers (modified from [112])

Siliceous	Non-siliceous
Aluminum silicate wool (ASW)—also called refractory ceramic fibers (RCFs)	Carbon fibers
Mullite fibers	Alumina fibers
Glass wool	Whiskers
Rock wool	Potassium titanate fibers
Slag wool	Others
Special purpose glass fibers	
Continuous filaments	

exposed [112]. Adequate personal protection gear needs to be provided according to the tasks performed [121].

- Another three chemical risks were identified as emerging with a view to allergies and sensitizing effects: (i) epoxy resins, (ii) isocyanates, and (iii) dermal exposure.
- Epoxy resins are important and widely used polymeric systems. They are used in adhesives, sealants, inks, varnishes, and reinforced polymer composite structure with glass fibers [61]. The continuous demand for always newer generations of epoxy resins and derived products with enhanced properties may introduce new, unknown adverse health effects. Epoxy resins have become one of the main causes of occupational allergic contact dermatitis. Skin sensitization of the hands, arms, face, and throat as well as photosensitization has also been reported [61]. Workers in the production of epoxy resins, workers in the manufacture of composite products, in the electrical and electronic industry, and painters may be at risk [61]. Epoxy resins skin sensitization is particularly problematic in the construction industry where a safe and healthy working environment (e.g., clean room) and the use of protective clothing (e.g., gloves) is less common and/or less practical [61]. The identification of the epoxy system involved in the process is essential for the selection of the appropriate prevention measure [61].
- Another emerging chemical risk is the increasing use of isocyanates. Exposure to these chemicals not only occurs at the production stage but also when polyurethane products containing isocyanates are used [e.g., when spraying], are processed (e.g., by grinding or welding), or when they undergo thermal or chemical degradation [61]. Isocyanates are powerful irritants to the mucous membranes of the eyes and of the gastrointestinal and respiratory tracts. Direct skin contact can cause serious inflammation and dermatitis [61]. Isocyanates are also powerful airways and skin sensitizing agents. Early recognition of sensitization, coupled with prompt and strict elimination of the source of exposure, is essential for the reduction of the risk of long-term or permanent respiratory problems and skin manifestation in sensitized workers.
- Dermal exposure is a major route of occupational exposure to dangerous substances. Chemicals are responsible for 80–90% of skin diseases. In the construction industry, chromate is the most important allergen, followed by epoxy resins and cobalt [61]. Particularly in the healthcare sector, glove materials may be the source of occupational allergens (rubber accelerators as Type-IV-allergens; natural rubber protein [latex] as a Type-I-allergen). Soaps, detergents, and solvents can cause dermatitis since they remove the surface lipids and dissolve the skin's natural protective barrier [61].
- Occupational risks related to global epidemics are the biggest "biological risk" issue identified in the EU-OSHA forecast on biological risks related to OSH [122]. Whereas earlier pandemics circled the globe in 6–9 months, today new biological agents can reach any continent in less than 3 months because of air travel [122]. Workers are certainly affected by these diseases and pathogens. It is difficult to identify the occupations most at risk, since sources of exposure vary and involve people, animals, plants, as well as goods. In the case of human-to-human transmissions, healthcare workers are most at risk. In the case of transmissions of zoonoses, workers in contact with live or dead infected animals or with aerosols, dust, or surfaces contaminated by animal secretions are at increased risk [122]. At-risk occupations thus include workers in farms, slaughterhouse facilities, workers involved in the disposal of carcasses, the cleaning and disinfection of contaminated areas, as well as veterinary services and research [122].
- Due to globalization, the risks of importing tropical disease has increased, e.g., with imported goods and particularly those in water [122]. Workers handling international trade containers are at risk of mosquito-

borne Dengue fever or other tropical fevers and encephalitis that are attributed to mosquitoes [61].

Traditionally, the focus of occupational safety and health has been on physical and chemical hazards in the workplace. Many of these are the subject of individual EU OSH Directives (as provided for under the Framework Directive 89/391/EEC [18] creating a common approach to hazards such as noise, vibration, and dangerous substances [123]. However, there has been a growing awareness that not all hazards have a physical presence. Psychosocial factors, shorthand for the psychological, economic, and social influences on workers, can also have an impact on both physical and mental health and well-being [123]. Furthermore, implications of the aging workforce in Europe are already starting to become apparent [124].

The occupational physician and the dermatologist need to take these factors into account when treating occupational dermatoses.

Disclaimer: The views expressed in this chapter are the personal views of the author and may not be understood or quoted as being made on behalf of or reflecting the position of the respective national competent authority, the European Medicines Agency, or one of its committees or working parties.

References

1. Alfonso JH, Bauer A, Bensefa-Colas L, Boman A, Bubas M, Constandt L, Crepy MN, Goncalo M, Macan J, Mahler V, Mijakoski D, Ramada Rodilla JM, Rustemeyer T, Spring P, John SM, Uter W, Wilkinson M, Giménez-Arnau AM. Minimum standards on prevention, diagnosis and treatment of occupational and work-related skin diseases in Europe - position paper of the COST Action StanDerm (TD 1206). J Eur Acad Dermatol Venereol. 2017;Suppl 4:31–43.
2. Mahler V, Aalto-Korte K, Alfonso JH, Bakker JG, Bauer A, Bensefa-Colas L, Boman A, Bourke J, Bubaš M, Bulat P, Chaloupka J, Constandt L, Danielsen TE, Darlenski R, Dugonik A, Ettler K, Gimenez-Arnau A, Gonçalo M, Johansen JD, John SM, Kiec-Swierczynska M, Koch P, Kohánka V, Krecisz B, Larese Filon F, Ljubojević S, Macan J, Marinović B, Matura M, Mihatsch PW, Mijakoski D, Minov J, Pace J, Pesonen M, Ramada Rodilla JM, Rast H, Reljic V, Salavastru C, Schuster C, Schuttelaar ML, Simon D, Spiewak R, Jurakic Tončić R, Urbanček S, Valiukevičienė S, Weinert P, Wilkinson M, Uter W. Occupational skin diseases: actual state analysis of patient management pathways in 28 European countries. J Eur Acad Dermatol Venereol. 2017;Suppl 4:12–30.
3. Marques PR, Soares RB. Reports of occupational dermatosis in the state of Espírito Santo from 2007 to 2016. Rev Bras Med Trab. 2021;19(1):60–7.
4. Commission Recommendation of 19 September 2003 concerning the European schedule of occupational diseases (Text with EEA relevance) (notified under document number C(2003) 3297). Official J. 2003;L 238:28–34.
5. EU-OSHA – European Agency for Safety and Health at Work, Skin diseases and dermal exposure: policy and practice overview, 2008. https://osha.europa.eu/en/publications/report-skin-diseases-and-dermal-exposure-policy-and-practice-overview; Last accessed: 6.8.2022.
6. Herloch V, Elsner P. The (new) occupational disease no. 5101: "Severe or recurrent skin diseases". J Dtsch Dermatol Ges. 2021;19(5):720–41.
7. Bauer A, Haufe E, Heinrich L, Seidler A, Schulze HJ, Elsner P, Drexler H, Letzel S, John SM, Fartasch M, Brüning T, Dugas-Breit S, Gina M, Weistenhöfer W, Bachmann K, Bruhn I, Lang BM, Brans R, Allam JP, Grobe W, Westerhausen S, Knuschke P, Wittlich M, Diepgen TL, Schmitt J, FB181 study group. Basal cell carcinoma risk and solar UV exposure in occupationally relevant anatomic sites: do histological subtype, tumor localization and Fitzpatrick phototype play a role? A population-based case-control study. J Occup Med Toxicol. 2020;15:28.
8. Communication from the Commission to the European parliament, the council, the European economic and social committee and the committee of the regions EU strategic framework on health and safety at work 2021–2027 Occupational safety and health in a changing world of work. As of 28.6.2021 (COM 2021; 323 final). https://eur-lex.europa.eu/legal-content/EN/TXT/PDF/?uri=CELEX:52021DC0323&from=EN; last accessed 31.7.2022.
9. Work-related skin diseases. (2017, June 1). http://oshwiki.eu/index.php?title=Work-related_skin_diseases&oldid=247465 (last visited July 31, 2022).
10. Diepgen TL. Occupational skin diseases. JDDG. 2012;10:297–315.
11. Oosterhaven JAF, Uter W, Aberer W, Armario-Hita JC, Ballmer-Weber BK, Bauer A, Czarnecka-Operacz M, Elsner P, García-Gavín J, Giménez-Arnau AM, John SM, Kręcisz B, Mahler V, Rustemeyer T, Sadowska-Przytocka A, Sánchez-Pérez J, Simon D, Valiukevičienė S, Weisshaar E, Schuttelaar MLA, ESSCA Working Group.

European Surveillance System on Contact Allergies (ESSCA): contact allergies in relation to body sites in patients with allergic contact dermatitis. Contact Dermatitis. 2019;80:263–72.

12. Rozas-Muñoz E, Gamé D, Serra-Baldrich E. Allergic contact dermatitis by anatomical regions: diagnostic clues. Actas Dermo-Sifiliográficas (English Edition). 2018;109:485–507.

13. Schnuch A, Szliska C, Uter W, IVDK. Facial allergic contact dermatitis. Data from the IVDK and review of literature. Hautarzt. 2009;60(1):13–21.

14. Eurostat. Occupational diseases statistics—European Commission (Data extracted in May 2022. Planned article update: June 2023.). 2022. Accessible at: https://ec.europa.eu/eurostat/statistic-sexplained/index.php?title=Occupational_diseases_statistics; last accessed 31.7.2022.

15. Diaz JH. The disease ecology, epidemiology, clinical manifestations, management, prevention, and control of increasing human infections with animal orthopoxviruses. Wilderness Environ Med. 2021;32(4):528–36.

16. Huong VT, Ha N, Huy NT, Horby P, Nghia HD, Thiem VD, Zhu X, Hoa NT, Hien TT, Zamora J, Schultsz C, Wertheim HF, Hirayama K. Epidemiology, clinical manifestations, and outcomes of Streptococcus suis infection in humans. Emerg Infect Dis. 2014;20(7):1105–14.

17. Consolidated version of the treaty on the functioning of the European Union—Part three: Union Policies and internal actions—Title X: Social Policy—Article 153 (ex Article 137 TEC).Official Journal *C115;* 9.5.2008, 114–116.

18. Council Directive 89/391/EEC of 12 June 1989 on the introduction of measures to encourage improvements in the safety and health of workers at work. Official Journal L 183, 29.6.1989, pp. 1–8. https://eur-lex.europa.eu/legal-content/EN/TXT/PDF/?uri=CELEX:31989L0391&from=EN, Current consolidated version: as of 11.12.2008: https://eur-lex.europa.eu/legal-content/EN/TXT/PDF/?uri=CELEX:01989L0391-20081211&from=EN; last accessed 31.7.2022.

19. Council Directive 89/654/EEC of 30 November 1989 concerning the minimum safety and health requirements for the workplace (first individual directive within the meaning of Article 16 (1) of Directive 89/391/EEC). Official Journal L 393, 30.12.1989, pp. 1–12. http://eur-lex.europa.eu/legal-content/EN/TXT/PDF/?uri=CELEX:31989L0654&qid=1456697023621&from=EN Current consolidated version: as of 26.07.2019: https://eur-lex.europa.eu/legal-content/EN/TXT/PDF/?uri=CELEX:01989L0654-20190726&from=EN; last accessed 31.7.2022.

20. Directive 2009/104/EC of the European Parliament and of the Council of 16 September 2009 concerning the minimum safety and health requirements for the use of work equipment by workers at work (second individual Directive within the meaning of Article 16(1) of Directive 89/391/EEC) (Text with *European Economic Area* (EEA) relevance). Official Journal *L 260, 3.10.2009, pp. 5–19.* https://eur-lex.europa.eu/legal-content/EN/TXT/PDF/?uri=CELEX:32009L0104&from=en; last accessed 31.7.2022.

21. Council Directive 89/656/EEC of 30 November 1989 on the minimum health and safety requirements for the use by workers of personal protective equipment at the workplace (third individual directive within the meaning of Article 16 (1) of Directive 89/391/EEC). Official Journal L 393, 30.12.1989, pp. 18–28. https://eur-lex.europa.eu/legal-content/EN/TXT/PDF/?uri=CELEX:31989L0656&from=EN Current consolidated version: as of 20.11.2019: https://eur-lex.europa.eu/legal-content/EN/TXT/?uri=CELEX%3A01989L0656-20191120; last accessed 31.7.2022.

22. Council Directive 90/269/EEC of 29 May 1990 on the minimum health and safety requirements for the manual handling of loads where there is a risk particularly of back injury to workers (fourth individual Directive within the meaning of Article 16 (1) of Directive 89/391/EEC). Official Journal L 156, 21.6.1990, pp. 9–13. http://eur-lex.europa.eu/legal-content/EN/TXT/PDF/?uri=CELEX:31990L0269&from=EN Current consolidated version: as of 26.07.2019: https://eur-lex.europa.eu/legal-content/EN/TXT/PDF/?uri=CELEX:01990L0269-20190726&from=EN; last accessed 31.7.2022.

23. Council Directive 90/270/EEC of 29 May 1990 on the minimum safety and health requirements for work with display screen equipment (fifth individual Directive within the meaning of Article 16 (1) of Directive 89/391/EEC). Official Journal L 156, 21.6.1990, pp. 14–18. https://eur-lex.europa.eu/legal-content/EN/TXT/PDF/?uri=CELEX:31990L0270&from=EN Current consolidated version: as of 26.07.2019: https://eur-lex.europa.eu/legal-content/EN/TXT/PDF/?uri=CELEX:01990L0270-20190726&from=EN; last accessed 31.7.2022.

24. Directive 2004/37/EC of the European Parliament and of the Council of 29 April 2004 on the protection of workers from the risks related to exposure to carcinogens or mutagens at work (Sixth individual Directive within the meaning of Article 16(1) of Council Directive 89/391/EEC) (codified version) (Text with EEA relevance). Official Journal *L 158, 30.4.2004, pp. 50–76.* https://eur-lex.europa.eu/legal-content/EN/TXT/PDF/?uri=CELEX:32004L0037&from=en Current consolidated version: as of 05.04.2022: https://eur-lex.europa.eu/legal-content/EN/TXT/PDF/?uri=CELEX:02004L0037-20220405&from=EN; last accessed 31.7.2022.

25. Directive 2000/54/EC of the European Parliament and of the Council of 18 September 2000 on the protection of workers from risks related to exposure to biological agents at work (seventh individual directive within the meaning of Article 16(1) of Directive 89/391/EEC). Official Journal *L 262,*

17.10.2000, pp. 21–45. https://eur-lex.europa.eu/legal-content/EN/TXT/PDF/?uri=CELEX:32000L0054&from=EN Current consolidated version: as of 24.06.2020: https://eur-lex.europa.eu/legal-content/EN/TXT/PDF/?uri=CELEX:02000L0054-20200624&from=EN; last accessed 31.7.2022.

26. Council Directive 92/57/EEC of 24 June 1992 on the implementation of minimum safety and health requirements at temporary or mobile construction sites (eighth individual Directive within the meaning of Article 16 (1) of Directive 89/391/EEC), Official Journal *L 245, 26.8.1992, pp. 6–22.* https://eur-lex.europa.eu/legal-content/EN/TXT/PDF/?uri=CELEX:31992L0057&from=EN Current consolidated version: as of 26.07.2019 https://eur-lex.europa.eu/legal-content/EN/TXT/PDF/?uri=CELEX:01992L0057-20190726&from=EN; last accessed 31.7.2022.

27. Council Directive 92/58/EEC of 24 June 1992 on the minimum requirements for the provision of safety and/or health signs at work (ninth individual Directive within the meaning of Article 16 (1) of Directive 89/391/EEC). Official Journal *L 245, 26.8.1992, pp. 23–42.* http://eur-lex.europa.eu/legal-content/EN/TXT/PDF/?uri=CELEX:31992L0058&from=EN Current consolidated version: as of 26.07.2019: https://eur-lex.europa.eu/legal-content/EN/TXT/PDF/?uri=CELEX:01992L0058-20190726&from=EN; last accessed 31.7.2022.

28. Council Directive 92/85/EEC of 19 October 1992 on the introduction of measures to encourage improvements in the safety and health at work of pregnant workers and workers who have recently given birth or are breastfeeding (tenth individual Directive within the meaning of Article 16 (1) of Directive 89/391/EEC). Official Journal *L 348, 28.11.1992, pp. 1–7.* https://eur-lex.europa.eu/legal-content/EN/TXT/PDF/?uri=CELEX:31992L0085&from=EN Current consolidated version: as of 26.07.2019: https://eur-lex.europa.eu/legal-content/EN/TXT/PDF/?uri=CELEX:01992L0085-20190726&from=EN; last accessed 31.7.2022.

29. Council Directive 92/91/EEC of 3 November 1992 concerning the minimum requirements for improving the safety and health protection of workers in the mineral- extracting industries through drilling (eleventh individual Directive within the meaning of Article 16 (1) of Directive 89/391/EEC). Official Journal *L 348, 28.11.1992, pp. 9–24.* https://eur-lex.europa.eu/legal-content/EN/TXT/PDF/?uri=CELEX:31992L0091&from=EN Current consolidated version: as of 27.06.2007: https://eur-lex.europa.eu/legal-content/EN/TXT/PDF/?uri=CELEX:01992L0091-20070627&from=EN; last accessed 31.7.2022.

30. Council Directive 92/104/EEC of 3 December 1992 on the minimum requirements for improving the safety and health protection of workers in surface and underground mineral-extracting industries (twelfth individual Directive within the meaning of Article 16 (1) of Directive 89/391/EEC). Official Journal L 404, 31.12.1992, pp. 10–25. https://eur-lex.europa.eu/legal-content/EN/TXT/PDF/?uri=CELEX:31992L0104&from=EN Current consolidated version: as of 27.06.2007: https://eur-lex.europa.eu/legal-content/EN/TXT/PDF/?uri=CELEX:01992L0104-20070627&from=EN; last accessed 31.7.2022.

31. Council Directive 93/103/EC of 23 November 1993 concerning the minimum safety and health requirements for work on board fishing vessels (thirteenth individual Directive within the meaning of Article 16 (1) of Directive 89/391/EEC). Official Journal L 307, 13.12.1993, pp. 1–17. https://eur-lex.europa.eu/legal-content/EN/TXT/PDF/?uri=CELEX:31993L0103&from=EN Current consolidated version: as of 27.06.2007: https://eur-lex.europa.eu/legal-content/EN/TXT/PDF/?uri=CELEX:01993L0103-20070627&from=EN; last accessed 31.7.2022.

32. Council Directive 92/29/EEC of 31 March 1992 on the minimum safety and health requirements for improved medical treatment on board vessels. Official Journal L 113, 30.4.1992, pp. 19–36. https://eur-lex.europa.eu/legal-content/EN/TXT/PDF/?uri=CELEX:31992L0029&from=en Current consolidated version: as of 20.11.2019: https://eur-lex.europa.eu/legal-content/EN/TXT/PDF/?uri=CELEX:01992L0029-20191120&from=EN; last accessed 31.7.2022.

33. Council Directive 98/24/EC of 7 April 1998 on the protection of the health and safety of workers from the risks related to chemical agents at work (fourteenth individual Directive within the meaning of Article 16(1) of Directive 89/391/EEC). Official Journal *L 131, 5.5.1998, pp. 11–23.* https://eur-lex.europa.eu/legal-content/EN/TXT/PDF/?uri=CELEX:31998L0024&from=EN Current consolidated version: as of 26.07.2019: https://eur-lex.europa.eu/legal-content/EN/TXT/PDF/?uri=CELEX:01998L0024-20190726&from=EN; last accessed 31.7.2022.

34. Directive 1999/92/EC of the European Parliament and of the Council of 16 December 1999 on minimum requirements for improving the safety and health protection of workers potentially at risk from explosive atmospheres (15th individual Directive within the meaning of Article 16(1) of Directive 89/391/EEC). Official Journal L 23, 28.1.2000, pp. 57–64. https://eur-lex.europa.eu/legal-content/EN/TXT/PDF/?uri=CELEX:31999L0092&from=EN Current consolidated version: as of 27.06.2007: https://eur-lex.europa.eu/legal-content/EN/TXT/PDF/?uri=CELEX:01999L0092-20070627&from=EN; last accessed 31.7.2022.

35. Directive 2002/44/EC of the European Parliament and of the Council of 25 June 2002 on the minimum health and safety requirements regarding the exposure of workers to the risks arising from physical agents (vibration) (sixteenth individual Directive within the meaning of Article 16(1) of Directive 89/391/EEC) - Joint Statement by the European Parliament and the Council.). Official Journal L 177, 6.7.2002, pp. 13–20. https://eur-lex.

europa.eu/resource.html?uri=cellar:546a09c0-3ad1-4c07-bcd5-9c3dae6b1668.0004.02/DOC_1&format=PDF Current consolidated version: as of 26.07.2019: https://eur-lex.europa.eu/legal-content/EN/TXT/PDF/?uri=CELEX:02002L0044-20190726&from=EN; last accessed 31.7.2022.

36. Directive 2003/10/EC of the European Parliament and of the Council of 6 February 2003 on the minimum health and safety requirements regarding the exposure of workers to the risks arising from physical agents (noise) (Seventeenth individual Directive within the meaning of Article 16(1) of Directive 89/391/EEC).). Official Journal L 42, 15.2.2003, pp. 38–44. https://eur-lex.europa.eu/legal-content/EN/TXT/PDF/?uri=CELEX:32003L0010&from=EN Current consolidated version: as of 26.07.2019: https://eur-lex.europa.eu/legal-content/EN/TXT/PDF/?uri=CELEX:02003L0010-20190726&from=EN; last accessed 31.7.2022.

37. Directive 2006/25/EC of the European Parliament and of the Council of 5 April 2006 on the minimum health and safety requirements regarding the exposure of workers to risks arising from physical agents (artificial optical radiation) (19th individual Directive within the meaning of Article 16(1) of Directive 89/391/EEC). Official Journal L 114, 27.4.2006, pp. 38–59. https://eur-lex.europa.eu/legal-content/EN/TXT/PDF/?uri=CELEX:32006L0025&from=EN Current consolidated version: as of 26.07.2019: https://eur-lex.europa.eu/legal-content/EN/TXT/PDF/?uri=CELEX:02006L0025-20190726&from=EN; last accessed 31.7.2022.

38. Directive 2013/35/EU of the European Parliament and of the Council of 26 June 2013 on the minimum health and safety requirements regarding the exposure of workers to the risks arising from physical agents (electromagnetic fields) (20th individual Directive within the meaning of Article 16(1) of Directive 89/391/EEC) and repealing Directive 2004/40/EC.). Official Journal L 179, 29.6.2013, pp. 1–21. https://eur-lex.europa.eu/legal-content/EN/TXT/PDF/?uri=CELEX:32013L0035&from=EN; last accessed 31.7.2022.

39. Council Directive 2010/32/EU of 10 May 2010 implementing the Framework Agreement on prevention from sharp injuries in the hospital and healthcare sector concluded by HOSPEEM and EPSU (Text with EEA relevance). Official Journal L 134, 1.6.2010, pp. 66–72. https://eur-lex.europa.eu/legal-content/EN/TXT/PDF/?uri=CELEX:32010L0032&from=EN, last accessed 31.7.2022.

40. Directive 2009/148/EC of the European Parliament and of the Council of 30 November 2009 on the protection of workers from the risks related to exposure to asbestos at work (Text with EEA relevance). Official Journal L 330, 16.12.2009, pp. 28–36. https://eur-lex.europa.eu/legal-content/EN/TXT/PDF/?uri=CELEX:32009L0148&from=en Current consolidated version: as of 26.07.2019: https://eur-lex.europa.eu/legal-content/EN/TXT/PDF/?uri=CELEX:02009L0148-20190726&from=EN; last accessed 31.7.2022.

41. Commission Directive 91/322/EEC of 29 May 1991 on establishing indicative limit values by implementing Council Directive 80/1107/EEC on the protection of workers from the risks related to exposure to chemical, physical and biological agents at work. Official Journal L 177, 5.7.1991, pp. 22–24. https://eur-lex.europa.eu/legal-content/EN/TXT/PDF/?uri=CELEX:31991L0322&from=en. Current consolidated version: as of 21.08.2018: https://eur-lex.europa.eu/legal-content/EN/TXT/PDF/?uri=CELEX:01991L0322-20180821&from=EN; last accessed 31.7.2022.

42. Commission Directive 2000/39/EC of 8 June 2000 establishing a first list of indicative occupational exposure limit values in implementation of Council Directive 98/24/EC on the protection of the health and safety of workers from the risks related to chemical agents at work (Text with EEA relevance). Official Journal L 142, 16.6.2000, pp. 47–50. https://eur-lex.europa.eu/legal-content/EN/TXT/PDF/?uri=CELEX:32000L0039&from=en Current consolidated version: as of 20/05/2021: https://eur-lex.europa.eu/legal-content/EN/TXT/PDF/?uri=CELEX:02000L0039-20210520&from=EN; last accessed 31.7.2022.

43. Commission Directive 2006/15/EC of 7 February 2006 establishing a second list of indicative occupational exposure limit values in implementation of Council Directive 98/24/EC and amending Directives 91/322/EEC and 2000/39/EC (Text with EEA relevance). Official Journal L 38, 9.2.2006, pp. 36–39. https://eur-lex.europa.eu/legal-content/EN/TXT/PDF/?uri=CELEX:32006L0015&from=EN; last accessed 31.7.2022.

44. Commission Directive 2009/161/EU of 17 December 2009 establishing a third list of indicative occupational exposure limit values in implementation of Council Directive 98/24/EC and amending Commission Directive 2000/39/EC (Text with EEA relevance). Official Journal L 338, 19.12.2009, pp. 87–89. https://eur-lex.europa.eu/legal-content/EN/TXT/PDF/?uri=CELEX:32006L0015&from=EN; last accessed 31.7.2022.

45. Commission Directive (EU) 2017/164 of 31 January 2017 establishing a fourth list of indicative occupational exposure limit values pursuant to Council Directive 98/24/EC, and amending Commission Directives 91/322/EEC, 2000/39/EC and 2009/161/EU (Text with EEA relevance.). Official Journal *L 27, 1.2.2017, pp. 115–120*. https://eur-lex.europa.eu/legal-content/EN/TXT/PDF/?uri=CELEX:32017L0164&from=EN; last accessed 31.7.2022.

46. Commission Directive (EU) 2019/1831 of 24 October 2019 establishing a fifth list of indicative occupational exposure limit values pursuant to Council Directive 98/24/EC and amending

Commission Directive 2000/39/EC (Text with EEA relevance). Official Journal L 279, 31.10.2019, p. 31–34. https://eur-lex.europa.eu/legal-content/EN/TXT/PDF/?uri=CELEX:31991L0322&from=en Current consolidated version: as of 31.10.2019 https://eur-lex.europa.eu/legal-content/EN/TXT/PDF/?uri=CELEX:02019L1831-20191031&from=EN; last accessed 31.7.2022.

47. Council Directive 91/383/EEC of 25 June 1991 supplementing the measures to encourage improvements in the safety and health at work of workers with a fixed- duration employment relationship or a temporary employment relationship. Official Journal L 206, 29.7.1991, pp. 19–21. https://eur-lex.europa.eu/legal-content/EN/TXT/PDF/?uri=CELEX:31991L0383&from=EN Current consolidated version: as of 28.06.2007: https://eur-lex.europa.eu/legal-content/EN/TXT/PDF/?uri=CELEX:01991L0383-20070628&from=EN; last accessed 31.7.2022.

48. Directive 2003/88/EC of the European Parliament and of the Council of 4 November 2003 concerning certain aspects of the organisation of working time. Official Journal L 299, 18.11.2003, pp. 9–19. https://eur-lex.europa.eu/legal-content/EN/TXT/PDF/?uri=CELEX:32003L0088&from=en; last accessed 31.7.2022.

49. Council Directive 94/33/EC of 22 June 1994 on the protection of young people at work. Official Journal L 216, 20.8.1994, pp. 12–20. https://eur-lex.europa.eu/legal-content/EN/TXT/PDF/?uri=CELEX:31994L0033&from=EN Current consolidated version: as of 26.07.2019: https://eur-lex.europa.eu/legal-content/EN/TXT/PDF/?uri=CELEX:01994L0033-20190726&from=EN; last accessed 31.7.2022.

50. European Commission on Employment, Social Affairs & Inclusion > policies and activities >Rights at work > Health and safety at work > Areas of activity; https://ec.europa.eu/social/main.jsp?catId=716&langId=en; last accessed: 5.8.2022.

51. Regulation (EC) No 1338/2008 of the European Parliament and of the Council of 16 December 2008 on Community statistics on public health and health and safety at work (Text with EEA relevance). Official Journal L 354, 31.12.2008, pp. 70–81.

52. Krohn S, Bauer A, Drechsel-Schlund C, Engel D, Fartasch M, John SM, Köllner A, Römer W, Wehrmann W, Weisshaar E, Skudlik C. DGUV Hautarztverfahren—Update Hautarztbericht 2021. Dermatologie Beruf Umwelt. 2021;69:97–100.

53. Union Européenne des Médecins specialists (UEMS) _European Union of medical specialists. Postgraduate training. https://www.uems.eu/areas-of-expertise/postgraduate-training; Last accessed 5.8.2022 https://www.uems.eu/areas-of-expertise/postgraduate-training/european-standards-in-medical-training; Last accessed 5.8.2022.

54. Directive 2005/36/EC of the European Parliament and of the Council of 7 September 2005 on the recognition of professional qualifications (Text with EEA relevance). Official Journal L 255, pp.22–142. https://eur-lex.europa.eu/legal-content/EN/TXT/PDF/?uri=CELEX:32005L0036&from=EN Current consolidated version: as of 10/12/2021. https://eur-lex.europa.eu/legal-content/EN/TXT/PDF/?uri=CELEX:02005L0036-20211210&from=EN; last accessed 31.7.2022.

55. UEMS. Training Requirements for the Specialty of Dermatology and Venereology European Standards of Postgraduate Medical Specialist Training. https://www.uems.eu/__data/assets/pdf_file/0010/52687/UEMS-2017.29-European-Training-Requirements-in-Dermatology-and-Venerology.pdf; Last accessed 5.8.2022.

56. UEMS. Training requirements for the specialty of occupational medicine European Standards of Postgraduate Medical Specialist Training. https://www.uems.eu/__data/assets/pdf_file/0005/44429/UEMS-2013.19-European-Training-Requirements-Occupational-Medicine.pdf; Last accessed 5.8.2022.

57. Turcu V, Seremet Caplanusi T, Kokkinakis I, Crepy MN, Zyska Cherix A, Rast H, Krief P. Occupational dermatoses: management for general practitioners and an interdisciplinary collaboration model. Rev Med Suisse. 2022;18(788):1322–8.

58. Krief P, Cohidon C, Turcu V, Rinaldo M, Kamara M, Koller M, Zyska Cherix A, Senn N, Peters S. Occupational cancers: essentials for the general practioners. Rev Med Suisse. 2022;18(788):1313–21.

59. Adisesh A, Robinson E, Nicholson PJ, Sen D, Wilkinson M, Standards of Care Working Group. U.K. standards of care for occupational contact dermatitis and occupational contact urticaria. Br J Dermatol. 2013;168:1167–75.

60. Johansen JD, Aalto-Korte K, Agner T, Andersen KE, Bircher A, Bruze M, Cannavó A, Giménez-Arnau A, Gonçalo M, Goossens A, John SM, Lidén C, Lindberg M, Mahler V, Matura M, Rustemeyer T, Serup J, Spiewak R, Thyssen JP, Vigan M, White IR, Wilkinson M, Uter W. European Society of Contact Dermatitis guideline for diagnostic patch testing—recommendations on best practice. Contact Dermatitis. 2015;73(4):195–221.

61. Monitoring new and emerging risks. (2017, June 1). OSHWiki. http://oshwiki.eu/index.php?title=Monitoring_new_and_emerging_risks&oldid=247462; last accessed 31.7.2022.

62. Steffens E, Zeidan H, Weisshaar E. Pitfalls in occupational dermatology. Hautarzt. 2021;72(6):502–8.

63. Mahler V, Schmidt A, Fartasch M, Loew TH, Diepgen TL. Value of psychotherapy in expert assessment of skin diseases. Recommendations and indications for additional psychotherapy evaluation in expert assessment from the viewpoint of dermatology. Hautarzt. 1998;49(8):626–33.

64. Mahler V. Hand dermatitis—differential diagnoses, diagnostics, and treatment options. J Dtsch Dermatol Ges. 2016;14(1):7–26.

65. Meneghini CL, Angelini G. Occupational dermatitis artefacta. Dermatologie Beruf Umwelt. 1979;27(6):163–5.

66. Larese Filon F, Pesce M, Paulo MS, Loney T, Modenese A, John SM, Kezic S, Macan J. Incidence of occupational contact dermatitis in healthcare workers: a systematic review. J Eur Acad Dermatol Venereol. 2021;35(6):1285–9.

67. Thyssen JP, Schuttelaar MLA, Alfonso JH, Andersen KE, Angelova-Fischer I, Arents BWM, Bauer A, Brans R, Cannavo A, Christoffers WA, Crépy MN, Elsner P, Fartasch M, Filon FL, Giménez-Arnau AM, Gonçalo M, Guzmán-Perera MG, Hamann CR, Hoetzenecker W, Johansen JD, John SM, Kunkeler ACM, Hadzavdic SL, Molin S, Nixon R, Oosterhaven JAF, Rustemeyer T, Serra-Baldrich E, Shah M, Simon D, Skudlik C, Spiewak R, Valiukevičienė S, Voorberg AN, Weisshaar E, Agner T. Guidelines for diagnosis, prevention, and treatment of hand eczema. Contact Dermatitis. 2022;86:357–78.

68. Lampel HP, Powell HB. Occupational and hand dermatitis: a practical approach. Clin Rev Allergy Immunol. 2019;56(1):60–71.

69. Pesonen M, Jolanki R, Larese Filon F, Wilkinson M, Kręcisz B, Kieć-Świerczyńska M, Bauer A, Mahler V, John SM, Schnuch A, Uter W, ESSCA network. Patch test results of the European baseline series among patients with occupational contact dermatitis across Europe—analyses of the European Surveillance System on Contact Allergy network, 2002-2010. Contact Dermatitis. 2015;72(3):154–63.

70. Bauer A, Geier J, Mahler V, Uter W. Contact allergies in the German workforce: data of the IVDK network from 2003-2013. Hautarzt. 2015;66(9):652–64.

71. De Groot AC. Patch testing—test concentrations and vehicles for 4900 chemicals (4th edition). acdegroot publishing; 2018.

72. Mahler V, Dickel H. Most important contact allergens in hand eczema. Hautarzt. 2019;70:778–89.

73. Patel K, Nixon R. Irritant contact dermatitis—a review. Curr Dermatol Rep. 2022;11(2):41–51.

74. Nosbaum A, Vocanson M, Rozieres A, Hennino A, Nicolas JF. Allergic and irritant contact dermatitis. Eur J Dermatol. 2009;19(4):325–32.

75. Ibler KS, Jemec GBE, Agner T. Exposures related to hand eczema: a study of healthcare workers. Contact Dermatitis. 2012;66(5):247–53.

76. Hamnerius N, Svedman C, Bergendorff O, Björk J, Bruze M, Pontén A. Wet work exposure and hand eczema among healthcare workers: a cross-sectional study. Br J Dermatol. 2018;178(2):452–61.

77. Menne T, Johansen J, Sommerlund M, Veien N. Hand eczema guidelines based on the Danish guidelines for the diagnosis and treatment of hand eczema. Contact Dermatitis. 2011;65(1):3–12.

78. Loman L, Uter W, Armario-Hita JC, Ayala F, Balato A, Ballmer-Weber BK, Bauer A, Bircher AJ, Buhl T, Czarnecka-Operacz M, Dickel H, Fuchs T, Giménez Arnau A, John SM, Kränke B, Kręcisz B, Mahler V, Rustemeyer T, Sadowska-Przytocka A, Sánchez-Pérez J, Scherer Hofmeier K, Schliemann S, Simon D, Spiewak R, Spring P, Valiukevičienė S, Wagner N, Weisshaar E, Pesonen M, Schuttelaar MLA, ESSCA Working Group. European Surveillance System on Contact Allergies (ESSCA): characteristics of patients patch tested and diagnosed with irritant contact dermatitis. Contact Dermatitis. 2021;85(2):186–97.

79. Hiller J, Vogel KE, Mahler V. Diagnosis and treatment of occupational hand eczema according to recommendations of the German guideline. ASU Arbeitsmed Sozialmed Umweltmed. 2014;49:834–43.

80. Pesonen M, Koskela K, Aalto-Korte K. Contact urticaria and protein contact dermatitis in the Finnish register of occupational diseases in a period of 12 years. Contact Dermatitis. 2020;83(1):1–7.

81. Li BS, Ale IS, Maibach HI. Contact urticaria syndrome: occupational aspects. In: John S, Johansen J, Rustemeyer T, Elsner P, Maibach H, editors. Kanerva's occupational dermatology. Cham: Springer; 2018. https://doi.org/10.1007/978-3-319-40221-5_208-2.

82. Mørtz CG, Bindslev-Jensen C. Skin tests for immediate hypersensitivity. In: Johansen JD, Mahler V, Lepoittevin JP, Frosch PJ, editors. Contact dermatitis. 6th edition. Cham: Springer; 2020. https://doi.org/10.1007/978-3-030-36335-2_28.

83. Mahler V. Prick and intracutaneous testing and IgE testing. In: John S, Johansen J, Rustemeyer T, Elsner P, Maibach H, editors. Kanerva's occupational dermatology, third edition. Cham: Springer; 2020. p. 1317–45.

84. Wakelin SH. Diagnostic methods: cutaneous provocation tests. In: Giménez-Arnau AM, Maibach HI, editors. Contact urticaria syndrome. Diagnosis and management. Cham: Springer; 2018. p. 123–30.

85. Helaskoski E, Suojalehto H, Kuuliala O, Aalto-Korte K. Prick testing with chemicals in the diagnosis of occupational contact urticaria and respiratory diseases. Contact Dermatitis. 2015;72:20–32.

86. Brockow K, Garvey LH, Aberer W, Atanaskovic-Markovic M, Barbaud A, Bilo MB, Bircher A, Blanca M, Bonadonna B, Campi P, Castro E, Cernadas JR, Chiriac AM, Demoly P, Grosber M, Gooi J, Lombardo C, Mertes PM, Mosbech H, Nasser S, Pagani M, Ring J, Romano A, Scherer K, Schnyder B, Testi S, Torres M, Trautmann A, Terreehorst I. Skin test concentrations for systemically administered drugs– an ENDA/EAACI Drug Allergy Interest Group position paper. Allergy. 2013;68:702–12.

87. Mayorga C, Celik G, Rouzaire P, Whitaker P, Bonadonna P, Rodrigues-Cernadas J, Vultaggio A, Brockow K, Caubet JC, Makowska J, Nakonechna A, Romano A, Montañez MI, Laguna JJ, Zanoni G, Gueant JL, Oude Elberink H, Fernandez J, Viel S, Demoly P, Torres MJ. In vitro tests for drug hypersensitivity reactions: an ENDA/EAACI Drug Allergy Interest Group position paper. Allergy. 2016;71:1103–34.

88. Walter A, Seegräber M, Wollenberg A. Food-related contact dermatitis, contact urticaria, and atopy patch test with food. Clin Rev Allergy Immunol. 2019;56:19–31.

89. Ortolani C, Ispano M, Pastorello EA, Ansaloni R, Magri GC. Comparison of results of skin prick tests (with fresh foods and commercial food extracts) and RAST in 100 patients with oral allergy syndrome. J Allergy Clin Immunol. 1989;83(3):683–90.

90. Leiter U, Heppt MV, Steeb T, Amaral T, Bauer A, Becker JC, Breitbart E, Breuninger H, Diepgen T, Dirschka T, Eigentler T, Flaig M, Follmann M, Fritz K, Greinert R, Gutzmer R, Hillen U, Ihrler S, John SM, Kölbl O, Kraywinkel K, Löser C, Nashan D, Noor S, Nothacker M, Pfannenberg C, Salavastru C, Schmitz L, Stockfleth E, Szeimies RM, Ulrich C, Welzel J, Wermker K, Garbe C, Berking C. S3 guideline for actinic keratosis and cutaneous squamous cell carcinoma (cSCC)—prevention and occupational disease. S3 guideline for actinic keratosis and cutaneous squamous cell carcinoma (cSCC)—short version, part 2: epidemiology, surgical and systemic treatment of cSCC, follow-up, prevention and occupational disease. J Dtsch Dermatol Ges. 2020;18(4):400–13.

91. Peris K, Fargnoli MC, Garbe C, Kaufmann R, Bastholt L, Seguin NB, Bataille V, Marmol VD, Dummer R, Harwood CA, Hauschild A, Höller C, Haedersdal M, Malvehy J, Middleton MR, Morton CA, Nagore E, Stratigos AJ, Szeimies RM, Tagliaferri L, Trakatelli M, Zalaudek I, Eggermont A, Grob JJ, European Dermatology Forum (EDF), the European Association of Dermato-Oncology (EADO), the European Organization for Research, Treatment of Cancer (EORTC). Diagnosis and treatment of basal cell carcinoma: European consensus-based interdisciplinary guidelines. Eur J Cancer. 2019;118:10–34.

92. Garbe C, Amaral T, Peris K, Hauschild A, Arenberger P, Bastholt L, Bataille V, Del Marmol V, Dréno B, Fargnoli MC, Grob JJ, Höller C, Kaufmann R, Lallas A, Lebbé C, Malvehy J, Middleton M, Moreno-Ramirez D, Pellacani G, Saiag P, Stratigos AJ, Vieira R, Zalaudek I, Eggermont AMM, European Dermatology Forum (EDF), the European Association of Dermato-Oncology (EADO), the European Organization for Research and Treatment of Cancer (EORTC). European consensus-based interdisciplinary guideline for melanoma. Part 1: diagnostics—update 2019. Eur J Cancer. 2020;126:141–58.

93. Rundle CW, Presley CL, Militello M, Barber C, Powell DL, Jacob SE, Atwater AR, Watsky KL, Yu J, Dunnick CA. Hand hygiene during COVID-19: recommendations from the American Contact Dermatitis Society. J Am Acad Dermatol. 2020;83(6):1730–7.

94. Greveling K, Kunkeler ACM. Hand eczema pandemic caused by severe acute respiratory syndrome coronavirus 2 hygiene measures: the set-up of a hand eczema helpline for hospital personnel. J Eur Acad Dermatol Venereol. 2020;34(10):e556–7.

95. Yu J, Chen JK, Mowad CM, Reeder M, Hylwa S, Chisolm S, Dunnick CA, Goldminz AM, Jacob SE, Wu PA, Zippin J, Atwater AR. Occupational der-matitis to facial personal protective equipment in health care workers: a systematic review. J Am Acad Dermatol. 2021;84(2):486–94.

96. Aguilera SB, De La Pena I, Viera M, Baum B, Morrison BW, Amar O, Beustes-Stefanelli M, Hall M. The impact of COVID-19 on the faces of frontline healthcare workers. J Drugs Dermatol. 2020;19(9):858–64.

97. Dowdle TS, Thompson M, Alkul M, Nguyen JM, Sturgeon ALE. COVID-19 and dermatological personal protective equipment considerations. Proc (Bayl Univ Med Cent). 2021;34(4):469–72.

98. Berufsgenossenschaft Holz und Metall (Hrsg.). BGHM-Information 102; Beurteilen von Gefährdungen und Belastung, Anleitungshilfe zur systematischen Vorgehensweise, sichere Schritte zum Ziel. Oktober 2021;18–20. https://www.bghm.de/fileadmin/user_upload/Arbeitsschuetzer/Gesetze_Vorschriften/Informationen/BGHM-I_102.pdf; last accessed: 6.12.2022.

99. Elsner P. Skin protection in the prevention of skin diseases. Curr Probl Dermatol. 2007;34:1–10.

100. Uter W, Kanerva L. Physical causes—heat, cold, and other atmospheric factors. In: John SM, Johansen J, Rustemeyer T, Elsner P, Maibach H, editors. Kanerva's occupational dermatology. Cham: Springer; 2018. https://doi.org/10.1007/978-3-319-40221-5_33-2.

101. International Atomic Energy Agency (IAEA). Radiation Protection and Safety in Medical Uses of Ionizing Radiation. Specific Safety Guide No. SSG-46. Vienna, 2018. https://www-pub.iaea.org/MTCD/publications/PDF/PUB1775_web.pdf; last accessed: 6.12.2022.

102. Landeck L., Wulfhorst B., John SM. Prevention in health-care professionals. In: John SM, Johansen J, Rustemeyer T, Elsner P, Maibach H (eds): Kanerva's occupational dermatology. Springer, Cham, 2018. https://doi.org/10.1007/978-3-319-40221-5_109-2

103. Smith T, Quencer K, Smith T, Agarwal D. Radiation effects and protection for technologists and other health care professionals. Radiol Technol. 2021;92(5):445–58.

104. Bauer A, Adam KE, Soyer PH, Adam KWJ. Prevention of occupational skin cancer. In: John SM, Johansen J, Rustemeyer T, Elsner P, Maibach H, editors. Kanerva's occupational dermatology. Cham: Springer; 2018. https://doi.org/10.1007/978-3-319-40221-5_115-2.

105. Rocholl M, Ludewig M, Skudlik C, Wilke A. Occupational skin cancer : prevention and recommendations for UV protection as part of the treatment approved by the public statutory employers' liability insurance. Hautarzt. 2018;69(6):462–70.

106. Harries MJ, Lear JT. Occupational skin infections. Occup Med (Lond). 2004;54(7):441–9.

107. Kreft B, Sunderkötter C. Occupational skin infections. In: John SM, Johansen J, Rustemeyer T, Elsner P, Maibach H, editors. Kanerva's occupational dermatology. Cham: Springer; 2019. https://doi.org/10.1007/978-3-319-40221-5_213-1.

108. GESTIS Biological Agents Database. www.dguv. de/ifa/gestis-biological-agents; last accessed: 6.12.2022.

109. Houle MC, Holness DL, DeKoven J. Occupational contact dermatitis: an individualized approach to the worker with dermatitis. Curr Dermatol Rep. 2021;10(4):182–91.

110. Ahlström MG, Dietz JB, Johansen JD, John SM, Brans R. Evaluation of the secondary and tertiary prevention strategies against occupational contact dermatitis in Germany: a systematic review. Contact Dermatitis. 2022;87(2):142–53.

111. Eurofound. Working conditions in sectors, Publications Office of the European Union, Luxembourg. 2020. https://www.eurofound.europa. eu/sites/default/files/ef_publication/field_ef_document/ef19005en.pdf; last accessed: 31.7.2022.

112. EU-OSHA – European Agency for Safety and Health at Work Expert forecast on emerging chemical risks related to occupational safety and health. 2009. http://osha.europa.eu/en/publications/reports/ TE3008390ENC_chemical_risks; last accessed: 31.7.2022.

113. Eurofound – European Foundation for the Improvement of Living and Working Conditions, Fourth European Working Conditions Survey (Résumé). Publications Office of the European Union, Luxembourg. 2008. https://www.eurofound. europa.eu/sites/default/files/ef_publication/field_ef_ document/ef0678en.pdf; last accessed: 31.7.2022.

114. Eurofound. Fifth European Working Conditions Survey (Overview report). Luxembourg: Publications Office of the European Union; 2012. https://www.eurofound.europa.eu/sites/default/files/ ef_publication/field_ef_document/ef1182en.pdf; last accessed: 31.7.2022

115. Roach KA, Stefaniak AB, Roberts JR. Metal nanomaterials: immune effects and implications of physicochemical properties on sensitization, elicitation, and exacerbation of allergic disease. J Immunotoxicol. 2019;16(1):87–124.

116. Smulders S, Golanski L, Smolders E, Vanoirbeek J, Hoet PH. Nano-TiO2 modulates the dermal sensitization potency of dinitrochlorobenzene after topical exposure. Br J Dermatol. 2015;172(2):392–9.

117. International Labour Organization (ILO), International Occupational Safety and Health Information Centre (CIS), Ceramic fibers (aluminisilicate) – ICSC:0123. March 1999. Available at: http://www.ilo.org/public/english/protection/ safework/cis/products/icsc/dtasht/_icsc01/icsc0123. htm; last accessed: 31.7.2022.

118. International Labour Organization (ILO), International Occupational Safety and Health Information Centre (CIS), Glass wool—ICSC:0157. March 1999. http://www.ilo.org/public/english/protection/safework/cis/products/icsc/dtasht/_icsc01/ icsc0157.htm; last accessed: 31.7.2022.

119. International Labour Organization (ILO), International Occupational Safety and Health Information Centre (CIS), Rock wool – ICSC:0194. April 2000. http://www.ilo.org/public/english/protection/safework/cis/products/icsc/dtasht/_icsc01/ icsc0194.htm; last accessed: 31.7.2022.

120. International Labour Organization (ILO), International Occupational Safety and Health Information Centre (CIS), Slag wool – ICSC:0195. April 2000. http://www.ilo.org/public/english/protection/safework/cis/products/icsc/dtasht/_icsc01/ icsc0195.htm; last accessed: 31.7.2022.

121. Bundesanstalt für Arbeitsschutz und Arbeitsmedizin (BAuA), „TRGS 521 - Abbruch-, Sanierungs- und Instandhaltungsarbeiten mit alter Mineralwolle", Ausschuss für Gefahrstoffe - AGS-Geschäftsführung, February 2008. http://www.baua.de/nn_16736/de/ Themen-von-A-Z/Gefahrstoffe/TRGS/pdf/TRGS-521.pdf?; last accessed: 31.7.2022.

122. EU-OSHA – European Agency for Safety and Health at Work, European Risk Observatory Report – Expert forecasts on emerging biological risks related to occupational safety and health, 2007. http://osha. europa.eu/en/publications/reports/7606488; last accessed: 31.7.2022.

123. Psychosocial issues. (2022, June 8). OSHWiki.. http://oshwiki.eu/index.php?title=Psychosocial_ issues&oldid=254526, last accessed 31.7.2022.

124. Ofenloch R, Oesterhelt A, Weisshaar E. Rehabilitation program for occupational skin diseases at the university hospital Heidelberg, Germany: increase in disease duration and age of patients. J Dtsch Dermatol Ges. 2021;19(5):746–9.

International Standards for Prevention of Occupational Dermatoses

José Hernán Alfonso

Introduction

Work-related and occupational dermatoses lead to frequent use of health care services, high occurrence of sick leave, job loss, job change, and mental distress [1]. Both occupational dermatoses and its consequences are highly preventable by eliminating and reducing exposure to occupational hazards.

Scope of Preventive Measures

Prevention can be defined as:

> "measures adopted by or practiced on persons not currently feeling the effects of a disease, intended to decrease the risk that disease will afflict them in the future" [2].

The ultimate goal for prevention in occupational dermatology is to maintain a healthy skin in a safe work environment. Thus, prevention focuses on human, organizational, and technical and organizational measures for avoidance and limitation of exposure to skin irritants, urticariogens, allergens, and carcinogens at the work-place according to legislation and the provision of regular training in the use of personal protective measures adapted to the needs of the employees [3].

Thus, from a public health perspective preventive measures comprise:

1. *Universal measures:* include strategies for health promotion to benefit the full population. Legislation regulating the availability of skin irritants, allergens, and urticarigens is the best example of universal measures. For instance, a significant decline of occupational contact urticaria attributed to latex in gloves was observed in Germany, France, and the United Kingdom after legislation to reduce occupational exposure [4–6]. Preservatives such as methylchloroisothiazolinone/methyl-isothiazolinone (CMIT/MIT, also known as MCI/MI, Kathon CG®), methyldibromo glutaronitrile (MDBGN), and several formaldehyde releasers are substances which have caused a rapid and alarming increase in contact allergy and dermatitis [7]. Liquid soaps, industrial hand cleansers, detergents, skin care products, paints, metal-working fluids, and their biocides, as well as fountain solution additives in printing work, are the most common sources of exposure to MIT or MCIT/MIT. Julander and a group of experts from the Nordic countries summarize important dates concerning legislation, classification, and

J. H. Alfonso (✉)
Department of Occupational Medicine and Epidemiology, National Institute of Occupational Health, Oslo, Norway

Department of Dermatology and Venereology, Oslo University Hospital, Oslo, Norway

© The Author(s), under exclusive license to Springer Nature Switzerland AG 2023
A. M. Giménez-Arnau, H. I. Maibach (eds.), *Handbook of Occupational Dermatoses*, Updates in Clinical Dermatology, https://doi.org/10.1007/978-3-031-22727-1_8

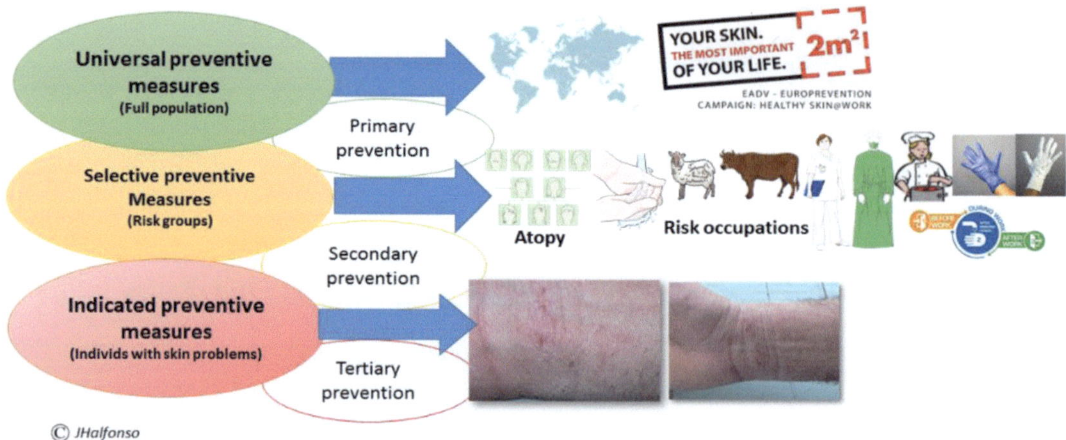

Servier Medical Art kindly provided graphic images for the design of this figure.

Fig. 8.1 Preventive measures according to population groups. Servier Medical Art kindly provided graphic images for the design of this figure

restriction of sensitizing preservatives in Europe [8].

2. ***Selective measures:*** include specific preventive actions focusing on specific risk factors and risk groups. Examples include education about risk factors for developing work-related skin problems, training on skin protection such as proper use of protective equipment, provision and training on use of moisturizers, and periodical health surveillance in risk occupations. The effectiveness of these measures to prevent work-related and occupational dermatoses depends on the knowledge, awareness, and motivation of both employers and employees. Firstly, employers should be aware about the risks at work to develop immediate contact reactions and provide the workers with proper skin education and protective elements. Secondly, workers should be motivated to carry out or seek out specific preventive measure. Occupational health professionals and health educators have an essential role to facilitate the effective design and implementation of these actions.

3. ***Indicated measures:*** comprise the application of specific diagnostic procedures in workers with already established skin problems. Indicated prevention is most commonly applied in the clinical setting, as indication is ordinarily one discovered through medical examination or laboratory testing, and many of the preventive measures require professional advice or assistance for optimal results [2]. The German "Dermatologist's procedure" serves as a model on how to identify early work-related skin problems by mandatory reporting and prevent its social, psychological, and economic consequences [9].

Figure 8.1 summarizes the scope of prevention based on a population approach for whom the measure is advisable according to scientific evidence and cost-benefit analysis.

International Standards for Prevention

Scientific evidence-based criteria and standards are necessary to assess workers at risk for developing work-related and occupational dermatoses and patients with these conditions in order to prevent and treat occupational dermatoses.

Evidence-based recommendations for the prevention, identification, and management of occupational contact dermatitis and urticaria were first developed by Nicholson et al. after a systematic review of the literature (Table 8.1) [10].

Minimum standards for effective prevention, diagnosis, and treatment of work-related and occupational skin diseases (Fig. 8.2 and Table 8.2) have been established by a consensus-based approach by means of the Delphi method with over 80 experts (dermatologists, occupational

Table 8.1 Evidence-based recommendations for the prevention of occupational contact dermatitis and urticaria. Adapted from [10]

Recommendations to health and safety personnel

1. Implement programs to remove or reduce exposure to agents that cause occupational contact dermatitis or occupational contact urticaria.
2. Provide appropriate gloves and cotton liners where the risk of developing occupational contact dermatitis or occupational contact urticaria cannot be eliminated by removing exposure to its causes.
3. Make after-work creams readily available in the workplace and encourage workers to use them regularly.
4. Not promote the use of pre-work (barrier) creams as a protective measure.
5. Provide workers with appropriate health and safety information and training.
6. Ensure that workers who develop occupational contact dermatitis or occupational contact urticaria are properly assessed by a physician who has expertise in occupational skin disease for recommendations regarding appropriate workplace adjustments.

Recommendations to health practitioners

1. Ask a worker who has been offered a job that will expose them to causes of occupational contact dermatitis whether they have a personal history of dermatitis, particularly in adulthood, and advise them of their increased risk, and to care for and protect their skin.
2. Ask the worker who has been offered a job that will expose them to causes of occupational contact urticaria whether they have a personal history of atopy and advise them of their increased risk, and to care for and protect their skin.
3. Take a full occupational history whenever someone of working age presents with dermatitis or urticaria, asking about their job, the materials with which they work, the location of the rash, and any temporal relationship with work (chap. 10).
4. Arrange for a diagnosis of occupational contact dermatitis or occupational contact urticaria to be confirmed objectively (patch tests and/or prick tests); not on the basis of a compatible history alone, because of the implications for future employment.

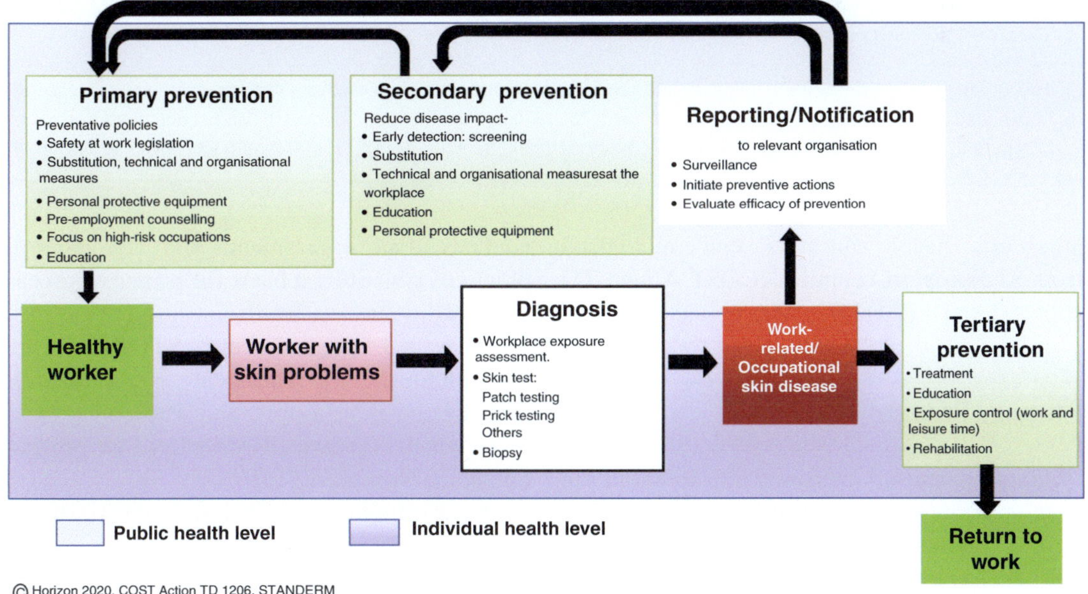

Fig. 8.2 Minimum European standards for primary, secondary, and tertiary prevention of work-related and occupational skin diseases [3]

Table 8.2 Standards for prevention, diagnosis, and treatment of work-related and occupational skin diseases [3]

Definition and classification

1. Work-related as well as occupational diseases comprise entities/conditions with an occupational contribution. However, occupational diseases are additionally defined by diverging national legal definitions. These definitions have an impact on prevention, management, and compensation.

2. The implementation of the proposed ICD-11 classification of WRSD/OSD is recommended. It will enable comprehensive identification of WRSD/OSD and thereby valid surveillance.

Diagnosis

1. Comprehensive and early diagnosis is key for prevention and management.

2. The diagnosis of WRSD/OSD should be based on existing guidelines and should include a multidisciplinary approach.

3. Patch testing is essential if contact dermatitis persists longer than 3 months or relapses.

Work exposure assessment

1. Workplace exposure assessment is an essential part of the assessment and management of patients with WRSD/OSD.

2. Minimum requirements for workplace exposure assessment in diagnosis of WRSD/OSD include worker's medical and occupational history, physical examination, and product labels/material safety data sheets assessment.

3. Full labeling of product ingredients should be made mandatory on MSDS in Europe.

Reporting

1. Current registries are usually incomplete. Accurate and complete reporting is important for monitoring and effective allocation of resources.

2. Reporting procedures should be transparent, simple, and easily accessible to provide optimal care for affected workers. They contribute to preventing chronic and relapsing disease courses.

3. The investment in reporting systems offers a substantial reduction of cost related to medical care, retraining, and compensation.

Treatment

1. The therapeutic treatment of work-related chronic hand dermatitis and skin cancers does not differ from the corresponding non-work-related dermatosis. In addition, avoidance of the trigger factors, e.g., skin contact with irritants and allergens or sun exposure at the workplace, by technical and/or organizational measures is essential.

2. The use of available guidelines for treatment of chronic hand dermatitis [11] and non-melanoma skin cancers is recommended.

Prevention

3. The aim of primary prevention is maintaining a healthy worker by by creating safe workplaces. This includes risk assessment and early intervention.

4. The aim of secondary prevention is to avoid disease chronicity and/or progression through early diagnosis and intervention.

5. The aim of tertiary prevention is medical and occupational rehabilitation of workers with an established disease.

6. Minimum requirements for the prevention of work-related/occupational hand dermatitis and occupational skin cancer include regular use of personal protective equipment and regular provision of health and safety information in vocational schools and workplaces.

physicians, health educators, epidemiologists) from 31 European countries (COST Action TD 1206, STANDERM) [3].

Primary Prevention

Primary prevention measures aim to avoid the development of work-related dermatoses in healthy workers [3]. The implementation of risk management processes involving risk analysis, risk assessment, and risk control practices constitute a basis for primary prevention [12].

Table 8.3 presents the **STOP** concept (**S**ubstitution, **T**echnical measures, **O**rganizational measures, and **P**ersonal protection), which is practically orientated for prevention at the workplace [13].

If substitution, technical and organizational prevention measures are not available or are insufficient, personal protective equipment (e.g.,

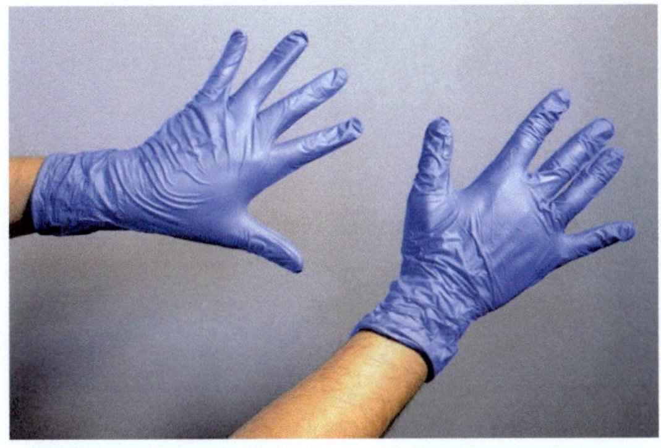

Fig. 8.3 Nitrile accelerator-free gloves. Photo: National Institute of Occupational Health, STAMI

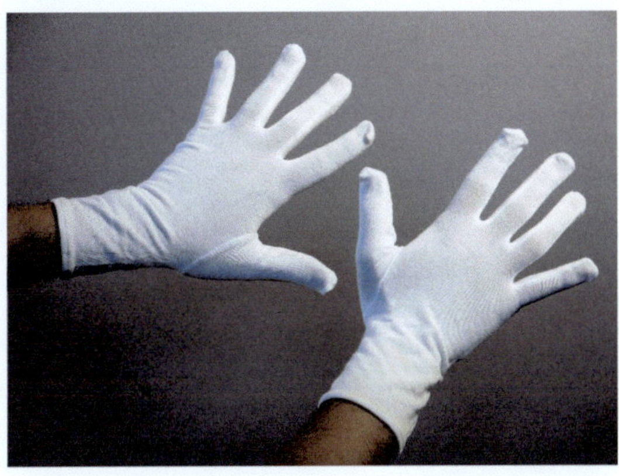

Fig. 8.4 Gloves made of bamboo viscose fiber. Photo: National Institute of Occupational Health, STAMI

Table 8.3 Preventive measures for work-related/occupational dermatoses Adapted from [3]

Preventive measure	
Substitution and replacement	Regulation of exposure by legislation on threshold values. Replacement, modification, or inactivation of hazardous substances [4, 5, 6, 16].
Technical measures	Proper labeling and storage of chemicals and regular maintenance of tools. Industrial measures to avoid direct skin contact with skin irritants, urticariogens, allergens, and carcinogens [13, 14]. Technical measures such as ventilation and automatization in work practices will reduce if not eliminate the risk of skin irritations, sensitization, and carcinogenesis.
Organizational measures	Reduce wet work to less than 2 h. Work tasks rotation and variation to reduce wet work. Skin protection programs providing information on healthy and diseased skin and skin care to facilitate a behavioral change regarding skin protection and decrease the occurrence of work-related skin problems. Such recommendations should be evidence-based [17]. They should be implemented in the curriculum of vocational schools and provided regularly at workplaces. These programs have been shown to be effective in primary, secondary, and tertiary prevention, but also in secondary and tertiary prevention [[18].
Personal protection	**Good hand hygiene regimes** should include: – Alcohol hand rubs. – Hand washing with lukewarm water, rinsing the liquid soap thoroughly, and drying hands carefully with single-use paper towels. *Protective gloves (powder and accelerator-free):* – Should be worn on dry and clean hands for wet work and work with hazardous substances for as short a time as possible. – Cotton glove liners should be used if gloves have to be worn longer than 10 min. – Single-use gloves should be worn only once. – Defect gloves must be removed immediately. *Moisturizers:* – Should be used to prevent and support the treatment of irritant hand dermatitis. – Should be applied all over the hands including the fingerwebs, fingertips, and back of the hand. – Should not contain fragrances, coloring agents, and preservatives [19–21].

gloves and moisturizers) must be available as well as regular training on correct application/use. Several studies have shown that protective strategies are applied insufficiently; therefore regular instructions on use and application are necessary [14, 15].

Recommendations for the Use of Protective Gloves

Accelerators-Free Gloves

Protective gloves can lead to skin irritation and allergy due to skin occlusion and the presence of allergens. For instance, while an effective reduction in the occurrence of occupational contact urticaria due to natural rubber latex has been registered [4–6], rubber additives are still causing occupational contact dermatitis and urticaria [22]. Low-protein rubber gloves, vulcanization accelerator-free, or gloves containing antimicrobial agents or moisturizers new technologies are now available [22]. These gloves are useful for primary prevention among healthy workers in risk occupations, and among workers with already established skin problems in terms of secondary prevention. Unfortunately, these gloves may be more expensive than regular non-accelerator-free gloves as cheaper options gloves are usually not tested for allergy and may still contain both allergens and urticariogens. Table 8.4 shows an overview of some available accelerator-free gloves.

It is highly recommended that food handlers do not use natural rubber latex gloves, as latex

Table 8.4 Accelerator-free gloves to prevent gloves-related skin allergies

Occupational group	Material	Manufacturer
Health workers Veterinarians	Low-protein latex gloves: Use of deproteinized and purified natural rubber latex is obtained by adding proteolytic enzymes and/or surfactants, chlorination, and high-temperature post-washing [22].	Ansell https://www.ansell.com/
	Non-latex surgical gloves. MEDI-GRIP® Made from synthetic neoprene and free from latex proteins and chemical accelerators.	
	GAMMEX® non-latex PI. Made of 100% synthetic polyisoprene. Safe for latex-sensitive (type I).	
	MICRO-TOUCH nitrile accelerator-free	
Surgical personnel (surgical gloves)	Biogel® NeoDerm® made of polychloroprene, without accelerators.	Mölnlycke http://www.molnlycke.us/
	Sempermed® Syntegra UV Polyisoprene photocross-linked (powder free, natural latex free, accelerator free)	Sempermed https://www.sempermed.com/en/
	Finessis corium® Styrene elastomer (SEBS) (powder free, natural latex free, accelerator free)	Finessis http://finessis.com/
Food handlers, catering, cleaners, hairdressers	Accelerators-free, powder-free, nitrile gloves	Granberg http://www.granberg.no/

proteins can be transferred to food [23, 24]. Subjects with known latex allergies can develop severe allergic reactions to foods handled by latex gloves [25]. The website of the American Latex Allergy Association provides an extensive list of alternative latex-free products at http://latexallergyresources.org/latex-free-products.

Practical Recommendations for Proper Glove Use

Table 8.5 summarizes practical recommendations for proper glove use to prevent the effects of glove occlusion on the skin barrier disruption and further development of work-related and occupational dermatoses [25, 26].

Table 8.5 Tips on proper glove use

1. Use the recommended gloves on the data safety material sheet of the chemical products you are handling. In case of doubt, contact the producer or ask for advice from occupational hygienists or safety engineers.
2. Use accelerator-free gloves.
3. Always choose gloves that are CE marked.
4. Protective gloves should be used when necessary, but for as short a time as possible.
5. Protective gloves should be intact and clean and dry inside.
6. Use gloves with long cuffs to avoid that water and chemical products coming inside the glove.
7. Hands must be washed after glove removal. Gloves have an imperfect barrier to infectious material.
8. Avoid finger rings and long nails inside when using gloves.
9. Use gloves made of cotton or bamboo viscose fiber under the protective glove, which will absorb moisture and sweat (Fig. 8.5). Gloves made of bamboo viscose fiber are softer and more comfortable. The fingertips of the glove can be cut in order to keep a good finger sensation.
10. Disposable gloves are gloves for single use. They should not be cleaned and reused.
11. Choose the right glove size.
12. Remove the gloves without touching the outer surface of the glove to avoid contact with substances that may cause allergy or irritation on the skin.
13. Use protective gloves when performing wet work during domestic or free time activities.

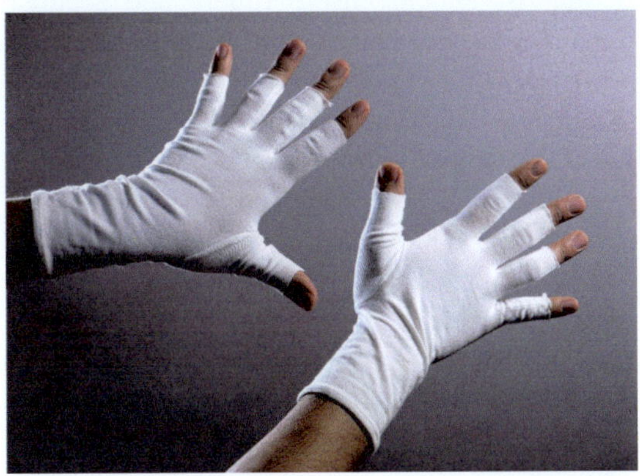

Fig. 8.5 Customized gloves made of bamboo viscose fiber to keep good sensation in the fingertips. Photo: National Institute of Occupational Health, STAMI

Moisturizers

A healthy skin assures protection against physical agents, chemicals, mechanical injuries, impact, light, UV radiation, cold, and heat. Extrinsic factors such as occupational exposure to chemical, physical, and mechanical exposures may threaten skin integrity and proper restoration leading to skin barrier disruption.

Skin barrier disruption leads to irritant contact dermatitis, facilitates the penetration of skin urticariogens and allergens with further sensitization. Proper use of moisturizers promotes regeneration and reparation of a disrupted skin barrier [27, 28] and contributes to keeping a healthy skin. A lipid-rich moisturizer free from fragrances and with preservatives and the lowest allergen potential is highly recommended [29].

Moderate evidence is available on preventive effect of the regular application of moisturizers to avoid the development of occupational contact dermatitis [10, 30]. Moreover, strong evidence, from high-quality independent studies, supports that the use of moisturizers before work ("premoisturizers") may help to prevent the development of occupational contact dermatitis. However, the denomination "barrier cream" is highly discouraged as it may provide with a false feeling of full skin protection.

After a literature review focusing on primary prevention through the use of skin creams in healthy populations, an expert panel suggested three moments, for skin cream application to prevent irritant contact dermatitis in the workplace: before work; during work after hand washing; and after work [31]. This suggestion can be applied to all industrial sectors, with evidence drawn from different workplace scenarios such as hairdressers, food handlers, timber, building trade, machinists, and metalworkers.

More randomized controlled trials including long-term controlled observations as well as intervention studies in risk occupations are needed to confirm the effectiveness of this suggestion.

It has to be emphasized that proper use of gloves and moisturizers should not be a substitute elimination, substitution, and reduction of hazardous skin exposures through legislation, risk assessment, and training on health and safety at the workplace.

Secondary Prevention

The aim of secondary prevention is to provide workers with accessible facilities for early diagnosis and intervention to avoid disease progression. Thus, secondary prevention measures are implemented to detect and treat early stages of the disease, to prevent relapses or chronicity by improvement of hazardous workplace situations, behavioral change, and proper skin protection at both work and free time.

Unfortunately, a significant delay between the onset of work-related skin problems and seeking health care varying from 9 months [32] to more than 30 months [33] often leads to a poorer prognosis [34].

Chapter 10 presents the basics of a proper diagnosis of work-related and occupational dermatoses and will not be repeated here. An individual approach to the worker with occupational dermatosis should ensure timely and accurate diagnosis as well as a better prognosis if early diagnosis and interventions are possible [35].

As Fig. 8.2 shows notification and surveillance systems for work-related and occupational dermatoses are necessary for early intervention, to initiate diagnostic, treatment, and interventions at the workplace.

Tertiary Prevention Measures

The aim of tertiary prevention is medical, occupational, and psychosocial rehabilitation of workers with an established disease. These measures aim to facilitate social rehabilitation and quality of life of workers who are at risk of losing their jobs or even had already suffered job loss because of their occupational dermatoses. Experiences from Germany suggest that tertiary individual programs including psychological interventions contribute to improving mental health in patients with severe occupational hand eczema [36].

Knowledge dissemination by Interdisciplinary teams composed of dermatologists, occupational physicians, allergists, safety engineers, and health educators are necessary for effective measures in all levels of prevention [37].

Conclusion

The most effective preventive measures to prevent occupational dermatoses include legislation, elimination, substitution, and reduction of exposure to skin hazardous substances. When substitution, technical, and organizational measures are not feasible, skin protection by the terms of proper use of protective gloves and moisturizers is highly encouraged.

Continuous training and education will contribute not only to keeping a healthy skin in safe workplaces, but also to recognizing early signs of skin disease and facilitate rehabilitation. Hence, early diagnosis and intervention will prevent a relapse and chronic disease course. When an occupational disease is already established, measures aim to facilitate medical, occupational, social, economic compensation and psychological rehabilitation should be available.

The practical implementation of the already developed standards for the prevention of work-related and occupational skin diseases is essential for effective prevention.

References

1. European Agency for Safety and Health at Work. Occupational skin diseases and dermal exposure in the European Union (EU-25): Policy and practice review; 2008. Available at: https://osha.europa.eu/en/publications/reports/TE7007049ENC_skin_diseases. Accessed 20 Nov 2017.
2. Gordon RS Jr. An operational classification of disease prevention. Public Health Rep. 1983;98:107–9.
3. Alfonso JH, Bauer A, Bensefa-Colas L, et al. Minimum standards on prevention, diagnosis and treatment of occupational and work-related skin diseases in Europe – position paper of the COST action StanDerm (TD 1206). J Eur Acad Dermatol Venereol. 2017;31(Suppl. 4):31–43.
4. Allmers H, Schmengler J, John SM. Decreasing incidence of occupational contact urticaria caused by natural rubber latex allergy in German health care workers. J Allergy Clin Immunol. 2004;114:347–51.
5. Bensefa-Colas L, Telle-Lamberton M, Faye S, et al. Occupational contact urticaria: lessons from the French National Network for occupational disease vigilance and prevention (RNV3P). Br J Dermatol. 2015;173:1453–61.
6. Turner S, McNamee R, Agius R, et al. Evaluating interventions aimed at reducing occupational exposure to latex and rubber glove allergens. Occup Environ Med. 2012;69:925–31.
7. Schwensen JF, Uter W, Bruze M, Svedman C, et a (2017). The epidemic of methylisothiazolinone: a European prospective study. Contact Dermatitis;76:272–279. https://doi.org/10.1111/cod.12733.
8. Julander A, Boman A, Johanson G, Lidén C. Occupational skin exposure to chemicals. Arbete och Hälsa (Work and Health) Scientific Serial. 2018; 52(3). http://hdl.handle.net/2077/56215. Accessed on 13 March 2022.
9. Voß H, Gediga G, Gediga K, et al. Secondary prevention of occupational dermatoses: first systematic evaluation of optimized dermatologist's procedure and hierarchical multi-step intervention. J Dtsch Dermatol Ges J Ger Soc Dermatol. 2013;11:662–71.
10. Nicholson PJ, Llewellyn D, English JS, on behalf of the Guidelines Development Group. Evidence-based guidelines for the prevention, identification and management of occupational contact dermatitis and urticaria. Contact Dermatitis. 2010;63:177–86.
11. Thyssen JP, Schuttelaar MLA, Alfonso JH, et al. Guidelines for diagnosis, prevention, and treatment of hand eczema. Contact Dermatitis. 2021; https://doi.org/10.1111/cod.14035. Epub ahead of print. PMID: 34971008
12. Council Directive 89/391/EEC of 12 June 1989 on the introduction of measures to encourage improvements in the safety and health of workers at work. OSHA. Available at https://oshwiki.eu/wiki/Occupational_safety_and_health_risk_assessment_methodologies Last accessed 19 Mar 2022.
13. Wulfhorts R, John SM, Strunk M. Worker's protection: gloves and cream. In: Duus Johansen J, Lepoittevin JP, Thyssen JP, editors. Quick guide to contact dermatitis. Berlin: Springer-Verlag; 2016. p. 275–87.
14. Diepgen TL, Andersen KE, Chosidow O, et al (2015) Guidelines for diagnosis, prevention and treatment of hand eczema--short version. J Dtsch Dermatol Ges J Ger Soc Dermatol JDDG; 13:77–85.
15. Oreskov KW, Søsted H, Johansen JD. Glove use among hairdressers: difficulties in the correct use of gloves among hairdressers and the effect of education. Contact Dermatitis. 2015;72:362–6. 215–220
16. Uter W, Pfahlberg A, Gefeller O, Schwanitz HJ. Hand dermatitis in a prospectively followed cohort of hairdressing apprentices: final results of the POSH study.

Prevention of occupational skin disease in hairdressers. Contact Dermatitis. 1999;41:280–6.

17. English J, Aldridge R, Gawkrodger DJ, et al. Consensus statement on the management of chronic hand eczema. Clin Exp Dermatol. 2009;34:761–9.

18. Held E, Mygind K, Wolff C, Gyntelberg F, Agner T. Prevention of work related skin problems: an intervention study in wet work employees. Occup Environ Med. 2002;59:556–61.

19. Korinth G, Geh S, Schaller KH, Drexler H. In vitro evaluation of the efficacy of skin barrier creams and protective gloves on percutaneous absorption of industrial solvents. Int Arch Occup Environ Health. 2003;76:382–6.

20. Korinth G, Lüersen L, Schaller KH, et al. Enhancement of percutaneous penetration of aniline and o-toluidine in vitro using skin barrier creams. Toxicol Vitro Int J Publ Assoc BIBRA. 2008;22:812–8.

21. Korinth G, Weiss T, Penkert S, et al. (2007) percutaneous absorption of aromatic amines in rubber industry workers: impact of impaired skin and skin barrier creams. Occup Environ Med. 2007;64:366–72.

22. Crepy MN. Rubber: new allergens and preventive measures. E J Dermatol. 2016;26:523–30.

23. Beezhold DH, Kostyal DA, Wiseman JS. The transfer of protein allergens from latex gloves. A study of influencing factors. AORN. 1994;59:605–14.

24. Palosuo T, Antoniadou I, Gottrup F, Phillips P. Latex medical gloves: time for a reappraisal. Int Arch Allergy Immunol. 2011;156:234–46.

25. Bernardini R, Novembre E, Lombardi E, et al. Anaphylaxis to latex after ingestion of a cream-filled doughnut contaminated with latex. J Allergy Clin Immunol. 2002;110:534–5.

26. Lind ML, Boman A, Sollenberg J, et al. Occupational dermal exposure to permanent hair dyes among hairdressers. Oxford J Ann Occup Hyg. 2005;49:473–80.

27. Held E, Agner T. Comparison between 2 test models in evaluating the effect of a moisturizer on irritated human skin. Contact Dermatitis. 1999;40:261–8.

28. Loden M, Andersson A. Effect of topically applied lipids on surfactant-irritated skin. Br J Dermatol. 1996;134:215–20.

29. Agner T, Held E. Skin protection programmes. Contact Dermatitis. 2002;47:253–6.

30. Winker R, Salameh B, Stolkovich S, et al. Effectiveness of skin protection creams in the prevention of occupational dermatitis: results of a randomized, controlled trial. Int Arch Occup Environ Health. 2009;82:653–62.

31. Hines J, Wilkinson SM, John SM, et al. The three moments of skin cream application: an evidence-based proposal for use of skin creams in the prevention of irritant contact dermatitis in the workplace. J Eur Acad Dermatol Venereol. 2017;31:53–64.

32. Rusca C, Hinnen U, Elsner P. 'Patient's delay' – analysis of the preclinical phase of occupational dermatoses. Dermatology. 1997;194:50–2.

33. Keegel T, Cahill J, Noonan A, Dharmage, et al. Incidence and prevalence rates for occupational contact dermatitis in an Australian suburban area. Contact Dermatitis. 2005;52(5):254–9.

34. DeKoven JG, DeKoven BM, Warshaw EM, et al. Occupational contact dermatitis: retrospective analysis of north American contact dermatitis group data, 2001 to 2016. J Am Acad Dermatol. 2021;86(4):782–90. https://doi.org/10.1016/j.jaad.03.042. Online ahead of print.

35. Houle MC, Holness DL, DeKoven J. Occupational contact dermatitis: an individualized approach to the worker with dermatitis. Curr Derm Rep. 2021;10:182–91. https://doi.org/10.1007/s13671-021-00339-0.

36. Breuer K, John SM, Finkeldey F, et al. Tertiary individual prevention improves mental health in patients with severe occupational hand eczema. J Eur Acad Derm. 2015;29:1724–31.

37. Wilke A, Bollmann U, Cazzaniga S, et al. The implementation of knowledge dissemination in the prevention of occupational skin diseases. J Eur Acad Dermatol Venereol. 2018;32(3):449–58. https://doi.org/10.1111/jdv.14653.

Diagnostic Methods of Eczema and Urticaria: Patch Test, Photopatch Test, and Prick Test

Alicia Cannavó and An Goossens

Patch Test

Background

Joseph Jadassohn was the first, in 1985, to publish about patch testing in a patient sensitized to mercury [1], a method used ever since to demonstrate contact allergy.

Definition

Patch testing is a standardized in vivo diagnostic procedure regarded as the gold method to confirm a delayed-type allergic skin reaction (contact allergy or skin sensitization) to a low-molecular chemical, i.e., a "hapten" or "incomplete allergen" but generally referred to as allergen. It is a simple and safe procedure that results, in a sensitized individual, in an eczematous skin reaction at the contact site with the allergen. It is the first step in the diagnosis of allergic contact dermatitis, for which it is necessary to determine the relationship between the allergen identified and the clinical history, anatomic location, time course, and sensitization source [2–4].

Indications

Patch testing should be considered for patients suspected to suffer from allergic contact dermatitis, dermatitis related to occupational origin, hand dermatitis, other types of chronic dermatitis resistant to topical therapy such as atopic dermatitis, and non-eczematous conditions potentially related to delayed-type hypersensitivity [3–5].

Who Should Not Be Patch Tested?

Patch test should not be performed in subjects:

- With active generalized dermatitis.
- Under high doses of systemic corticosteroids or immune-suppressive agents.
- With a recent sunburn.
- With dermatitis on the patch test area.
- When test sites were recently treated with corticosteroids [2, 5].

A. Cannavó (✉)
Contact Unit and Occupational Dermatoses,
Dermatology Department Hospital de Clínicas
"José de San Martín", Buenos Aires University,
Buenos Aires, Argentina

A. Goossens
Department of Dermatology, Faculty of Medicine,
Katholieke Universiteit Leuven, Leuven, Belgium

© The Author(s), under exclusive license to Springer Nature Switzerland AG 2023
A. M. Giménez-Arnau, H. I. Maibach (eds.), *Handbook of Occupational Dermatoses*, Updates in
Clinical Dermatology, https://doi.org/10.1007/978-3-031-22727-1_9

Patient Information

It is important to explain the patch testing procedure to the patient using a written or digital sheet, to minimize the incidence of false negative patch test results [6].

Patch Test Procedure

The patch test procedure has been standardized by the International Contact Dermatitis Research Group (ICDRG) and the European Society of Contact Dermatitis (ESCD) [2, 3].

The European Academy of Dermatology and Venereology Task Force on Contact Dermatitis recommends that the informed consent form must contain a brief explanation about patch test procedure including purpose, possible risks, adverse reactions, and legally relevant privacy issues [7].

Materials

Patch Test System

There are different patch test systems available on the market, among which Finn Chambers (www.Smartpractice.com), IQ Ultra ®, and IQ Ultimate® (www.chemotechnique.se) [5, 8], which are the most common ones.

Finn chambers are circular and made of aluminum, the 8-mm inner diameter providing a 50-mm² area. IQ chambers are square and made of polyethylene. In both systems, the allergens must be placed in the chambers by the dermatologist, technician, or nurse (Fig. 9.1). There also exist preloaded systems, i.e., the True test system (www.Smartpractice.com) and Epiquick® (Hermal, Reinbek, Germany), the units which already contain the allergens [2, 4, 5].

Preloaded systems with standardized allergens are easy to use [8].

Allergens

The allergens are generally available on the market. They must be chemically pure and safe [2]. More than 5.200 contact allergens have been

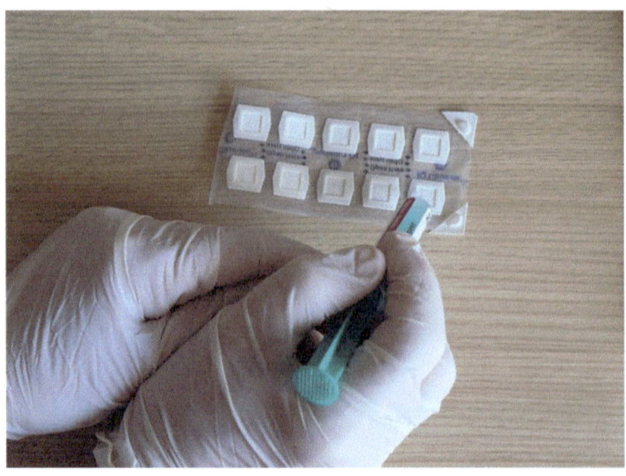

Fig. 9.1 Applying allergens

described, however, only a limited amount of them is available on the market. Sometimes, one needs to dilute potential allergens in the dermatological practice, according to concentrations and vehicles listed in the literature [9]. In practice, all patients are tested with a baseline (standard) screening series, which has been updated through the years, though may differ from country to country, certain allergens being added (or withdrawn) according to the advice of expert dermatologists in the field [8] (Table 9.1). Besides, path testing is often also performed with additional series, the content of which is related to certain occupations (e.g., hairdressers), specific skin sites (e.g., eyelids), or sensitization sources (e.g., cosmetics) [4, 10].

Most of the allergens are diluted in petrolatum as a vehicle, while some of them are present in an aqueous solution, the latter for which the use of a micropipette is advised for application onto the chambers. The baseline screening series contains also mixes of certain allergens, for example, of fragrances and parabens [5, 11, 12] (Table 9.1).

Allergens must be kept in the dark and in the refrigerator, and some of them even in the freezer, such as, for example, isocyanates that are very unstable [3].

Testing the Products Contacted by the Patients, Including Work-Environmental Products

To keep skin testing safe and efficient, the availability of information regarding the content of the

Table 9.1 International Standard Series Chemotechnique®

Allergen	Concentration
Potassium dichromate	0.5% pet
Neomycin sulfate	20.0% pet
Thiuram mix	1.0% pet
P-phenylenediamine	1.0% pet
Formaldehyde	2.0% aq
Colophonium	20.0% pet
Peru balsam	25.0% pet
Lanolil alcohol	30.0% pet
Mercapto mix	3.5% pet
Epoxy resin, bisphenol A	1.0% pet
4-tert-Butylphenolformaldehyde resin (PTBP)	1.0% pet
Fragrance mix I	8.0% pet
Nickel(II)sulfate hexahydrate	2.5% pet
Textile dye mix	6.6% pet
Budesonide	0.01% pet
Quaternium-15	2.0% pet
Methylisothiazolinone+Methylchloroisothiazolinone	0.215% aq
Imidazolidinyl urea	2.0% pet
Tixocortol-21-pivalate	0.1% pet
Methyldibromo glutaronitrile	0.3% pet
Carba mix	3.0% pet
Cobalt(II)chloride hexahydrate	1.0% pet
Compositae mix II	5.0% pet
Diazolidynil urea	2.0% pet
Fragrance mix II	14.0% pet
Phenol formaldehyde resin (PFR2)	1.0% pet
Hydroxyisohexyl 3-cyclohexene carboxaldehyde	5.0% pet
N-isopropyl-N-phenyl-4-phenylenediamine (IPPD)	0.1% pet
Paraben mix	16.0% pet
Sesquiterpene lactone mix	0.1% pet

aq: aqueous
pet: petrolatum

products is crucial to the dermatologist or technician performing patch testing [13, 14]. Fortunately, the ingredients of topical pharmaceutical and cosmetic products are labeled, and regarding occupational products material safety data sheets (MSDS) may be helpful, although the information is most often limited to chemicals present in high concentrations and, unfortunately, not always correct [3, 15].

Adhesive Tape

For practical reasons, patch test chambers must be occluded with tape, which, sometimes, may induce an irritant or even an allergic reaction [2, 16].

Location

Generally, patch tests are applied on the back but, if this is not possible, the upper arm can also be a suitable site. The patients should not apply corticosteroids or calcineurin inhibitors at least seven days before patch testing, and recent sunburn excludes the application of patch tests as well [11, 17].

Reading Time

Patch tests must be removed after two days of occlusion, preferably waiting 30 minutes following their removal to perform the first reading [18]. A second reading will be performed after 4 days, no significant differences having been found between a second reading at 3 instead of 4 days. Moreover, also a third reading after 5–7 days is recommended in order not to miss late positives, such as, for example, in the case of p-phenylenediamine, neomycin, nickel sulfate, gold sodium thiosulfate, palladium chloride, potassium dichromate, and corticosteroids [18, 19].

A retrospective study indeed revealed that 13.6% of the positive reactions observed to allergens of the baseline series would have been missed if a D/7 reading had not been performed [20].

Interpretation of Patch Test Results

As the ESCD, the ICDRG recommends the following criteria: no reaction (−); irritant reaction (IR), characterized by various morphologies (e.g., soap effect, bulla, necrosis); doubtful reaction (+?) which is characterized by weak erythema; weak positive reaction (+) characterized by erythema, infiltration, and possibly papules; strong positive reaction (++) characterized by erythema, infiltration, papules, and vesicles, and extreme positive reaction (+++) characterized by intense erythema, infiltrate, vesicles, and coalescing vesicles (Table 9.2) [21]. Usually, irritative reactions tend to vanish after the first reading and are strictly limited to the areas tested, while allergic reactions tend to increase after the first reading and expand outside the patch test area [22] (Table 9.2) (Fig. 9.2a, b).

Table 9.2 Interpretation of Patch test result according to ICDRG

? +	Doubtful reaction faint erythema only
+	Weak positive reaction; erythema, infiltration papules
++	Strong positive reaction; erythema, infiltration, papules, vesicles
+++	Extreme positive reaction; intense erythema, infiltration, and coalescing vesicles
−	Negative reaction
IR	Irritant reaction
NT	Not tested

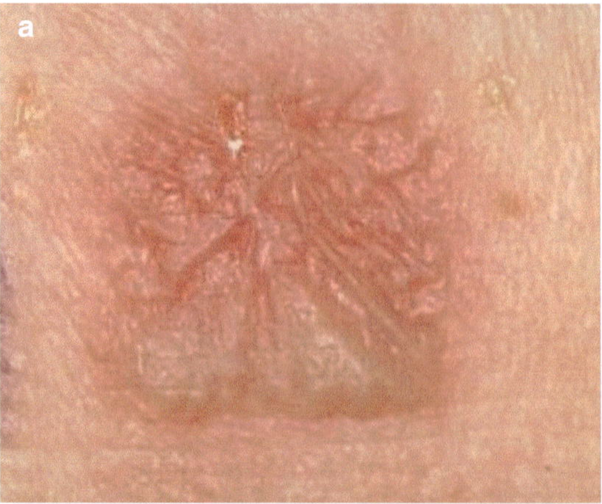

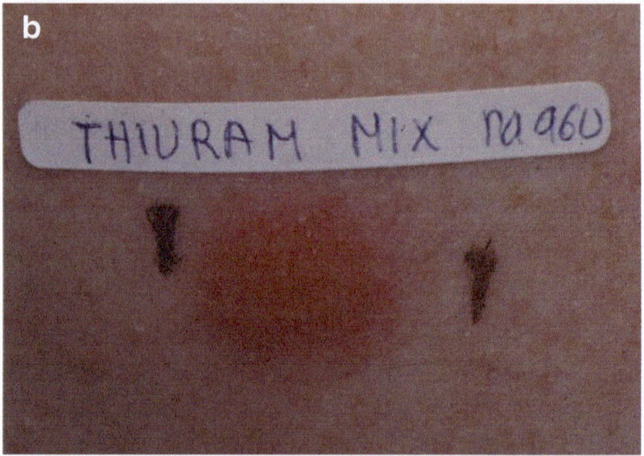

Fig. 9.2 (a) Patch test reading: Irritant reaction. (b) Patch test reading: Allergic reaction

Patch Test Relevance

A positive patch test reaction means contact allergy or sensitization to a specific chemical, but its relevance for the patient's dermatitis needs to be determined to obtain the diagnosis of allergic contact dermatitis. Past relevance refers to previous exposures to the specific allergen identified [23–25].

False Positive Reactions

False positive or irritant reactions may occur when a too high concentration of a chemical is applied when patch tests are applied onto a dermatitis site or in case of generalized dermatitis, or if there are pressure effects [17].

False Negative Reactions

False negative reactions occur when a too low dose or a too low concentration of allergen is applied, in case an inappropriate vehicle was used, a reading was performed too early, or because of an insufficient occlusion time [17, 26].

Adverse Effects

Some of the following adverse effects have been described: patch test sensitization, reactivation of previous allergen-contact sites, hyper or hypopigmentation at the test site, bacterial and viral infections, Koebner phenomenon, granulomas, generalized subjective symptoms, and more exceptionally anaphylactoid reactions [27–28].

Prognosis of Patch Testing

The prognosis of allergic contact dermatitis is better when patients remember the allergens that caused contact dermatitis and when they can avoid contact with them [29, 30].

> *Core message*
> Patch testing is the gold standard procedure for patients suffering from contact dermatitis.
> Interpretation of the results and the determination of relevance are crucial for the management of contact dermatitis.

Photopatch Test

Background

Photopatch testing is a screening tool to detect photo-contact allergy [31].

Definition

Photopatch testing is an in vivo diagnostic procedure (not completely standardized yet) regarded as the gold method to confirm a delayed-type photoallergic skin reaction (photo-contact allergy) to a low-molecular chemical (i.e., a "photo-hapten" or "incomplete photoallergen" but generally referred to as Photoallergen) [32]. It is defined as a combination of the patch test technique followed by UV radiation to induce the formation of a photoallergen [33].

Indications

Photopatch tests should be considered basically for patients who are suspected of photoallergic contact dermatitis and photoallergic drug eruptions. This technique is also indicated in patients with dermatitis in photo-exposed areas, immunologically mediated photo-dermatoses, such as chronic actinic dermatitis, skin intolerance to sunscreens and in all eczematous diseases located on photo-exposed areas and polymorphous light eruption (PMLE), it might indeed be interesting to do phototesting in order to exclude photoallergy [34–36].

Who Should Not Be Photopatch Tested?

- See Patch testing.

Patient Information

See patch testing.

Photopatch Test Procedure

Methodology

Several methodologies have been proposed through the years, for example, one in 1982 by the Scandinavian Photodermatitis Research group [37]. In 2000, a Multicentre Photopatch Test Taskforce (EMCPPTS) was created by the ESCD and the European Society for Photodermatology, who established a European Multicentre Photopatch test study resulting in recommendations [38]. Even though there is consensus about the procedure, the UVA dose, and the occlusion time (1 or 2 days) may still vary from Center to Center [39].

Materials

Photoallergens

Photoallergens are most often diluted with petrolatum or in an aqueous solution and are provided by the same companies (see Patch testing).

Based on the Photopatch test study mentioned previously [38], the EMCPPTS recommended a European photopatch baseline series consisting of 20 photoallergens as well as an extended series of 15 additional chemicals [38, 40–42] (Table 9.3), both prone to updates over time [43].

Such series are commercialized as the European Photopatch and Extended Series, "Photoallergen Series" by Dormer Laboratories Inc. (Toronto, Ontario, Canada), "North American Photopatch Series," "Sunscreen Series", "Plant Series". Besides, lists of test agents for AllergEAZE are "Photoallergen Series," "Sunscreen Series," and AllergEAZE "Photochemical Series" by SmartPractice Canada (Calgary, Alberta, Canada) [42]. Photopatch series are also provided by Chemotechnique (www.chemotechnique.se).

Testing Patients' Own Products

Any product used by the patients that may have induced photoallergic contact dermatitis should be tested [38] (cf. Patch testing).

Methodology of Photopatch Testing

Photoallergens are tested on the patient's back in duplicate. The sites are covered with a UV-impermeable and opaque material for 1 day or 2 days to prevent any UV exposure. Then one of the two sets is irradiated with UVA, 5 Joules/cm^2 or 50% of the MED-A in case the patient has a low MED-A. The panel not irradiated remains covered with opaque material. The reading must be performed previous and post-irradiation in both panels. Further readings should be performed 2- and 4 days following irradiation, and preferably also on day 7 [3, 4, 35].

Table 9.3 Photopatch Series Chemotechnique®

Allergen	Concentration
Benzophenone-3	10.0% pet
Benzophenone-4	2.0% pet
4-Methylbenzylidene camphor	10.0% pet
Ethylhexyl methoxycinnamate	10.0% pet
Octocrylene	10.0% pet
Isoamyl p-methoxycinnamate	10.0% pet
Paba	10.0% pet
Butylmethoxydibenzoylmethane	10.0% pet
Bis-Ethylhexylphenol methoxyphenol triazine	10.0% pet
Drometriazole Trisiloxane	10.0% pet
Ketoprofen	1.0% pet
2-(4-Diethylamino-2-hydroxybenzoyl)-benzoic acid hexylester	10.0% pet
Ethylhexyl Triazone	10.0% pet
Methylene bis-benzotriazolyl tetramethylbutylphenol	10.0% pet
Etofenamate	2.0% pet
Diethylhexyl Butamido Triazone	10.0% pet
Piroxicam	1.0% pet
Decyl Glucoside	5.0% pet
Benzophenone-10	10.0% pet
Phenylbenzimidazole Sulfonic Acid	10.0% pet
Homosalate	10.0% pet
Ethylhexyl Salicylate	10.0% pet
Polysilicone-15	10.0% pet
Disodium phenyl dibenzimidazole tetrasulfonate	10.0% pet
Triclosan	2.0% pet
Diclofenac sodium salt	5.0% pet
Thiourea	0.1% pet
Hexachlorophene	1.0% pet
Methyl Antranilate	5.0% pet
Triclocarban	1.0% pet

aq: aqueous
pet: petrolatum

Interpretation of Photopatch Test

Photo-contact allergy is confirmed if a positive (eczematous) reaction occurs at the irradiated site only. If a positive reaction is visible on both sites (radiated and unirradiated), then it concerns contact allergy (Fig. 9.3). In the case of photo-aggravation, both test sites present a positive reaction, which is stronger at the irradiated site [34]. The photoallergen series may thus vary from country to country [43, 44] influencing the reported frequency of the photopatch test results obtained [45].

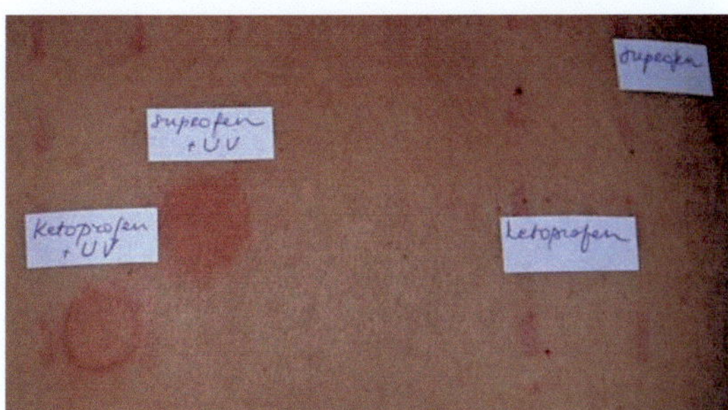

Fig. 9.3 Positive Photopatch test to ketoprofen and the chemically related suprofen, both NSAIDS

The scores used for reading as well as the determination of relevance are the same as for patch testing.

Core Message
Photopatch testing is the gold standard method to diagnose photo-contact allergy.
Need for standardizing and periodic updates of the photoallergens.
Interpretation of the results and determination of the relevance are crucial for the management of photo-contact Dermatitis.

Skin Prick Test

Historical Aspects

The skin prick test (SPT), first performed by Charles Blackley in 1865, is the common diagnostic procedure for detecting immediate-type sensitivity [46, 47].

Definition

Skin Prick Testing is recommended as a standardized simple and fast screening method to detect type I Immunoglobulin E (IgE)-mediated allergy [48].

Indications

SPT should be considered for patients suspected of contact urticaria, protein contact dermatitis, allergic rhinitis, asthma, atopic dermatitis, insect stings, food allergy and immediate-type drug allergy [49].

Patient Information

It is very important for patients to be informed on the nature of this test (see Patch testing). Clinical relevance must be determined because detecting sensitization does not necessarily mean that the patient is suffering from an immediate-type of disease [50].

SPT Procedure

Methodology
This procedure consists of the application of a small amount of allergen, a drop, onto the skin (usually the volar surface of the forearm) that subsequently is punctured with a special needle to contact the skin mast cells (Fig. 9.4). Several allergens are often tested simultaneously. In case of sensitization, a wheal and flare response caused by histamine liberation will appear on the skin, which is marked with a pen.

The results are compared with histamine solution as a positive and physiologic solution as a negative control [51, 52].

Allergens for SPT

The allergens for SPT concern either molecules with a low or high molecular weight (proteins). Standardized extracts are provided by various companies and mainly include major inhalant allergens, food, drugs, and insects, but freshly prepared materials can be tested as well [49, 51].

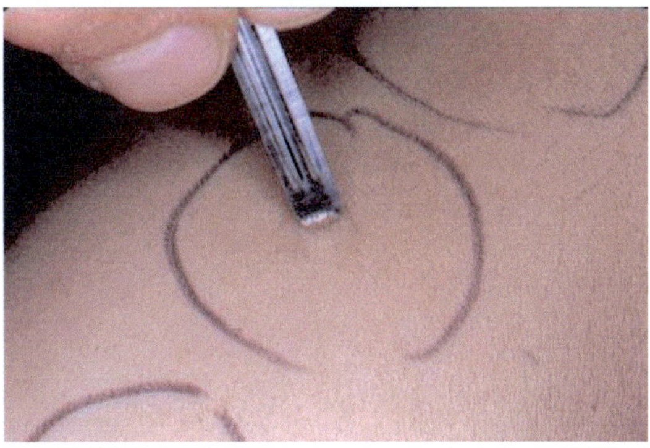

Fig. 9.4 Skin Prick Test procedure

Moreover, certain occupational allergens may be involved, such as the low-molecular chemicals chlorhexidine, para-phenylenediamine, and acrylic monomers, and proteinic allergens, such as jellyfish and latex, which all have caused immediate-type allergic reactions [51, 53].

A Skin Prick Test System Tape (SPT tape), a preloaded system with four chambers [54], has more recently been introduced.

Test Conditions

To avoid false negative reactions, before prick testing, H1-antihistamines must be suspended for 4–5 days, ideally for 7 days, and H2-antihistamines should be suspended for 24 hours [55].

Besides, the use of corticosteroids is not recommended either, for example, a single randomized study showed that treatment with a topical high-potency steroid significantly inhibited the response to SPT for 36 hours, though less than 3 days [56].

Reading Time

Readings must be performed 15–20 minutes following application of the allergen [53, 57].

Interpretation of SPT

The size of the wheal is interpreted as positive depending on its diameter, which usually is 3 mm [58] (Figs. 9.5 and 9.6).

To make diagnosis on wheal dimension independent of human interpretation some technologies have been developed like a wide-field 3D imaging system for the 3D reconstruction of the SPT, computational determination of the wheal area, and a study of the temperature variation of the patient's skin in the puncture region [59, 60].

Adverse Reactions

Even though systemic adverse reactions have been reported, SPT is considered a safe diagnos-

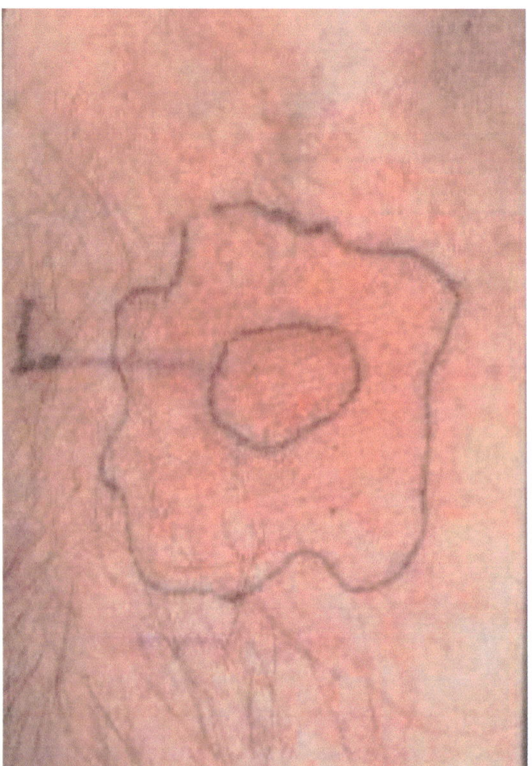

Fig. 9.5 Positive Skin Prick Test

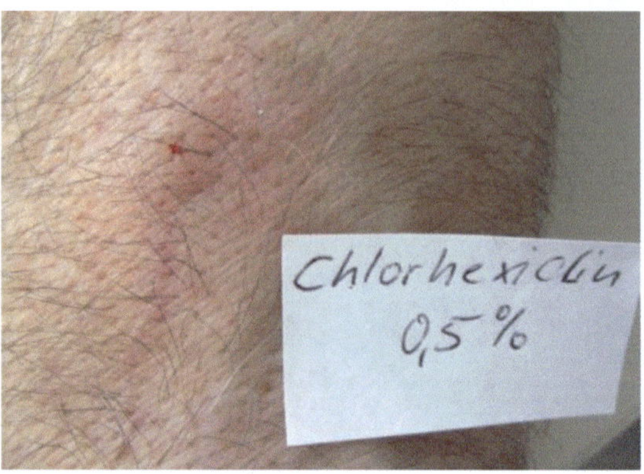

Fig. 9.6 Positive Prick test to chlorhexidine

tic tool to detect type I Immunoglobulin E (IgE)-mediated allergy [61, 62].

> **Core Message**
> Skin Prick testing is the gold standard to diagnose type I Immunoglobulin E (IgE)-mediated allergy.
> It is a simple and relatively economic and safe test method.
> A positive test means sensitization but not necessarily a disease. The test results must be correlated with the clinical history.

References

1. Lachapelle JM. Historical aspects of contact Dermatitis. In: Johansen JD, Mahler V, Lepoittevin JP, Frosch P, editors. Contact Dermatitis. 6th ed. Cham: Springer Nature; 2021. p. p1–10.
2. Lachapelle JM, Maibach HI. Patch testing methodology. In: Lachapelle JM, Maibach H, editors. Patch testing and prick testing. A practical guide. 4th ed. Springer; 2021. p. p35–78.
3. Johansen JD, Aalto-Corte K, Agner T, et al. European Society of Contact Dermatitis guideline for diagnostic patch test – recommendations on best practice. Contact Dermatitis. 2015;73:195–221.
4. Johnston GA, Exton LS, Mohd Mustapa MF, et al. British Association of Dermatologists' guidelines for the management of contact dermatitis 2017. Br J Dermatol. 2017;176:317–29.
5. Svedman C, Bruze M. Patch testing. Technical details and interpretation. In: Johansen JD, Mahler V, Lepoittevin JP, Frosch P, editors. Contact dermatitis. 6th ed. Cham: Springer Nature; 2021. p. 515–50.
6. Wu PA. The importance of education when patch testing. Dermatol Clin. 2020;38:351–60.
7. Balato A, Scala E, Ayala F, et al. Patch test informed consent form: position statement by European academy of dermatology and venereology task force on contact Dermatitis. J Eur Acad Dermatol Venereol. 2021;35:1957–62.
8. Uyesugui BA, Sheehan MP. Patch testing pearls. Clinic Rev Allerg Immunol. 2019;56:110–8.
9. De Groot AC. Patch testing-test concentrations and vehicles for 4900 chemicals. 4th ed. Wapserveen: Ac de Groot publishing. 2018.
10. Tagka A, Katsarou A. Patch testing. In: Katsambas AD, Lotti TM, Dessinioti C, D'Erme AM, editors. European handbook of dermatological treatments. Berlin, Heidelberg: Springer; 2015. https://doi.org/10.1007/978-3-662-45139-7_124.
11. Foti C, Bonamonte D, Filoni A, Angelini G. Patch Testing. Clinical Contact Dermatitis: A Practical Approach. 2021;499–527.
12. Bruze M, Isaakson M, Gruvberger B, Frick-Engfeldt M. Recommendations of appropriate amounts of petrolatum preparation to be applied on patch testing. Contact Dermatitis. 2007;56:281–5.
13. Cohen DE. Contact dermatitis emerging trends. Dermatol Clin. 2019;37:21–8.
14. Siegel PD, Law BF, Warshaw EM. Chemical identification and confirmation of contact allergens. Dermatitis. 2020;31:99–105.
15. Keegel T, Saunders H, LaMontagne AD, Nixon R. Are material safety data sheets (MSDS) useful in the diagnosis and management of occupational contact dermatitis? Contact Dermatitis. 2007;57:331–6.
16. Daevos SA, der Valk V. Epicutaneous patch testing. Euro J Dermatol. 2002;12:506–14.
17. Fornacier L. A practical guide to patch testing. J Allergy Immunol Pract. 2015;3:669–75.
18. Fornacier L. Contact dermatitis and patch testing for the allergist. Ann Allergy Asthma Immunol. 2018;120:592–8.
19. Beltrani VS, et al. Contact Dermatitis: a practice parameter. Ann Allergy Asthma Immunol. 2015;97:1–38.
20. van Amegoren CCA, Ofenloch R, Ditmar D, Schuttelaar MLA. New positive patch test reactions on day 7- the additional value of the 7-patch test reading. Contact Dermatitis. 2019;81:280–7.
21. Ljubojević Hadžavdić S, Nives P, Žužul K, Švigir A. Contact allergy: an update. G Ital Dermatol Venereol. 2018;153:419–28.
22. Bains SN, Nash P, Fonacier L. Irritant contact Dermatitis. Clinic Rev Allerg Immunol. 2019;56:99–109. https://doi.org/10.1007/s12016-018-8713-0.
23. Rashid RS, Ngee TN. Contact dermatitis. BMJ. 2016;30:1–12.
24. DeKoven JG, Warshaw EM, Zug KA, Maibach H, Belsito DV, Sasseville D, Taylor JM, Fowler JF, Mathias CGT, Marks JG, Pratt MD, Zirwas J, De Leo V. North American contact dermatitis group patch test results: 2015-2016. Dermatitis. 2018;29:297–309.
25. Goossens A. Art and science of patch test. Indian J Dermatol Venereol Leprol. 2007;73:1–4.
26. Ophaug S, Schwarzenberger K. Pitfalls in patch testing. Minimizing risks of avoidable false-negative reactions. Dermatol Clin. 2020;38:293–300.
27. Vaibhav Garg BS, Brod B, Gaspari AA. Patch testing: uses, systems, risks/benefits, and its role in managing the patients with contact dermatitis. Clin Dermatol. 2021;39(4):580–90.
28. Kamphof WG, Kunkeler L, Bikkers SCE, Bezemer PD, Bruynzeel DP. Patch-test-induced subjective complaints. Dermatology. 2003;207:28–32.
29. Korkmaz P, Boyvat A. Effect of patch testing on the course of allergic contact Dermatitis and prognostic factors that influence outcomes. Dermatitis. 2019;30:135–41.
30. Goossens A. Recognizing and testing allergens. Dermatol Clin. 2009;27:219–26.
31. Bruze M. Thoughts on the interpretation of positive photopatch tests. Eur J Dermatol. 2020;30:541–4.
32. Aşkın Ö, Cesur SK, Engin B, Tüzün, Y. Photoallergic Contact Dermatitis. Current Dermatology Reports. 2019;8:157–63.
33. De Leo VA. Photocontact dermatitis. Dermatol Ther. 2014;17:279–88.
34. Gonçalo M. Photopatch testing In: Contact Dermatitis. Johansen JD, Mahler V, Frosch PJ. (eds). Springer Nature. 2021; p. 594–604.
35. Jiang A and Lim HW. Phototherapy (2020) In the evaluation and management of photodermatoses. Dermatol Clin 38:71–77.
36. Lachapelle JM, Goossens A. Photopatch testing. In: Lachapelle JM, Maibach H, editors. Patch testing and prick testing. A practical guide. 4th ed. Berlin: Springer; 2021. p. 95–101.
37. Jansen CT, Wennersten G, Tystedt I, et al. The Scandinavian standard photopatch test procedure. Contact Dermatitis. 1982;8:155–8.

38. Gonçalo M, Ferguson J, Bonevalle A, Bruynzeel DP, Gimenez-Arnau A, Goossens A, Kerr A, Lecha M, Neumann N, Pigatto P, Rhodes LE, Rustemeyer T, Sarkany R, Thomas P, Wilkinson M. Photopatch testing: recommendations for a European photopatch test baseline series. Contact Dermatitis. 2013;68:239–43.

39. Kerr A, Ferguson J. Photoallergic contact Dermatitis. Photoderm Photoimmunol Photomed. 2010;26:56–65.

40. Hinton AN, Goldminz AM. Feeling the burn phototoxicity and Photoallergy. Dermatol Clin. 2020;38:165–75.

41. Kerr AA, European Multicentre Photopatch Test Study. The European multicentre Photopatch test study (EMCPPTS) taskforce. Br J Dermatol. 2012;166:1002–9.

42. Kim T, Taylor JS, Maibach H, Chen JK, Honari G. Photopatch testing among members of the American contact Dermatitis society. Dermatitis. 2020;31:59–67.

43. Asemota E, Crawford G, Kovarik C, Brod BA. A survey examining photopatch test and phototest methodologies of contact dermatologists in the United States: platform for developing a consensus. Dermatitis. 2017;24(4):265–69.

44. García Castro R, Velasco Tirado V, Alonso Sardón M, González de Arriba M. Standard photopatch test battery? Proposal based on current epidemiology and experience in our skin allergy unit. Photodermatol Photoimmunol Photomed. 2021;37(5):449–53. https://doi.org/10.1111/phpp.12680.

45. Greenspoon J, Ahluwalia R, Juma N, Rosen CF. Allergic and Photoallergic Dermatitis: a 10-year experience. Dermatitis. 2013;24(1):29–32.

46. Dreborg SKG. Skin testing in allergen standardization and research. Immunol Allergy Clin N Am. 2001;21:329–54.

47. Eigenmann PA, Oh JW, Beyer K. Diagnostic Testing in the evaluation of food allergy. Pediatr Clin North Am. 2011;58(2):351–62.

48. Shokouhi Shoormasti R, Mahloujirad M, Sabetkish N, Kazemnejad A, Ghobadi Dana V, Tayebi B, Moin M. The most common allergens according to skin prick test: The role of wheal diameter in clinical relevancy. Dermatologic Therapy. 2021;34(1):e14636.

49. Ansotegui et al. (2020) IgE allergy diagnostics and other relevant tests in allergy, a world allergy organization position paper. World Allergy Organization J 13:1–50.

50. Patel G, Saltoun C. Skin testing in allergy. Allergy Asthma Proc. 2019;40:366–8.

51. Gotthard Mørtz C, Bindslev-Jensen C. Skin test for immediate hypersensitivity. In: Johansen JD, Mahler V, Frosch PJ, editors. Contact Dermatitis. 6th ed. Cham: Springer Nature. p. 609–18.

52. Heinzerling L, Mari A, Bergmann KC, et al. The skin prick test – European standards. Clin Transl Allergy. 2013;3:3. https://doi.org/10.1186/2045-7022-3-3.

53. Lachapelle JM, Maibach H. Spectrum of Diseases for Wich Prick Testing and Open (Non-prick) Testing Are Recommended: Patients Who Should Be Investigated. In: Lachapelle JM, Maibach H (eds) Patch testing and Prick Testing. A practical guide. 3rd ed. Springer. 2012;p. 147–57.

54. Gong A, Yang Z, Wu R, Jia M. Comparison of a new skin prick test tape with the conventional skin prick test. J Aller Immunol. 2019;143:424–7.

55. Jakka S. Skin prick testing in children. Karnataka Pediatr J. 2020;35:67–71.

56. Ebsen A, Riis L, Gradman J. Effect of topical steroids on skin prick test: a randomized controlled trial. Dermatol Ther. 2018;(8):285–90.

57. Bousquet J, Heinzerling L, Bachert C, Papadopoulos NG, Bousquet PJ, Burney PG, Demoly P. Practical guide to skin prick tests in allergy to aeroallergens. Allergy. 2011;67(1):18–24.

58. Bernstein IL, Li JT, Bernstein DI, Hamilton R, Spector SL, Tan R, Weber R. Allergy diagnostic testing: an updated practice parameter. Annals of allergy, asthma & immunology. 2008;100(3):S1–S148.

59. Pineda J, Vargas R, Lenny A, Romero J, Marrugo J, Meneses J, Marrugo AG. Robust automated reading of the skin prick test via 3D imaging and parametric surface fitting. PLoS ONE. 2019. https://doi.org/10.1371/journal.pone.0223623.

60. Mendes Almeida ML, Pontes Perger EL, Marting Gomex RH, dos Santos SG, Hecker Vasques LH, Olbrich RJEP, Neto J, Plana Simões R. Objective evaluation of immediate reading skin prick test applying image planimetric and reaction thermometry analyses. J Immunol Methods. 2020. https://doi.org/10.1016/j.jim.2020.112870.

61. Bagg A, Chacko T, Lockey R. Reactions to prick and intradermal test. Ann Allergy Asthma Immunol. 2009;102:400–2.

62. Liccardi G, Salzillo A, Spadaro G, Senna G, Canonina WG, D´Amato G, Passalacqua G. Anaphylaxis caused by skin prick testing with aeroallergens: Case report and evaluation of the risk in Italian allergy services. J Allergy Clin Immunol. 2003;111(6):1410–12.

Work-Related and Occupational Hand Eczema (OHE), Diagnosis and Treatment

Juan Pedro Russo, José Hernán Alfonso, and Andrea Nardelli

Introduction

Work-related and occupational hand eczema (or hand dermatitis) consist of an inflammatory skin condition localized to the hands, wrists, or lower forearms partially or fully caused by exposures at work [1, 2].

The definition of occupational hand eczema (OHE) is different across countries as it includes specific national legal requirements that define when and how work-related hand eczema (HE) should be recognized as an occupational disease. This has an impact on surveillance, prevention, management, and compensation [1].

Work-related HE should be suspected at onset/worsening or exacerbation of eczema at work and improvement during holidays, sick leave periods, and/or weekends [1]. Early clinical suspicion is essential for diagnosis, prevention of chronic hand eczema (CHE) as well as for primary prevention among non-affected workers in the same factory or plant.

J. P. Russo (✉)
Dermatology Unit at Hospital Vithas 9 de Octubre, Valencia, Spain

Framingham Medical Center, La Plata, Buenos Aires, Argentina

J. H. Alfonso
Department of Occupational Medicine and Epidemiology, National Institute of Occupational Health, Oslo, Norway

Department of Dermatology and Venerology, Oslo University Hospital, Oslo, Norway

A. Nardelli
Department of Medicine, Farncombe Family Digestive Health Research Institute, McMaster University, Health Sciences Centre, Hamilton, ON, Canada

Epidemiology

Frequency and Burden of Disease

HE is not only a common skin condition in the general population (1 year prevalence of at least 9.1) [3], but also the most common occupational skin disease reaching a prevalence of up to 40% in risk occupations [1]. The higher prevalence among women (10.5%) compared to men (6,4%) is explained by a difference in the distribution of exposure, domestically and occupationally [3–7]. Self-reported HE in women is more prevalent in the age range 19–29 years, and decreases with age, while in men there is an opposite trend [3, 5]. The prevalence of self-reported work-related HE in the general population was up to 5% according to a Norwegian study [8].

The main risk occupations include health personnel, hairdressers, cleaners, metal workers, dental technicians, plumbers, machine operators, workers in metal surface processing, bakers, butchers, florists, cashiers, and electroplaters [1, 8].

OHE has often a chronic and relapsing course with a poor prognosis in the long term leading to a significant burden in terms of sick leave,

© The Author(s), under exclusive license to Springer Nature Switzerland AG 2023
A. M. Giménez-Arnau, H. I. Maibach (eds.), *Handbook of Occupational Dermatoses*, Updates in Clinical Dermatology, https://doi.org/10.1007/978-3-031-22727-1_10

reduced work productivity, early work retirement, and unemployment [9, 10].

Risk Factors

The development of work-related and occupational HE is influenced by an interplay between endogenous risk factors (individual susceptibility), and exogenous risk factors (environmental exposures). Occupational skin exposure to hazardous substances such as physical factors and chemical factors at work is a sine qua non-*condition* to develop occupational HE and can explain up to 59% of the etiology [11, 12]. On the other hand, individual susceptibility makes some individuals more prone to develop HE.

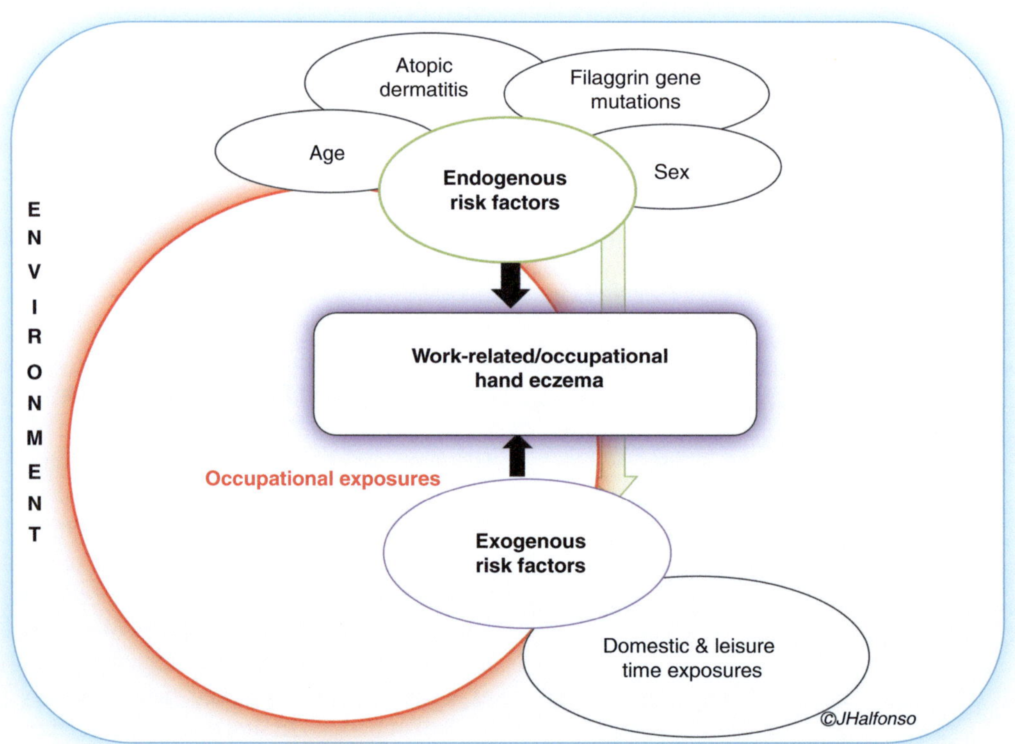

Endogenous Risk Factors

Atopic dermatitis (AD) as a child [13, 14], persistent or severe AD [3, 15] are consistent risk factors. Additionally, filaggrin gene mutations (FLG), a barrier protein in the skin, lead to dry skin, being strongly associated with early onset of HE and CHE in individuals with AD [16–18]. Additionally, FLG mutations are associated with incident (new cases of) HE among such as metal workers apprentices [19] and irritative contact dermatitis (ICD) among nurses, metal and construction, hairdressing, food and catering, and cleaning [20–23]. It may be difficult to provide evidence of an association between FLG mutations and risk of HE for all risk occupations due to a small number of study participants of some studies, or because of the healthy worker effect, which implies that workers with poorer skin health avoid hazardous occupational exposures. For instance, evidence on avoidance of occupa-

Table 10.1 Wet work definition

Wet work is work in which the skin (especially of the hands, wrists or forearms):
• is in contact with water for two hours or more per day,
• is washed more than 20 times per day, or
• is covered by tight gloves for two hours or more per day

tional exposure to irritants in adulthood among carriers of FLG mutations is available [24]. Strong contact allergens such as p-Phenylenediamine (PPD) may lead to downregulation and expression of FLG among occupationally exposed workers such as hairdressers [25].

Exogenous Risk Factors

Exposure to "wet work" (Table 10.1) [26, 27], chemical exposures (other irritants than wet work, allergens, or mixed exposures), physical exposures such and cold/dry weather conditions and low indoor humidity [28] are the main occupational risk factors.

Lifestyle factors such as high levels of stress and tobacco smoking are associated with a poorer prognosis of OHE [29–31], while a high level of exercise and change of profession is associated to a better prognosis and healing of OHE [30, 31].

Clinical Picture and Classification

The clinical manifestations of HE includes erythema, edema, vesicles, crusting, scaling, lichenification, hyperkeratosis, and fissures.

Proper classification of HE is the first step toward effective and efficient treatment. Several classification systems based on clinico-morphologic features and etiologic factors have been proposed. The relationship between these systems, however, is complex, as disease presentation and progression are often dynamic. Currently, there is no universally accepted classification system. However, we will focus on a practical classification for general practitioners [32].

Firstly, HE can be classified as acute HE (< 3 months' duration), which usually presents as erythema, edema, vesicles, and papules. It usually begins with pruritic millimeter-sized vesicles, often located on the palms and on the sides of the fingers. Hand eczema is considered chronic when it lasts for at least 3 months or relapses at least twice a year despite adequate treatment and treatment adherence [33]. Typical manifestations include edema, erythema, lichenification, hyperkeratosis, and fissures.

Occupational contact dermatitis is a general term that encompasses irritant contact dermatitis (ICD), allergic contact dermatitis (ACD), contact urticaria (CU), protein contact dermatitis, and/or a combination of several types. ICD, ACD, and CU account for approximately one-third of all occupational-related medical complaints and 90%–95% of occupation-related skin complaints [34] Each variant of contact dermatitis is the result of activation of distinct immune response, thus resulting in their unique clinical presentations.

Irritant Contact Dermatitis (ICD)

It is the result of a physical injury to the stratum corneum, resulting in barrier dysfunction typically caused by repetitive friction, water, or chemical products. The compromised skin barrier and damage to keratinocytes lead to cytokine release and activation of the innate immune system. Approximated 80% of OCD is caused by ICD. Clinically is characterized by erythema, scaling/hyperkeratosis, fissuring, burning, and pain. ICD was most frequent in chronic, dry fissured hand eczema (44.3%), pulpitis (41.7%), and nummular hand eczema (40.9), whereas ACD dominated in vesicular types of hand eczema, with recurrent (35%) and rare (24.4%) eruptions, which fits with the overall experience, but also shows that patch testing and exposure analysis are necessary to achieve an etiological classification [35].

Allergic Contact Dermatitis (ACD)

A delayed type IV hypersensitivity reaction to an allergen or hapten, which elicits an adaptive immune response, specifically allergen-specific CD4 T lymphocytes. After the initial exposure or sensitization, cutaneous re-exposure to the allergen will elicit a brisk T-lymphocyte response that results in the typical erythema, vesiculation, pruritus, and/or scaling observed in ACD (Figs. 10.1, 10.2, and 10.3).

Protein contact dermatitis (PCD) is a subtype of contact eczema. It is triggered by skin contact with a protein that initiates an IgE-mediated immunological response (type I) with subsequent development of eczema. The patient will report stinging, itching, and burning seconds to minutes after exposure to the relevant protein. PCD occurs in occupations involving wet work and frequent skin contact with proteins from food, animals and/or plants. Vulnerable occupational groups include chefs, fishermen, bakers, veterinarians, and veterinary nurses [1]

Atopic Dermatitis (AD)

People with atopic dermatitis have a significantly increased risk for development of hand eczema when exposed to irritants at work or at home. Preventive measures are taken to inform young

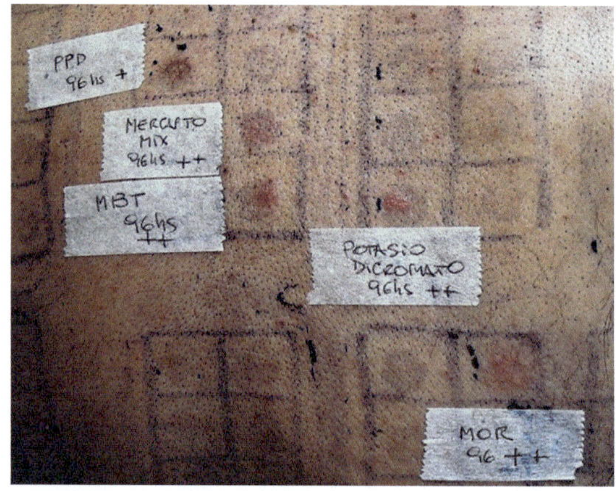

Fig. 10.3 Reading at 96 hours of the patch test with sensitizations to chromium salts (cement) and rubber additives (gloves)

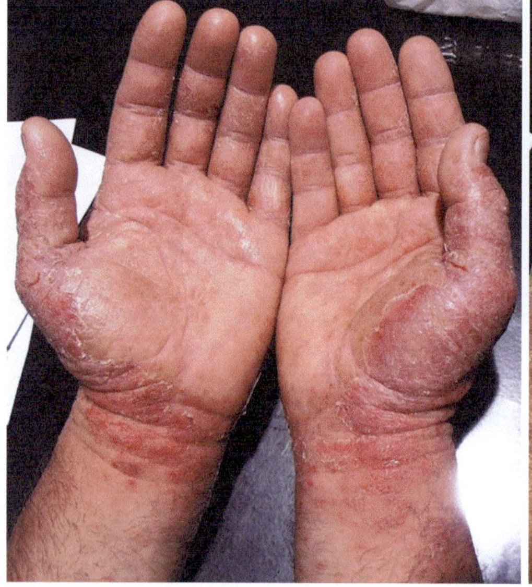
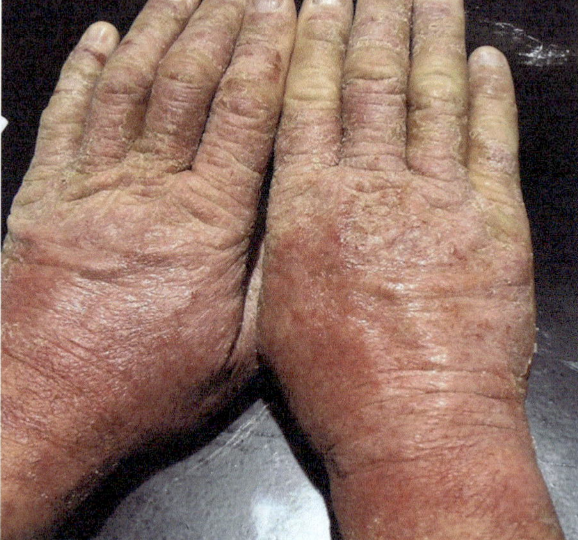

Figs. 10.1 and 10.2 OHE in construction worker

people with atopic dermatitis to avoid professions including wet or dirty work or food handling. Hand eczema in atopic patients often takes a chronic course, and a change of job seems to improve the prognosis less for atopic population than for others. Cellular immunity in atopic patients is decreased, and contact dermatitis seems to occur in a smaller number of patients with past or present atopic disease than in non-atopic subjects. Positive patch tests, often related to topical treatments, are, however, sometimes found in atopic patients. Therefore, patch test should be performed as in other patients with hand eczema.

Contact Urticaria (CU)

A type I hypersensitivity reaction that can be accompanied by systemic symptoms such as rhinitis, conjunctivitis, wheezing and in rare but severe cased anaphylactic shock.

Endogenous Forms

- *Acute and Recurrent Vesicular Hand Eczema (Pompholyx)*: is a morphological description of typically intensely pruritic hand eczema seen at the characteristic sites. The eruption may also extend to the periungual area, and there may be simultaneous, similar eruptions on the soles. The dermatitis is usually symmetrical and on both hands. There is little or no inflammation unless frequent eruptions occur. In such cases, inflammation may gradually develop, in which case dermatitis may mimic chronic hand eczema. Crops of tiny vesicles usually occur without external contact with allergens or irritants, and close inspection may be required in order to see the vesicle [36].

Hyperkeratotic Hand Eczema: this condition seemed to constitute a special category, mostly being seen in older men and with less relationship to etiological groups.

Even though each variant of contact dermatitis represents a distinct entity with its own patho-

physiology, a single patient can be affected by multiple types of contact dermatitis. A Danish study demonstrated that ICD was responsible for 70% of cases of OCD, ACD constituted 15%, whereas an additional 10% was caused by a combined presence of ICD and ACD [37].

Diagnosis

It is interesting that in most of the patients, one or more additional diagnoses were given. This reflects the fact that, in most cases, HE is a multifactorial disease, and this becomes even more prominent in severe and long-lasting cases.

Medical History

The occupational anamnesis maps the patient's occupational exposure to skin irritants and allergens in order to identify any association between occupational exposure and disease onset/exacerbation and any improvement during time off work. The occupational anamnesis and systemic review of safety data sheets can often permit the diagnosis of work-related allergic hand eczema [38]

The environmental anamnesis focuses on risk factors associated with home and leisure activities. Cosmetics and personal hygiene products may contain allergenic substances. Hobbies can involve the handling of glue, paint, plants, and tropical hardwoods. In various sporting activities such as handball, weightlifting, golf and tennis, players may encounter rubber-based allergens or resins. Climate conditions such as humidity, heat, cold, and UV light can also be contributing factors.

Clinical Examination and Supplementary Testing

The hands must be examined for signs of acute or chronic eczema. The patient may be tested using procedures such as epicutaneous testing, skin prick testing and/ or blood IgE assays. Hand Eczema is work-related when occupational exposure, in whole or in part, is the cause of the disorder [1].

It is highly recommended diagnostic patch tests be performed in all patients with HE of more than 3 months' duration or irresponsive to adequate treatment or clinical suspicion of contact allergy [32].

Positive patch test reaction were found in one-third of patient with diagnosis different form ACD as the main diagnosis, indicating that in these cases the finding of a positive patch test was not considered to be of current relevance [37]

Although mandatory before establishing a correct diagnosis, a positive patch test needs further interpretation, and may not be relevant to present dermatitis. Moreover, a negative patch test result, if the correct allergen was not tested, cannot determine ACD.

One of the great challenges is to refine the definition of ICD. This diagnosis is based on the presence of risk factors that are generally present in the environment. In a recent Swedish investigation, 20% of the population of working age acknowledged occupational skin exposure to water [4]. The lack of a diagnostic test increased the risk of misclassification. In twin studies, it has been shown that wet work is only a risk factor if a certain genetic disposition is present [11, 12]. Work should be performed to identify this genotype and eventually develop a diagnostic test, which could be a combination of genotypes and immunological markers, of this disease category as a new basis for an etiological classification.

In rare cases, a skin biopsy may be necessary to rule out other inflammatory skin diseases such as psoriasis. An asymmetric pruritic rash raises clinical suspicion of dermatophytosis. Other common differential diagnoses include scabies and palmoplantar pustulosis.

It is generally agreed that no simple relationships between clinical patterns and etiological diagnosis can be found. The classification system should include both morphological patterns as well as etiological causes for HE.

Differential Diagnosis

With respect to psoriasis, it is well known that the distinction between hyperkeratosis endogenous HE and palmar psoriasis can sometimes be difficult [39] and sometimes only the development of eczema or psoriasis over time will solve this dilemma. However, no statistical difference between the groups was found with respect to previous or current symptoms of psoriasis elsewhere on the body.

The increased frequency of atopic dermatitis in patients with PCD/CU as the main diagnosis is not surprising, since atopic patients are more prone to develop type I allergies and PCD/CU [40].

With respect to concomitant eczema on the feet, there is little data on this subject in the literature. It is well known that HE is related to eczema on the feet, and resent study found additional foot eczema in a total of 30% of the patients [37]. However, in-patient with endogenous eczema as the main diagnosis (vesicular and hyperkeratosis endogenous HE), the frequency was as high as 50%, while in patients with ICD the frequency of foot eczema was significantly lower.

Factors Influencing Prognosis for OHE: New Trends

Variables traditionally reported to influence the prognosis of occupational hand eczema (OHE) are atopic dermatitis (AD) and contact sensitization. However, recent studies indicated that lifestyle factors might be of major importance. Indeed, a recent Danish study indicates those lifestyle factors are important factors associated with poor prognosis of OHE. They reported that an increased level of stress is associated with persistence of hand eczema and a poor prognosis. The reason for this potential "new trend" is presumed to be improved counseling of patients with AD in Scandinavian countries, in relation to the choice of profession and other preventive strategies. Although further studies are needed to elucidate the relationship between lifestyle factors and the prognosis of OHE, it is recommended to increase the focus on lifestyle factors in the counseling of patients [30, 31].

Treatment

Standard Treatment

Detection and Removal of the Causative Agent

In the beginning, it must be done an exhaustive interrogation about manipulated substances, protection measures and personal hygiene products in the work and non-work environment that can trigger ICD or ACD. A correct physical examination must be assessed, and we must observe the environment and work activity that the patient develops [41].

Patch testing is the gold standard for the workup of allergic contact dermatitis, may require an extended allergen series and thus determine how to avoid contact [42]. It will be key that the occupational doctor determines the avoidance measures, such as protective material (special gloves) and change of job.

Astringent and Antisepsis Treatment

For vesiculous or bullous exudative lesions should be treated with astringent and antiseptic substances such as lotions or baths with copper sulfate or 1% zinc sulfate [41], potassium permanganate 1/5000 or solutions of silver nitrate 1–10%; applying them 2–3 times a day until the exudation disappears.

In addition, in cases of chronic eczema with fissures both antiseptics and topical antibiotics may be required. Never use topical anesthetics or antihistamines as well as the risk of contact sensitization. Avoid products that have perfumes or preservatives with a high risk of sensitization [43].

Anti-inflammatory Therapy

To treat the inflammatory process and improve the symptoms of the patient with hand eczema must be use topical treatment and if necessary, phototherapy or systemic treatment.

As a first line, we have topical corticosteroids (TCs) from medium to highest potency, formulated in cream or ointment. Recently its effectiveness in acute contact irritative eczema has been questioned due to the difficulty of penetration through the vesicles having to resort in several cases to oral corticosteroids but in the short term [44].

Clobetasol 0.05% cream has been evaluated in a meta-analysis as treatment for chronic HE achieves a 75% improvement in signs and symptoms, as well as the quality of life of patients [45].

On the other hand, using TCs in the long term (3–4 weeks) can delay the repair of the skin barrier due to its effect on the epidermal cellular turn over, decrease in lipid lamellar bodies and its atrophying effect. In addition, TCs could generate other long-term adverse effects such as infections or tachyphylaxis. When comparing the schemes of 1 against 2 daily applications of betamethasone, long-term benefits of one application per day over twice are observed in the long term.

Regarding topical calcineurin inhibitors (TCIs), tacrolimus 0.1% in ointment twice daily is an effective and safe treatment for mild to moderate HE or as long-term maintenance without modifying skin barrier or generating atrophy. Pimecrolimus 1% cream is not effective for the management of hand eczema [46]. Calcipotriol could be considered as a corticoid saver only as maintenance.

Both TCs and TCI's may adjust to maintenance 2–3 times a week after the first month of controlled eczema. In patients with keratoderma, it will be necessary to use simultaneously of keratolytic such as salicylic acid up to 20% or urea 10% cream [47].

In refractory cases it is necessary to turn to NB-UVB or PUVA phototherapy, which in addition to the anti-inflammatory effect will give us a positive effect on the repair of the skin barrier. On the other hand, there would be a synergistic effect in the combination of some treatments, for example, oral retinoids and PUVA, or calcipotriol and Excimer laser [48].

Second-generation antiH1 antihistamines are only used in case of control of symptoms such as pruritus.

In cases of more severe and refractory chronic OHE that do not respond to topical treatment or phototherapy, must be used systemic treatment such as oral corticosteroids, oral retinoids, and oral immunosuppressants.

Oral corticosteroids only for flare-ups with anti-inflammatory doses and short-term (up to 2 weeks); oral retinoids such as alitretinoin: 30 mg/day being considered the best second-line treatment for its long-term anti-inflammatory and antiproliferative effect [49]; acitretin reserved for keratoderma refractory at 30 mg/day for 4–12 weeks. As a third line, we can use cyclosporine, methotrexate, mycophenolate mofetil, and even azathioprine [50].

Reconstitution of the Skin Barrier

Once the inflammation of both chronic and acute processes of hand eczema has been controlled, the fundamental skin barrier for protection against irritants, sensitizers, and pathogens must be reconstituted. Studies showed that the use of emollients in patients who have suffered from occupational hand eczema, especially where there are more than 15 daily washes, significantly reduce relapses [51].

In cases of health, cleaning and gastronomy workers who are exposed to washing and using detergents permanently, barrier or occlusive creams based on silicone or petroleum jelly are recommended.

These products are intended to decrease hand dryness and restore the lipid bilayer of the stratum corneum [52], should have moisturizing substances (glycerol, hyaluronic acid, panthenol), emollients (ceramides, fatty acids, cholesterol) formulated in creams or emulsions oil in water without fragrances or preservatives that are linked to patient sensitization (Kathon CG, Formaldehyde, Quaternium 15). The application should be done constantly during and outside of work and after each washed hand.

Emergency Trends or New Drug Therapy

Dupilumab, an anti-IL4 and IL 13 monoclonal antibody used in Atopic Dermatitis is being evaluated for the treatment of chronic HE refractory to treatment with topical corticosteroids, in a randomized, double-blind phase 2 study. Case reports of hyperkeratotic hand eczema treated with dupilumab have demonstrated a good therapeutic response [53].

Delgocitinib, a topical JAK inhibitor, has been studied in a phase 2 study for hand eczema observing a significant response compared to placebo.

Prevention

Work-related and OHE are highly preventable by elimination, substitution, or reduction of occupational skin exposure to irritants and allergens (primary prevention). Early recognition, diagnosis, treatment, and reporting to work-health authorities are the main secondary preventive measures to avoid a chronic, recurrent and recalcitrant course. Moreover, tertiary preventive measures include medical, occupational, and social rehabilitation such as recognition of occupational skin disease and compensation, change of occupation, or early retirement when the other measures are not enough to avoid CHE and sick leave.

Health education strategies focusing on skin care and protection are essential in primary, secondary, and tertiary prevention. Chapter: *"Standards for prevention of work-related and occupational hand eczema"* presents available international consensus-based minimum standards to prevent occupational skin diseases that are applicable for OHE.

Occupational Hand Eczema in Time of COVID-19 (JPR)

There has been a significant increase in the prevalence of reported occupational dermatoses due to the enhanced infection prevention measures adopted by both healthcare workers and the general public in response to the COVID-19 pandemic. Irritant and allergic contact dermatitis are the most common occupational dermatitis reported and most often due to excessive hand washing and wearing personal protective equipment (PPE) such as latex gloves [54].

Healthcare workers in COVID-19 care units developed HE more frequently associated with increased hand hygiene practices than no COVID-19 patient care units (48.3% vs 12.7%, $P < 0.001$). A majority increased the frequency of moisturizer use, instead of using topical corticosteroids, after the development of HE for the purpose of treating eczema [55]. Risk factors of OHE in pandemic COVID-19 were studied: atopic dermatitis, male sex, younger age, longer working hours and having children younger than 4 years in the household were proposed to associate with hand eczema [56]. Healthcare workers who have washed their hands more than 10 times per day have a double risk of HE [57].

Conclusion

OHE is an entity that affects a large part of the working population, being a complex pathology due to having multiple risk factors both exogenous and endogenous, as well as a very variable clinical presentation.

This entails always carrying out an exhaustive clinical evaluation that requires a high training in Occupational Dermatology, even knowing how to determine the relevance of the results of the epicutaneous tests.

The management of these patients is usually difficult, where the patient must avoid causal agents and education is key in the improvement, repair of the skin barrier, and prevention of relapses.

Finally, the COVID-19 pandemic has increased the number of cases of OHE, and healthcare workers should be alert and emphasize prevention measures to control this work-related pathology.

References

1. Alfonso JH, Bauer A, Bensefa-Colas L, et al. Minimum standards on prevention, diagnosis and treatment of occupational and work-related skin diseases in Europe - position paper of the COST Action StanDerm (TD 1206). J Eur Acad Dermatol Venereol. 2017;31(4):31–43.
2. Lachapelle JM. Clinical subtypes and categorization of hand eczema: an overview. In: Alikhan A, Lachapelle JM, Maibach H, editors. Textbook of hand eczema. Berlin: Springer-Verlag, Berlin; 2014. p. 25–36.
3. Thyssen JP, Johansen JD, Linneberg A, Menné T. The epidemiology of hand eczema in the general population--prevalence and main findings. Contact Dermatitis. 2010;62:75–87.
4. Anveden Berglind I, Alderling M, Järvholm B, et al. Occupational skin exposure to water: a population-based study. Br J Dermatol. 2009;160(3):616–21.
5. Meding B, Järvholm B. Incidence of hand eczema— a population-based retrospective study. J Invest Dermatol. 2004;122(4):873–7.
6. Meding B, Lindahl G, Alderling M, et al. Is skin exposure to water mainly occupational or nonoccupational? A population-based study. Br J Dermatol. 2013;168(6):1281–6.
7. Mollerup A, Veien NK, Johansen JD. An analysis of gender differences in patients with hand eczema - everyday exposures, severity, and consequences. Contact Dermatitis. 2014;71(1):21–30.
8. Vindenes HK, Svanes C, Lygre S, et al. Prevalence of, and work-related risk factors for, hand eczema in a Norwegian general population (The HUNT Study). Contact Dermat. 2017;77:214–23.
9. Augustin M. Pharmacoeconomics of occupational diseases. In: Kanerva's occupational dermatology. T. Rustemeyer T (ed), Elsner P (ed), John SM (ed), Maibach H (ed). 2nd edn springer-Verlag. Ther Ber. 2012;2:19–25.
10. Cvetkovski RS, Zachariae R, Jensen H, et al. Prognosis of occupational hand eczema: a follow-up study. Arch Dermatol. 2006;142:305–11.
11. Lerbaek A, Kyvik KO, Mortensen J, et al. Heritability of hand eczema is not explained by comorbidity with atopic dermatitis. J Invest Dermatol. 2007a;127(7):1632–40.
12. Lerbaek A, Kyvik KO, Ravn H, et al. Incidence of hand eczema in a population-based twin cohort: genetic and environmental risk factors. Br J Dermatol. 2007b;157(3):552–7.
13. Meding B, Wrangsjö K, Järvholm B. Fifteen-year follow-up of hand eczema: predictive factors. J Invest Dermatol. 2005;124(5):893–7.
14. Yngveson M, Svensson A, Johannisson A, Isacsson A. Hand dermatosis in upper secondary school pupils: 2-year comparison and follow-up. Br J Dermatol. 2000;142(3):485–9.
15. Meding B, Wrangsjö K, Järvholm B. Hand eczema extent and morphology--association and influence on long-term prognosis. J Invest Dermatol. 2007;127(9):2147–51.
16. Heede NG, Thyssen JP, Thuesen BH, et al. Anatomical patterns of dermatitis in adult filaggrin mutation carriers. J Am Acad Dermatol. 2015;72(3):440–8.

17. Heede NG, Thyssen JP, Thuesen BH, et al. Predictive factors of self-reported hand eczema in adult Danes: a population-based cohort study with 5-year follow-up. Br J Dermatol. 2016;175(2):287–95.

18. Lagrelius M, Wahlgren C-F, Bradley M, et al. Filaggrin gene mutations in relation to contact allergy and hand eczema in adolescence. Contact Dermatitis. 2020;82(3):147–52.

19. Reich A, Wilke A, Gediga G, et al. Health education decreases incidence of hand eczema in metal work apprentices: results of a controlled intervention study. Contact Dermatitis. 2020;82(6):350–60.

20. Kezic S, Visser MJ, Verberk MM. Individual susceptibility to occupational contact dermatitis. Ind Health. 2009;47:469–78.

21. Timmerman J, Heederik D, Spee T, et al. Contact dermatitis in the construction industry: the role of loss-of-function mutations. Br J Dermatol. 2016;174:348–55.

22. Visser MJ, Landeck L, Campbell LE, McLean WH, Weidinger S, Calkoen F, et al. Impact of atopic dermatitis and loss-of-function mutations in the gene on the development of occupational irritant contact dermatitis. Br J Dermatol. 2013;168:326–32.

23. Visser MJ, Verberk MM, Campbell LE, McLean WH, Calkoen F, Bakker JG, et al. Filaggrin loss-of-function mutations and atopic dermatitis as risk factors for hand eczema in apprentice nurses: part II of a prospective cohort study. Contact Dermatitis. 2014;70:139–50.

24. Bandier J, Ross-Hansen K, Carlsen BC, et al. Carriers of filaggrin gene (FLG) mutations avoid professional exposure to irritants in adulthood. Contact Dermatitis. 2013;69(6):355–62.

25. Meisser SS, Altunbulakli C, Bandier Jet al (2020) Skin barrier damage after exposure to paraphenylenediamine. J Allergy Clin Immunol 145(2):619–631

26. Carøe TK, Ebbehøj N, Agner T. A survey of exposures related to recognized occupational contact dermatitis in Denmark in 2010. Contact Dermatitis. 2014;70(1):56–62.

27. Lund T, Petersen SB, Flachs EM, et al. Risk of work-related hand eczema in relation to wet work exposure. Scand J Work Environ Health. 2020;46(4):437–45.

28. Rycroft RJ, Smith WD. Low humidity occupational dermatoses. Contact Dermatitis. 1980;6(7):488–92.

29. Brans R, Skudlik C, Weisshaar E, et al. Association between tobacco smoking and prognosis of occupational hand eczema: a prospective cohort study. Br J Dermatol. 2014;171(5):1108–15.

30. Olesen CM, Agner T, Ebbehøj NE, Carøe TK. Factors influencing prognosis for occupational hand eczema: new trends. Br J Dermatol. 2019a;181(6):1280–6.

31. Olesen CM, Agner T, Ebbehøj NE, Carøe TK. Factors influencing prognosis for occupational hand eczema: new trends. Br J Dermatol. 2019b;181(6):1280–6.

32. Thyssen JP, Schuttelaar LA, Alfonso JH, et al. Guidelines for diagnosis, prevention and treatment of hand eczema. Contact Dermatitis. 2021;86:357. https://doi.org/10.1111/cod.14035.

33. Diepgen TL, Andersen KE, Chosidow O, et al. Guidelines for diagnosis, prevention and treatment of hand eczema. J Dtsch Dermatol Ges. 2015;13(1):1–22.

34. Kersh AE, Johansen M, Ojeaga A, de la Feld S. Hand dermatitis in the time of COVID-19: a review of occupational irritant contact dermatitis. Dermatitis. 2021;32(2):86–93.

35. Johansen JD, Hald M, Andersen BL, et al. Danish contact dermatitis group. Classification of hand eczema: clinical and aetiological types. Based on the guideline of the Danish Contact Dermatitis Group. Contact Dermatitis. 2011;65(1):13–21.

36. Veien NK. Acute and recurrent vesicular hand dermatitis. Dermatol Clin. 2009;27(3):337–53.

37. Agner T, Elsner P. J Eur Acad Dermatol Venereol. 2020;34(1):4–12.

38. Friis UF, Menné T, Flyvholm MA, et al. Occupational allergic contact dermatitis diagnosed by a systematic stepwise exposure assessment of allergens in the work environment. Contact Dermatitis. 2013;69(3):153–63.

39. Hersle K, Mobacken H. Hyperkeratotic dermatitis of the palms. Br J Dermatol. 1982;107(2):195–201.

40. Wollenberg A, Feichtner K. Atopic dermatitis and skin allergies - update and outlook. Allergy. 2013;68(12):1509–19.

41. García Pérez A, Conde-Salazar Gómez L, Giménez Camarasa J. In: Tratado de dermatosis profesionales. Giménez Camarasa J (ed). 1st edn Eudema Universidad. Madrid. 1987;5:517–28.

42. Lampel HP, Powell HB. Occupational and hand dermatitis: a practical approach. Clin Rev Allergy Immunol. 2019;56(1):60–71.

43. Gonzalez de Domingo MA, Conde-Salazar Gómez L. Tratamiento de las dermatosis laborales. In: Conde-Salazar Gómez L, editor. Dermatología Profesional, vol. 35. 1st ed. Madrid: Aula Médica; 2003. p. 491–500.

44. Maghfour J, Maibach H. Are topical corticosteroids effective for chronic irritant contact dermatitis? Dermatitis. 2021;32(6):148–50.

45. Jing M, Yu Q, Zhu B, et al. Topical 0.05% clobetasol cream in the treatment of chronic hand eczema. A protocol for systematic review and meta-analysis. Medicine. 2021;100(10):e24418.

46. Bauer A, Lange N, Matterne U, et al. Efficacy of pimecrolimus 1% cream in the long-term management of atopic hand dermatitis. A double-blind RCT. J Dtsch Dermatol Ges. 2012;10:426–33.

47. Diepgen TL, Elsner P, Schliemann S, et al. Guideline on the management of hand eczema ICD-10 code: L20. L23. L24. L25. L30. J Dtsch Dermatol Ges. 2009;7(3):1–16.

48. Juntongjin P, Chunhakham P. Synergistic effects of the 308-nm excimer light and topical Calcipotriol for the treatment of chronic hand eczema: a randomized controlled study. Dermatology. 2021;237(1):31–8.

49. Ruzicka T, Lynde CW, Jemec GB, et al. Efficacy and safety of oral alitretinoin (9-cis retinoic acid) in patients with severe chronic hand eczema refractory to topical corticosteroids: results of a randomized,

double-blind, placebo-controlled, multicentre trial. Br J Dermatol. 2008;158:808–17.

50. Menne T, Johansen JD, Sommerlund M, Veien NK. Hand eczema guidelines based on the Danish guidelines for the diagnosis and treatment of hand eczema. Contact Dermatitis. 2011;65(1):3–12.

51. Williams C, Wilkinson SM, McShane P, Lewis J, et al. A double-blind, randomized study to assess the effectiveness of different moisturizers in reventing dermatitis induced by hand washing to simulate healthcare use. Br J Dermatol. 2010;162(5):1088–92.

52. Lodén M. Effect of moisturizers on epidermal barrier function. Clin Dermatol. 2012;30(3):286–96.

53. Loman L, Diercks G, Schuttelaar M. Three cases of non-atopic hyperkeratotic hand eczema treated with dupilumab. Contact Dermatitis. 2021;84(2):124–7.

54. Abdali S, Yu J. Occupational dermatoses related to personal protective equipment used during the COVID-19 pandemic. Dermatol Clin. 2021;39:555–68.

55. Erdem Y, Inal S, Sivaz O, et al. How does working in pandemic units affect the risk of occupational hand eczema in healthcare workers during the coronavirus disease-2019 (COVID-19) pandemic: a comparative analysis with nonpandemic units. Contact Dermatitis. 2021;1:1–10.

56. Araghi F, Tabary M, Gheisari M, et al. Hand hygiene among health care WorkersDuring COVID-19 pandemic: challenges and recommendations. Dermatitis. 2020;31(4):223–37.

57. Lan J, Song Z, Miao X, Li H, et al. Skin damage among healthcare workers managing coronavirus disease-2019. J Am Acad Dermatol. 2020;82(5):1215–6.

Airborne Occupational Contact Dermatoses

Andac Salman

Introduction

Airborne contact dermatoses are caused by exposure to particles hanging in the air. They are classified as airborne irritant contact dermatitis, airborne allergic contact dermatitis, and airborne contact urticaria based on the pathomechanism (Type I or IV hypersensitivity) and the particle characteristics (allergic or irritant). They mostly occur in occupational settings. In this chapter, the epidemiology, pathophysiology, clinical features, diagnosis, and management of airborne occupational contact dermatoses will be addressed.

Epidemiology

The most common form of airborne contact dermatoses is airborne allergic contact dermatitis (AbACD). Although AbACD might also occur in non-occupational settings, the vast majority of the related allergens are occupational [1]. Those allergens include adhesives, rubbers, metals, drugs, and preservatives. In a previous study, 81 of the 1410 patients with at least one positive patch test reaction had airborne dermatitis.

Among those, 54 were women and 45 were occupationally related. The most common causes were fragrances, preservatives, and drugs [2]. In a study from Turkey, 63 of the 294 patients with occupational ACD had AbACD. The most common allergens were potassium dichromate, ammonium persulfate, epoxy resin, MCI/MI and MI, thiurams, and sesquiterpene lactone mix [3]. In a retrospective analysis of 201,344 patients who were patch tested, 0.6% of them had airborne contact dermatitis and 35% of these were occupational. The most frequent allergens in occupational cases were adhesives, plastics, construction materials, paints, and varnishes [4]. The same study reported that airborne contact dermatitis was more frequently occupational in men, patients younger than 40 years, and patients with hand dermatitis [4].

Risk Factors

Healthcare and pharmaceutical industry workers are at increased risk for drug-induced airborne allergic contact dermatitis because they might develop sensitization during crushing tablets for patients with swallowing difficulties, production, or machine maintenance [5, 6]. The most frequent occupations in a series of 63 patients were house builder/bricklayer, hairdresser, shipwright, house painter, florist/gardener, aircraft mechanic, and nurse [3]. In a larger series of patients with

A. Salman (✉)
Department of Dermatology, Acıbadem Mehmet Ali Aydınlar University School of Medicine, Istanbul, Turkey

© The Author(s), under exclusive license to Springer Nature Switzerland AG 2023
A. M. Giménez-Arnau, H. I. Maibach (eds.), *Handbook of Occupational Dermatoses*, Updates in Clinical Dermatology, https://doi.org/10.1007/978-3-031-22727-1_11

Table 11.1 Professions at increased risk for occupational airborne contact dermatitis [4]

Healthcare workers (nurses, nursing assistants, dental assistants)
Painters
Mechanics, machine operators, toolmakers
Construction workers
Florists, gardeners
Farmers
Engineers, technicians
Janitorial services
Plastic processors

AbCD, occupational relevance was more frequent in some professions (Table 11.1) [4].

In addition, a dry environment, repeated (micro)trauma to the skin, excessive heat, and sweating might increase the risk of AbACD by either barrier disruption or increased adhesion and absorption of allergens [7]. Personal history of atopy or atopic dermatitis also increases the risk of airborne contact dermatitis because the already impaired skin barrier allows easier penetration of the airborne particles to the skin [7].

Pathophysiology and Clinical Features

Occupational airborne contact dermatoses can be grouped into allergic and irritant reactions [8]. Allergic reactions may be caused by either type I hypersensitivity or type IV hypersensitivity, whereas irritant reactions are caused by mechanical and frictional effects of airborne particles (Table 11.2). Type I hypersensitivity reactions require the presence of allergen-specific IgE and may present as airborne contact urticaria or contact urticaria syndrome. Type IV, or delayed-type, hypersensitivity reactions are the most common form of airborne contact dermatoses and usually present as airborne allergic contact dermatitis. On the other hand, airborne irritant contact dermatitis does not involve immunologic mechanisms and might occur in any individual without prior sensitization. It occurs due to frictional and/ or mechanical effects of fibers, dust particles, vapors, or gases [9].

The body parts directly exposed to air, i.e., face, neck, upper chest, forearms, and hands, are frequently affected in airborne contact dermatoses. Because the skin in the upper eyelids is very thin, the allergen penetration is easier, thus airborne contact dermatoses involve this area very often. In addition to exposed skin areas, covered areas can also be affected because airborne particles are sometimes trapped under clothing [2, 10–12]. Genital involvement might also occur, particularly in men, through the transportation of airborne materials by the hands [2]. The nose can be spared due to the high sebaceous content leading to the appearance of the so-called "beak sign" [13].

Other than the airborne contact dermatitis and urticaria, airborne contact dermatoses of various clinical patterns have been reported in the literature (Table 11.3) [1, 2]. Physicians managing occupational skin disorders should recognize those to prevent possible delays in diagnosis.

Table 11.2 Airborne contact dermatoses

Classification		Pathophysiology	Diagnostic tests
Allergic	Contact Urticaria Contact Urticaria syndrome	Type I hypersensitivity	Skin prick testing, scratch test, in vitro serologic tests, provocation tests
	Allergic contact dermatitis	Type IV hypersensitivity	Patch testing
Irritant	Irritant contact dermatitis	Mechanical, frictional effects, non-immunologic	(−)

Table 11.3 Airborne occupational contact dermatoses [1, 22]

Occupational airborne contact urticaria (syndrome)
Occupational airborne irritant contact dermatitis
Occupational airborne allergic contact dermatitis
Occupational airborne phototoxic contact dermatitis
Occupational airborne photoallergic contact dermatitis
Other clinical variants (pigmented contact dermatitis, erythema-multiforme-like eruption, lichenoid eruption, exacerbation of atopic dermatitis by aeroallergens)

Airborne Contact Urticaria

Among the three types of contact urticaria syndrome (CUS) (immunologic, non-immunologic, and CUS of uncertain cause), immunologic CUS usually occur in occupational settings. The clinical findings of CUS can be observed in four stages: localized urticaria (stage 1), generalized urticaria (stage 2), allergic asthma, and/or allergic rhinitis (stage 3), anaphylaxis or anaphylactoid reactions (stage 4) [14]. The clinical findings and the severity of the symptoms vary depending on the route (skin or mucosa) and amount of exposure [15].

Natural rubber latex (NRL) proteins are major causes of occupational airborne contact urticaria. NRL allergens are present on the surfaces of rubber materials (e.g., medical gloves) and also in the cornstarch powder in the powdered NRL gloves. They can be aerosolized, might cause sensitization through skin and mucosa, and result in CUS [16, 17]. Despite a decrease in NRL sensitivity following regulatory measures in the last decades, NRL-related occupational airborne CUS can still be a problem for healthcare workers, food handlers, construction workers, and painters [18, 19].

In addition to NRL, occupational airborne contact urticaria, asthma and anaphylaxis have been reported following exposure to dried peas infested with *Bruchus pisorum*. Agronomists, cooks, farmers, and grocery workers are at increased risk for such exposures [20].

Airborne Contact Dermatitis

Contact dermatitis is an acute or chronic inflammatory cutaneous reaction occurring following exposure to an irritant and/or allergen substance. Contact dermatitis can be classified depending on the underlying pathomechanism as, irritant contact dermatitis (ICD) and allergic contact dermatitis (ACD). Airborne contact dermatitis is the form of contact dermatitis caused by contact allergens and irritants available in the air as fibers, dust particles, spray, vapor, and gas [4]. Table 11.4 shows the most common causes of airborne contact dermatitis.

Table 11.4 The causes of occupational airborne contact dermatitis. (Adapted from [4])

Adhesives	Construction materials	Metalworking fluids
Plastics	Gloves (leather, rubber, fabric)	Metals
Disinfectants	Rubber	Topical drugs
Cosmetics	Plants	Fragrances
Paints, varnishes	Cleaning products	Hair cosmetics (e.g., dyes)

Airborne Irritant Contact Dermatitis

A variety of fiber particles, including fiberglass, rockwool, glasswool, carbon fibers, and plastic fibers, might cause airborne irritant contact dermatitis (AbICD). However, the typical and the most common example of occupational AbICD is fiberglass dermatitis [9]. Fiber particles are usually chemically inert and provoke symptoms through their mechanical and frictional effects on the skin. Itching, burning, and stinging sensation are almost always present on the face and flexural areas. Dermatological examination usually shows excoriations, small papules, and sometimes a maculopapular eruption. Construction workers, electronic industry workers, fiberglass factory workers, wind energy industry workers, and marine industry workers are at increased risk for the development of fiberglass dermatitis [21].

In addition to fiber particles, dust particles, spray, vapors, and gasses (e.g., organic solvents, ammonia, formaldehyde) may also induce airborne irritant contact dermatitis. Dust particles may irritate the skin through either their frictional/mechanical or chemical properties. Dust particles can accumulate under the ill-fitted masks or clothes (e.g., sleeves), thus the clinical findings may be more prominent over these areas [22]. Fibers and dust particles may also affect the covered body parts, thus may complicate the diagnosis [9].

Airborne Allergic Contact Dermatitis

The lesions usually involve exposed skin areas, thus differentiation from photocontact dermatoses is critical. In airborne ACD, the shaded areas, including the upper eyelids, retro auricular areas, nasolabial folds, submandibular region, and skin creases, are involved, unlike the latter. Standard patch testing (may be positive in Airborne ACD) and photopatch testing may also help to differentiate these conditions [2, 7, 9, 11].

Common Allergens

The most frequent cause of AbACD is the allergens of plant origin [7]. AbACD due to allergen of plant origin are usually associated with two plant families: the Compositae and the Anacardiaceae [2, 7]. In addition to outdoor plants, exposure to edible forms of Compositae plants, e.g., chamomile tea vapor, lettuce, artichoke, may result in AbACD [23]. Occupational AbACD induced by plant-derived allergens has been also reported in a driver due to car fragrance diffusers (Balsam of Peru), in a bakery worker due to cinnamon, and beekeepers due to propolis [24–26]. Another source of plant-related occupational AbACD is *Parthenium hysterophorus* (Parthenium dermatitis), which is very common in India. The associated allergen, parthenin, is a sesquiterpene lactone. It may sometimes present with lichenified plaques on exposed skin areas resembling chronic actinic dermatitis [27].

Although airborne contact dermatoses were initially thought to be caused by plant-derived allergens, a vast array of allergens (of plant or non-plant origin) and irritants associated with airborne contact dermatoses have been recognized now [7, 12].

Epoxy resins, mainly found in plastics, glues, and adhesives, are frequent causes of ArACD in occupational settings. It frequently affects patients working as floorers, bricklayers, and repairmen [28, 29]. Methacrylates, also used as adhesives, have been reported to cause occupational ArACD in dental nurses and nail technicians applying acrylic nails [30, 31].

Thiurams are used as accelerators in the manufacturing process of rubber products. Occupational ArACD has been reported in healthcare workers due to thiurams released from medical gloves [32, 33].

Nickel, cobalt, and gold are among the metal allergens that are associated with occupational ArACD. The reported sources included nickel dust in a laboratory and metal sprays at factories [34–36].

Isothiazolinones are preservatives frequently found in cosmetics, household products, and water-based paints. The most commonly used isothiazolinones (ITs) are methylisothiazolinone (MI), methylchloroisothiazolinone (MCI)/MI, benzisothiazolinone (BIT), and, octylisothiazolinone (OIT) [37]. Water-based paints are important sources of isothiazolinone-related occupational AbACD in painters [38]. In a series of 44 patients with AbACD caused by isothiazolinones, 20.5% of the cases were occupational. In 70% of the patients, skin findings were limited to non-covered skin parts. Interestingly, 22.7% of the patients had also mucosal symptoms, i.e., breathing difficulties and/or rhinoconjunctivitis. The symptoms led to sick leave and hospitalization in 20% and 9.1% of the patients, respectively. The symptoms were long-lasting with a median duration of 6.9 weeks, moreover, it took a median of 5.5 weeks of delay until the patients were able to enter into a freshly painted room without exacerbation of the symptoms [39]. This is in line with a previous study that showed MI emission from water-based paints lasted up to 42 days [40]. Another common problem for patients sensitized with ITs is the lack of adequate labeling on paint containers [39].
Medications are another important cause of AbACD in pharmaceutical industry workers, healthcare workers, and patients. Exposure to airborne drug particles can occur during the manufacturing processes and drug preparation [7]. Proton pump inhibitors (omeprazole, lansoprazole, and pantoprazole) have been reported to cause occupational airborne allergic contact

dermatitis in three workers (production and maintenance) in the pharmaceutical industry [41]. Occupational airborne allergic contact dermatitis involving hands, face, and neck have been reported in nurses due to crushing benzodiazepine tablets [5]. AbACD due to budesonide aerosols has been also reported in healthcare workers [42].

Airborne Phototoxic/ Photoallergic Contact Dermatitis

Substances causing phototoxic and photoallergic contact dermatitis can also be airborne, although it is usually impossible to differentiate direct and airborne contact reactions. Relative sparing of the shaded areas in the former can be used as a diagnostic clue. Occupational airborne phototoxic or photoallergic substances include coal tar and derivatives, fragrances, and drug molecules [22].

Diagnosis

History

The diagnosis of airborne occupational contact dermatoses requires a detailed history, workplace visits, and patch testing with standard series and patients' own products. A previously proposed systematic stepwise exposure assessment can be used to identify occupational allergens not included in the standard series but available in the patients' workplace [43]. The followings should be emphasized during the history taking:

- Subjective symptoms
- Occupation, occupational exposures
- Concomitant medications, non-occupational exposures
- Presence of other risk factors
- Distribution of the lesions (airborne pattern, differentiation from photocontact dermatoses)
- Extracutaneous symptoms
- Relationship between exposure and onset of lesions

In addition to a detailed history, in vivo and in vitro tests can be used to aid the diagnosis of occupational airborne contact dermatoses.

In Vitro Testing

In the case of airborne CUS, in vitro diagnosis is possible with the use of serum-specific IgE level measurement and Basophil activation tests. The clinical relevance of the in vitro tests should be carefully assessed before confirming a diagnosis [14, 20, 44].

In Vivo Testing

Skin surface biopsy and tape stripping can be used to demonstrate the fibers within the epidermis if fiberglass dermatitis is suspected [45–47]. Patch testing (standard, photopatch, and patch testing with patients' own products) is the gold standard for the diagnosis of occupational AbACD.

In case of possible drug-induced airborne contact dermatitis,, patch testing with all drugs the patient is exposed to and possible cross-reacting molecules should be done [5]. According to a proposed diagnostic algorithm for CUS, an open application test should be done initially and if negative, occlusive application tests can be applied. Those tests should be done on normal skin. If there is no positive reaction in open application tests, then invasive methods including prick testing, prick by prick testing, scratch tests, and intradermal testing can be performed [14].

Management

The best and most effective strategy to manage airborne contact dermatoses is the identification and avoidance of the triggering substances [23]. In addition to better and continuing education of patients, proper labeling and stricter regulatory measures on the use of preservatives and other allergens are important to prevent further recurrences and to reduce the need for systemic treatments, sick leave, and job loss [39].

Strict use of protective equipment is essential for all patients. Patients should be recommended to wear masks, gloves, and industrial goggles at work. Clothing with sealed cuffs and necks can be preferred [20, 23]. In patients with drug-induced occupational AbACD, the use of drug-crushing devices and personal protective equipment (masks and gloves) should be encouraged [5]. Bathing after known exposures and frequent laundering of work clothes can sometimes be helpful [23]. The use of barrier creams before exposure has been reported to be helpful in selected cases [48].

Topical emollients, topical corticosteroids, and topical calcineurin inhibitors can be used for the acute treatment of occupational airborne dermatoses. In addition, systemic corticosteroids can be given for short-term use. In recalcitrant and severe cases changing occupations may be needed [23]. The use of systemic immunosuppressives may also be required to control the symptoms in the long term, particularly in patients with occupational AbACD. Azathioprine, methotrexate, and cyclosporine have been used successfully in the treatment of occupational AbACD, particularly in Parthenium dermatitis [49–51].

References

1. Huygens S, Goossens A. An update on airborne contact dermatitis. Contact Dermatitis. 2001;44:1–6.
2. Swinnen I, Goossens A. An update on airborne contact dermatitis: 2007-2011. Contact Dermatitis. 2013;68:232–8.
3. Özkaya E, Elinç Aslan MS. Occupational allergic contact dermatitis: a 24-year, retrospective cohort study from Turkey. Contact Dermatitis. 2021;85:503–13.
4. Breuer K, Uter W, Geier J. Epidemiological data on airborne contact dermatitis - results of the IVDK. Contact Dermatitis. 2015;73:239–47.
5. Swinnen I, Ghys K, Kerre S, Constandt L, Goossens A. Occupational airborne contact dermatitis from benzodiazepines and other drugs. Contact Dermatitis. 2014;70:227–32.
6. Ferran M, Giménez-Arnau A, Luque S, Berenguer N, Iglesias M, Pujol RM. Occupational airborne contact dermatitis from sporadic exposure to tetrazepam during machine maintenance. Contact Dermatitis. 2005;52:173–4.
7. Schloemer JA, Zirwas MJ, Burkhart CG. Airborne contact dermatitis: common causes in the USA. Int J Dermatol. 2015;54:271–4.

8. Lachapelle JM. Industrial airborne irritant or allergic contact dermatitis. Contact Dermatitis. 1986;14:137–45.

9. Lachapelle J-M. Environmental airborne contact dermatoses. Rev Environ Health. 2014;29:221–31.

10. Goossens A. Airborne dermatosis. Acta Dermatovenerol Croat. 2006;14:153–5.

11. Bonamonte D, Romita P, Filoni A, Angelini G, Foti C. Airborne contact dermatitis. Open Dermatol J. 2020;14:31–7.

12. Ghosh S. Airborne-contact dermatitis of non-plant origin: an overview. Indian J Dermatol. 2011;56:711–4.

13. Staser K, Ezra N, Sheehan MP, Mousdicas N. The beak sign: a clinical clue to airborne contact dermatitis. Dermat Contact Atopic Occup Drug. 2014;25:97–8.

14. Giménez-Arnau AM. Contact urticaria syndrome: how it is clinically manifested and how to diagnose it. In: Gimenez-Arnau AM, Maibach HI, editors. Contact Urticaria. 1st ed. CRC Press; 2014. p. 21–8.

15. Amaro C, Goossens A. Immunological occupational contact urticaria and contact dermatitis from proteins: a review. Contact Dermatitis. 2008;58:67–75.

16. Charous BL, Schuenemann PJ, Swanson MC. Passive dispersion of latex aeroallergen in a healthcare facility. Ann Allergy Asthma Immunol. 2000;85:285–90.

17. Swanson MC, Bubak ME, Hunt LW, Yunginger JW, Warner MA, Reed CE. Quantification of occupational latex aeroallergens in a medical center. J Allergy Clin Immunol. 1994;94:445–51.

18. Bensefa-Colas L, Telle-Lamberton M, Faye S, Bourrain J-L, Crépy M-N, Lasfargues G, Choudat D, RNV3P members M, Momas I. Occupational contact urticaria: lessons from the French National Network for occupational disease vigilance and prevention (RNV3P). Br J Dermatol. 2015;173:1453–61.

19. Valks R, Conde-Salazar L, Cuevas M. Allergic contact urticaria from natural rubber latex in healthcare and non-healthcare workers. Contact Dermatitis. 2004;50:222–4.

20. Armentia A, Alvarez R, Moreno-González V, et al. Occupational airborne contact urticaria, anaphylaxis and asthma in farmers and agronomists due to Bruchus pisorum. Contact Dermatitis. 2020;83:466–74.

21. Camacho I, Rajabi-Estarabadi A, Eber AE, Griggs JW, Margaret SI, Nouri K, Tosti A. Fiberglass dermatitis: clinical presentations, prevention, and treatment - a review of literatures. Int J Dermatol. 2019;58:1107–11.

22. Lachapelle J-M. Airborne contact dermatitis. In: John SM, Johansen JD, Rustemeyer T, Elsner P, Maibach HI, editors. Kanerva's occupational dermatology. 3rd ed. Cham: Springer Nature; 2020. p. 229–40.

23. Kimyon RS, Warshaw EM. Airborne allergic contact dermatitis: management and responsible allergens on the American contact dermatitis society Core series. Dermatitis. 2019;30:106–15.

24. Perper M, Cervantes J, Eber AE, Tosti A. Airborne contact dermatitis caused by fragrance diffusers in Uber cars. Contact Dermatitis. 2017;77:116–7.

25. Ackermann L, Aalto-Korte K, Jolanki R, Alanko K. Occupational allergic contact dermatitis from cinnamon including one case from airborne exposure. Contact Dermatitis. 2009;60:96–9.

26. Garrido Fernández S, Fernández SG, Arroabarren Alemán E, et al. Direct and airborne contact dermatitis from propolis in beekeepers. Contact Dermatitis. 2004;50:320–1.

27. Bhatia R, Sharma VK. Occupational dermatoses: an Asian perspective. Indian J Dermatol Venereol Leprol. 2017;83:525–35.

28. Geier J, Krautheim A, Fuchs T. Airborne allergic contact dermatitis in a parquet fitter. Contact Dermatitis. 2012;67:106–8.

29. Geier J, Lessmann H, Reinecke S. Occupational airborne allergic contact dermatitis in a concrete repair worker. Contact Dermatitis. 2009;60:50–1.

30. Hickey JR, Sansom JE. Allergic contact dermatitis following airborne exposure to methacrylates used in the manufacture of artificial skin. Contact Dermatitis. 2003;49:221.

31. Maio P, Carvalho R, Amaro C, Santos R, Cardoso J. Allergic contact dermatitis from sculptured acrylic nails: special presentation with an airborne pattern. Dermatology reports. 2012;4:e6.

32. Schwensen JF, Menné T, Johansen JD, Thyssen JP. Persistent periorbital allergic contact dermatitis in a dental technician caused by airborne thiuram exposure. Contact Dermatitis. 2015;73:321–2.

33. Jensen P, Menné T, Thyssen JP. Allergic contact dermatitis in a nurse caused by airborne rubber additives. Contact Dermatitis. 2011;65:54–5.

34. Kanerva L, Alanko K, Jolanki R, Estlander T. Laboratory assistant's occupational allergic airborne contact dermatitis from nickel presenting as rosacea. Eur J Dermatology. 1999;9:397–8.

35. Handfield-Jones S, Boyle J, Harman RR. Contact allergy caused by metal sprays. Contact Dermatitis. 1987;16:44–5.

36. Estlander T, Kari O, Jolanki R, Kanerva L. Occupational allergic contact dermatitis and blepharoconjunctivitis caused by gold. Contact Dermatitis. 1998;38:40–1.

37. Zirwas MJ, Hamann D, Warshaw EM, et al. Epidemic of isothiazolinone allergy in North America: prevalence data from the north American contact dermatitis group, 2013-2014. Dermatitis. 2017;28:204–9.

38. Lundov MD, Mosbech H, Thyssen JP, Menné T, Zachariae C. Two cases of airborne allergic contact dermatitis caused by methylisothiazolinone in paint. Contact Dermatitis. 2011;65:176–9.

39. Amsler E, Aerts O, Raison-Peyron N, et al. Airborne allergic contact dermatitis caused by isothiazolinones in water-based paints: a retrospective study of 44 cases. Contact Dermatitis. 2017;77:163–70.

40. Lundov MD, Kolarik B, Bossi R, Gunnarsen L, Johansen JD. Emission of isothiazolinones from water-based paints. Environ Sci Technol. 2014;48:6989–94.

41. Alarcón M, Herrera-Mozo I, Nogué S, Sanz-Gallen P. Occupational airborne contact dermatitis from pro-

ton pump inhibitors. Immunol: Curr. Allergy Clin; 2014. p. 27.

42. Corazza M, Baldo F, Osti F, Virgili A. Airborne allergic contact dermatitis due to budesonide from professional exposure. Contact Dermatitis. 2008;59:318–9.

43. Friis UF, Menné T, Flyvholm MA, Bonde JPE, Johansen JD. Occupational allergic contact dermatitis diagnosed by a systematic stepwise exposure assessment of allergens in the work environment. Contact Dermatitis. 2013;69:153–63.

44. Higuero NC, Igea JM, de la Hoz B. Latex allergy: position paper. J Investig Allergol Clin Immunol. 2012;22:313–30.

45. Liu C, Ko M-J, Lin R-Y, Lee M-S. Fiberglass (glass wool) dermatitis: rapid diagnoses using simple polarized microscope. Dermatologica Sin. 2020;38:256.

46. Company-Quiroga J, Alique-García S, Esteban-Garrido E, Rojas-Farias FE, Garrido-Ríos AA, Córdoba S, Borbujo J. Skin stripping technique: a diagnostic clue for fiberglass dermatitis. J Am Acad Dermatol. 2019;80:e141–2.

47. Marks R, Dawber RP. Skin surface biopsy: an improved technique for the examination of the horny layer. Br J Dermatol. 1971;84:117–23.

48. Walls AC, Silvestri DL. Prevention of airborne propolis-induced allergic contact dermatitis with barrier cream. Dermat contact, atopic, Occup drug. 2012;23:128–9.

49. Verma KK, Sethuraman G, Kalavani M. Weekly azathioprine pulse versus daily azathioprine in the treatment of Parthenium dermatitis: a non-inferiority randomized controlled study. Indian J Dermatol Venereol Leprol. 2015;81:251–6.

50. Sharma VK, Bhat R, Sethuraman G, Manchanda Y. Treatment of parthenium dermatitis with methotrexate. Contact Dermatitis. 2007;57:118–9.

51. Verma KK, Bhari N, Kutar BMRN. Rapid response to ciclosporin in patients with Parthenium dermatitis: a preliminary study. Contact Dermatitis. 2021;84:134–6.

Occupational Contact Dermatitis and Photodermatosis in the Agricultural Environment

Patricia Pérez-Feal [iD]
and Virginia Fernández-Redondo [iD]

Abbreviations

ACD	allergic contact dermatitis
CAD	actinic chronic dermatitis
CD	contact dermatitis
CU	contact urticaria
EHO	Environmental Health Officer.
EU	European Union
IARC	International Agency for Research on Cancer
ICD	irritant contact dermatitis
ICD-10	International Statistical Classification of Diseases and Related Health Problems
ISO	Internationals Organization for Standardization
NMSC	nonmelanoma skin cancer
OSC	occupational skin cancer
PCC	professional cutaneous cancer
PCD	protein contact dermatitis
US EPA	US Environmental Protection Agency
UVR	ultraviolet radiation
WHO	World Health Organization

P. Pérez-Feal (✉) · V. Fernández-Redondo
Complexo Hospitalario Universitario de Santiago de
Compostela, A Coruña, Spain

Introduction

Occupational Dermatosis are, by definition, skin diseases directly caused or aggravated by work. They are defined by the legislation of each country [1, 2]. They are one of the most frequent occupational diseases, constituting 50% of them [3].

The agricultural sector is divided into several subsectors, such as crops, forestry, cereal production or beekeeping, combination with livestock or forestry work, among others [4]. Therefore, there are plenty of dermatosis due to different triggers such as the use of pesticides and fertilizers, sun exposure, infections and the toxic or allergic power of the plants themselves [5]. Likewise, endogenous factors -such as atopic dermatitis- and exogenous factors -humidity, cold, heat, or friction- contribute in their appearance [6].

In this chapter, we will describe **Contact Dermatitis (CD)** mainly caused by production, harvesting and handling of vegetables. In addition, a brief reference will be made to the forestry / timber sector and **Photodermatoses**.

The incidence is not as well-known as in other professions due to the inherent characteristics of this work, whether if it is carried out on large automated farms or on smaller ones [3]. In the study by Park et al. [3] an incidence of 9.6% in male farmers and 14.4% in women is described. Moreover, difficult access to specialized healthcare units in the rural environment may have an

© The Author(s), under exclusive license to Springer Nature Switzerland AG 2023
A. M. Giménez-Arnau, H. I. Maibach (eds.), *Handbook of Occupational Dermatoses*, Updates in
Clinical Dermatology, https://doi.org/10.1007/978-3-031-22727-1_12

influence on it. In addition, the negative economic impact they have on both the individual and society must be taken into account [6].

Contact Dermatitis (CD)

Occupational contact dermatitis (OCD) is an eczematous acute or chronic inflammatory response. It predominantly affects the hands or body surface not covered by clothing. OCD can be **irritative or toxic (ICD)** when it appears after contact with a specific substance at a specific concentration and for a sufficient time to cause injury. It is the most common type of CD. On other occasions, this response is the result of a type IV-immune reaction and we will call it **allergic contact dermatitis (ACD)**. In both cases, the substances depending on their physicochemical characteristics can be dispersed in the air causing **airborne dermatitis**.

Irritants or allergens can be found anywhere in plants and can be modified by pesticides, soil composition and climatic influence.

Identification through the healthcare provider is not easy due to lack of botanical knowledge, ignorance of popular names, and chemical products used alone or in combination. We must add the ignorance on the part of the worker and the system of application of these products in powder, solution, or fumigation. An example is the sensitization to popular resin used to seal cracks in hives described in beekeepers.

It is of special interest the relationship between health and pesticide use. Considered as persistent organic pollutants resistant to degradation, their use is regulated worldwide. Side effects are well-known in people exposed to them, which include systemic processes, (such as neurotoxicity and endocrine disorders) and dermatological processes.

Contact Dermatitis by Pesticides

Under this denomination are included the products mentioned in Table 12.1, categorized in a specific way according to the desired protection

Table 12.1 Pesticides. Modified from Lidén, C. (2011) [7]

Pesticides	Products included
Herbicides and desiccants	– Glyphosate: Agriculture, public areas, domestic use. – Paraquat: Non-selective. Employed in weed control. – 2,4D and 2,4,5-T: Phenoxy acid herbicides. Broad-leaved and defoliant plants.
Insecticides	– Pyrethrins: Botanical pesticides obtained from *chrysanthemum cinerariaefolium*. – Pyrethroids: Synthetic. Longer duration and less toxic. – Organophosphorous pesticides: Malathion and parathion. – DDT and lindane: Chlorinated hydrocarbons. – Nicotine: Less used. – Rotenone: Acaricidal properties. – Arsenic.
Fungicides	– Benomil: Fruits, nuts, vegetables, crops and ornamental flowers. – Captan. – Chlorothalonil: Vegetables, fruits, flowers, trees, bananas. – Difolatan. – Fluazinam. – Mancozeb[a] – Maneb[a] – Thiram[a] – Zineb[a] – Sulfur: Also acaricide. – Triphenyltin hydroxide. – Tributyltin oxide. – Copper sulfate.
Repellent	– N,N-diethyl-m-toluamide (DEET): Mosquito repellent.
Rodenticides	– Warfarine y ANTU: Rat y mice.
Preservantives	– Dimethyl fumarate: Wood protector. – Chlorothalonil: Wood and paint protector. – Glutaraldehyde: Limicide and additive for the production of paper. – 5-chloro-2-methylisothiazole-3-1 / 2-methylisothiazole-3-1 (MCI / MI): Used with arsenic, chromium and copper for wood preservation. Limicidal. – Tributilin oxide: Wood preservative, antifouling paints. – Silver and silver salts.
Fumigants	– Ethylene oxide/epoxy ethane: Also sterilizing. – Methyl bromide. – Acrylonitrile. – Metam sodium/methylisocyanate.

[a] Part of the dithiocarbamate group

for the crops. Most are chemicals used to control pests and plants and seeds diseases. They are usually synthetic products, although some may have a biological origin. Their actives principles are often designated with respect to the International Organization for Standardization (ISO).

Currently, up to 750 active ingredients are used as pesticides on plant crops [7]. There are regulations in different countries on the substances that can compose them, methods, indications, application periods, education and protective equipment for workers -for instance, European Union, Directive 91/414 / EEC on plant protection products and Directive 98/8 / EC on biocidal products.

The most exposed workers are those in intensive agriculture in greenhouses and large surfaces, as well as flower and tree growers [7]. However, the incidence is unknown due to the working conditions of farmers and ranchers, seasonality, climatic differences and diversity between countries in terms of health care. Workers' contact with these products is usually accidental, with the skin being the main route of absorption and it is favored by occlusion, skin damage, concentration, contact time, area, humidity, and temperature [5, 7]. It should be noted that some pesticides can persist on the skin for a considerable period of time. An example is chlordane and dieldrin, which can last up to 2 years [8].

Skin reactions can be irritative, allergic (mainly due to fungicides and insecticides), airborne and photoallergic [5]. They especially affect areas devoid of clothing. For this reason, the most frequent location is the face, followed by the neck, forearms, hands, trunk, and extremities [9]. In addition, they can contaminate clothing and cause widespread reactions. Moreover, through transcutaneous absorption or inhalation, pesticides can cause very serious conditions (e.g., paraquat and organophosphates).

Furthermore, the WHO and IARC define a probable carcinogenic effect in the case of the glyphosate herbicide commonly used in genetically modified crops. Malathion, diazinon, tetrachlorvinphos, and parathion have also been linked to non-Hodgkin lymphoma and prostate neoplasms, but have been banned or restricted for more than 30 years [7]. Notably, chlorpyrifos, an organophosphate insecticide, has been shown to promote obesity by inhibiting diet-induced thermogenesis in brown adipose tissue [10].

Ecological Agriculture consists on optimal use of natural resources without using synthetic chemicals or genetically modified organisms either for compost or to combat pests, achieving organic products while preserves the fertility of the land and respects the environment. In Europe, it is expected in 2030, 25% of the land will be dedicated to organic crops. By that date, it is suggested to use 20% less chemical fertilizers and 50% less phytosanitary products, especially herbicides, bactericides, or fungicides.

Contact Dermatitis by Plants and Flowers

EU represents more than 50% of the world's flowers intake, being Germany the largest consumer, followed by the UK, France, and Italy. The Netherlands is the main supplier of flowers and foliage to other EU member countries. Other major flower suppliers to the EU are Kenya, Colombia, Ecuador and Israel.

Chemical composition and the maintained contact with water favor **irritant contact dermatitis (ICD). Hypersensitivity reactions (ACD)** are less common. More than 300,000 species of plants are known, but the identification of allergens can be complex because they are found in different parts of them and are modified by environmental changes, such as the composition of the soil or the climate. According to DeKoven and Houle [11], we consider a basic knowledge of botany necessary.

In the primary sector, self-employed farmers, gardeners, intensive greenhouse cultivation, the development of ornamental floriculture, the floristry sector, forestry workers, and food handlers are the most frequently affected professionals.

Therefore, we must differentiate food and ornamental plants.

A frequently asked question is whether there is a risk of a systemic contact dermatitis after ingestion of plants in which ADC has previously been diagnosed. In the literature there are several examples, especially referred to sesquiterpene lactones present in lettuce, infusions derived from Asteraceae. In their study of 45 patients with sensitization to sesquiterpene lactones, Lundh et al. [12] did not find a reactivation of the skin condition after an oral challenge with German chamomile. Paulsen [4] carried out a study with the intake of *Taraxacum Officinalis* in sensitized people and the reactivation of hand eczema. She defends that in patients sensitized to plants or their components there may be cross reactions, so there is an unsuspected risk of possible adverse reactions.

If the lesions are caused by insect bites, cereal mites, or waxes, it is called **Pseudophytodermatitis** [13]. A specific case of occupational disease is the intensely itchy, urticarial-looking rash caused by caterpillars, which particularly affects forestry workers. Occasionally, irritation and sensitivity can coexist. For example, the nickel composition of certain Euphorbia species, which usually causes irritative reactions, can give ACD in previously sensitized patients.

Irritative Contact Dermatitis

A large number of plants (wild, alimentary and flowers) can cause "macrotraumatic" injuries by mechanical elements such as thorns, hairs or spicules or trichomes in the ends of their leaves [13]. However, other plants can cause "microtraumas" from their quills. In addition, plants have highly irritating chemical compounds such as calcium oxalate [13]. Cleaning materials, fertilizers, pesticides, plants, woods, and animal secretions are most frequently described. For all these reasons, Frosch & Kügler [14] described the professions related to floriculture, horticulture and food handling as high risk for ICD, especially in greenhouses and food handling.

Clinically (Fig. 12.1), the lesions are usually monomorphic and limited to the area of contact, such as the hands or forearms [15, 16]. It shows as cutaneous xerosis, cracks, hyperkeratosis, edema, erythema, papules, and vesicles. It is characterized by pain, rather than itching. Individual susceptibility, the time of action of the

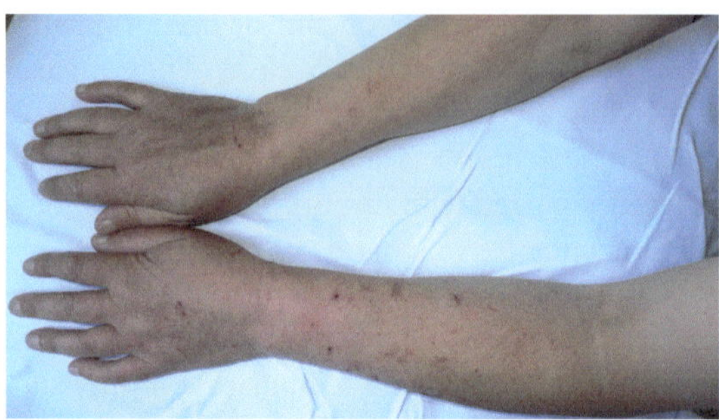

Fig. 12.1 ICD by plants. The lesions are monomorphic and limited to the area of contact

stimulus and the integrity of the epidermis play a fundamental role, favoring the appearance of epidermal necrosis.

Table 12.2 lists the most irritating substances and the species and families most commonly implicated are described below [15].

Amaryllidaceae

The Amaryllidaceae family -more than 1100 plant species from 85 genera- are cultivated for showy flowers. Among them, daffodils are the most common. The so-called "daffodil itch" is caused by calcium oxalate crystals contained in the external scales of the bulbs, leaves, petals, and in the sap obtained after cutting the stems. It develops on the pads, back of the hands (simulating a "tulip finger" but with less severity) and anterior face of the wrist, and can affect the neck, face, and genitals. Symptoms increase during planting and flowering. Its cause is mainly irritative, but allergic reactions can be involved.

Anacardiaceae

The best known is Poison ivy, especially in the USA. They grow on other trees, walls, or rocks. The symptoms appear a few hours or days after contact, and are characteristic: redness, papules, lesions of liquid content with a tendency to linear arrangement on the face and exposed areas [16].

Asparagaceae

This family is known for its irritating power due to calcium oxalate, saponins, and proteases.

Recently, Goméz Torrijos et al. [17] have described a gardener with a facial rash due to

Table 12.2 Most common plants implicated in contact dermatitis

Spe	Species	Family	Sensitizing/Irritative
Garlic	*Allium sativum*	Amarylidaceae	Sensitizing
Potato	*Solanum tuberosum; L.*	Solanaceae	Sensitizing
Carrot	*Daucus carota*	Apiaceae	Sensitizing
Celery	*Apium graveolens*	Apiaceae	Sensitizing
Parsnip	*Pastinaca sativa*	Apiaceae	Sensitizing
Tomato	*Solanum lycopersicum*	Solanaceae	Sensitizing
Pepper	*Capsicum annuum*	Solanaceae	Sensitizing
Kiwi	*Actinidia deliciosa*	Actinidiaceae	Sensitizing
Apple	*Malus domestica*	Rosaceae	Sensitizing
Pineapple	*Ananas cosmosus*	Bromeliaceae	Irritant
Strawberry	*Fragaria*	Rosaceae	Sensitizing
Prickly pear	*Opuntia ficus*	Cactaceae	Irritant
Cayenne	*Capsicum frutescens L.*	Solanaceae	Irritant
Mustard	*Bassica nigra*	Brassicaceae	Irritant
Tulip	*Tulipa spp*	Liliaceae	Sensitizing
Ivy	*Hedera helix*	Araliaceae	Sensitizing
Daffodil	*Narcissus*	Amarylidaceae	Irritant
Ficus benjamina	*Ficus benjamina*	Moraceae	Sensitizing
Poinsettia	*Euphorbia pulcherrima*	Euphorbiaceae	Irritant
Wicker	*Salix vimminalis.*	Salicaceae	Irritant
Agave	*Agave Americana*	Asparagaceae	Irritant
Hyacinth	*Hyacinthus orientalis L.*	Asparagaceae	Irritant
Anemone	*Anemone pavonina*	Ranunculaceae	Irritant
Poison ivy	*Toxicodendron radicans*	Anacardiaceae	Irritant

contact with *Agave americana L* (The Century Plant) after pruning with a chainsaw. They detected positivity by patch test a solution of 30% sap in aqueous solution and in pet. This reaction had not been previously described.

We highlight the genus *Hyacinthus L.*, which has calcium oxalate crystals in the bulb and causes very itchy lesions, also known as "hyacinth scabies".

In addition, it has s."sitizing power in the oil extracted from its flowers for cosmetic uses, due to its content in eugenol.

Cactaceae

Prickly pear (*Opuntia ficus indica*), cultivated in temperated areas, presents brush-forming cactys spines. Its pads and fruit have shorter tufts of hair called glochids causing mechanical trauma. It can produce the so-called sabra dermatitis, characterized by asymptomatic papules of 2–5 millimeters with a central pointed black dot at the site of the lesion, with subsequent formation of pustules and vesicles, which can be confused with scabies.

Cannabinaceae

It is well-known the hop picker rash, *Humulus lupulus L.*, a widely cultivated product. They usually cause irritative dermatitis, occasionally allergic, especially when the hop cones are separated from the stem. In wet climates, the spines become firmer and the skin is macerated, so that the mechanical abrasion caused by the hairs of the plant stem is necessary for the development of a vesicular dermatitis of the exposed skin: hands, wrists, face, and genitalia. A purpuric rash on the legs has also been described.

Euphorbiaceae

The members of this family can produce irritative dermatitis with vesicles, ulcers, or necrosis. About 2000 species are known [18, 19], like Poinsettia.

Allergic Contact Dermatitis (ACD)

The prevalence of ACD caused by plants is a reflection of the geographical distribution of wild and cultivated plants, as well as their use for ornamental, culinary, or medicinal purposes [18]. Sensitizing substances can be found in the leaves, flower petals or in the bulb. For this reason, farmers, florists, gardeners or woodworkers are the professions most exposed. Acute reactions frequently occur with involvement of exposed areas (hands, forearms, eyelids, and sometimes genitalia if the allergen is carried on clothing or hands). The lesions are diffuse, but they can spread to the unexposed area. After the initial maculopapular or vesicular involvement, blisters or even erythroderma can develop.

Chronically, it can present as a fissured and hyperkeratotic dermatitis that predominantly affects the fingertips, more painful than itchy. It is typical of tulip, narcissus, or Alstroemeria pickers (Fig. 12.2). It can involve the nails.

It is important to differentiate the most affected sectors, such as production, collection, and handling. Likewise, the recognition of specific patterns and the most frequent sensitizing substances that are exposed in the Tables 12.2 and 12.3 will facilitate a diagnosis.

Alliaceae

Garlic (*Allium sativum*) is used as a food condiment or for medical purposes. Its main allergen is diallyl sulfur. It mainly affects the first three fingers of the non-dominant hand (Fig. 12.3), so chefs and kitchen assistants are the most affected workers -especially in the Mediterranean area.

Alstroemeriaceae

Alstroemeria and Liliacea families contain the same allergen, tulipalin A, present in the bulbs

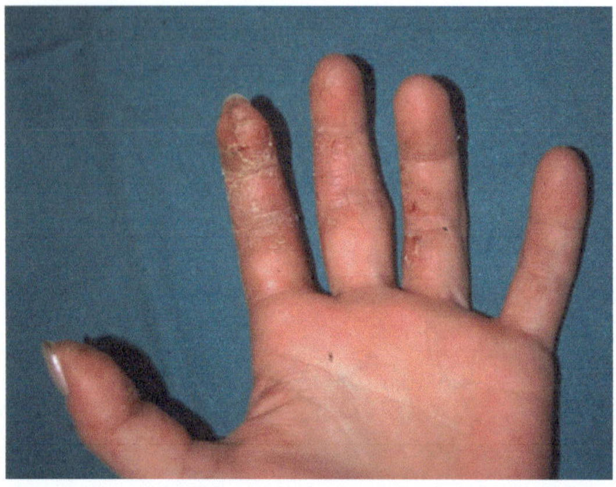

Fig. 12.2 ACD by Alstroemeria: lesions on the fingertips, preferably in the non-dominant hand

Table 12.3 Allergens in plants with sensitizing power

Chemical Group	Family	Allergen	Uses
Hidroquinone/ Benzoquinone	Hidrofoliaceae Primulaceae Orquideaceae Litraceae	Geranylhydroquinone Geranylbenzoquinone Primine	Wild Ornamental Woods Cosmetic
Sesquiterpenic lactones	Compositae (Asterraceae) Frunalliaceae	Alfa-metilen-gamma-butirolactone Frunalolide Costunolide	Wild Ornamental Food Mosses Lichens
Phenols	Anacardiaceae Ginkgcoaceae Araceae Ptroteaceae	Catechol Resorcinal	Wild Ornamental Food
Tulipalines	Liliaceae Alstroemeriaceae	Tulipaline A Tulipaline B	Ornamental
Disulfides	Aliaceae	Diallyldosulfide Allicin	Food
Flavoring	Lamiaceae Mirtaceae Fabaceae Laureaceae	Geraniol Linalol Eugenol Citral Basalm of Peru Própolis	Cosmetics Fragrances Food Topical drugs

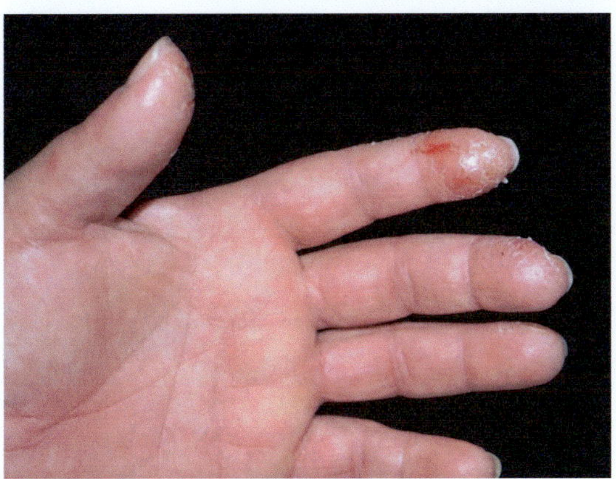

Fig. 12.3 ACD by garlic. It is a chronic, fissured and scaly, pruritic pulpitis that affects the fingers of the hand that hold the garlic cloves to be cut (thumb, index and middle of the non-dominant hand)

and petals, rich in alpha-methylene-gamma-butyrolactone.

It presents with lesions on the fingertips that cause functional impotence, preferably in the non-dominant hand.

Compositae

More than 25,000 species belong to this family of decorative, wild and food plants. The most common allergen are dehydrocostus lactone, alantolactone, costunolide, and parthenolide.

Chronic exposure induces a dermatitis with outbreaks and it can lead to lichenified dermatitis. In addition, it can cause airborne dermatitis that simulates photodermatitis, especially ragweed, for which certain environmental conditions such as arid and hot climates are needed. Other clinical forms described are seborrhea and seborrheic dermatitis [20].

Among the affected workers, flower growers stand out (those dedicated to the cultivation of chrysanthemums [21], horticulturists, cooks and peasants stand out.

Another relevant factor is the cultivation and use of herbs for medicinal use, frequent in folk medicine or in herbal shops. *Artemisia* (300 species, Compositae family) is used as an anti-inflammatory. However, this plant is also found in North America and Europe, being used as an antipruritic and astringent. Another example is *Calendula*, used as an ingredient in different products to treat eczema.

Paulsen & Andersen [22] propose in their review to use of the specific series of plants confirm diagnosis, in addition to specific ethereal extracts incorporated into 3% pet. That was motivated by the wide cultivation of these ornamental plants. These authors specify the allergens to study if there is a suspicion of an allergy to Compositae are: sesquiterpene lactone mix 0.1 pet., Parthenolide, 0.1% pet and compositae mix 6% pet.

Liliacea

Tulipalin A is rich in alpha-methylene-gamma-butyrolactone, an allergen in this family. It is found mainly in flowers and leaves. In bulb workers, the prevalence is up to 30% [23]. Activities with the highest risk of suffering from contact dermatitis are during the planting and harvesting of bulbs. Exposure to sap in these processes is the cause of the symptoms, worsened by continuous maceration [23].

They can cause a hyperkeratotic, fissured and painful eczema that affects the free edge of the nails, extending to the fingertips and periungual region, giving rise to the pattern known as "tulip finger". Characteristically, it is located on the first three fingers of the hand, although it can affect other body regions such as the face, always frequently affecting the eyelids or the entire body (tulip fire).

Aloe vera (*Aloe barbadensis Miller*) belongs to the Liliaceae family. The bark of the leaves contains aloin, Aloe-emodin and barbaloin, anthraquinones with properistaltic and antibiotic properties.

Primulaceae

Within this family, the *Primula obconcica L.*, cultivated as a decorative plant, stands out. It was a frequent cause of ADC in Europe, although it has decreased in frequency in recent years due to genetic modification.

The clinic is characterized by linear and vesicular dermatitis on fingers, hands, and forearms, also affecting other exposed surfaces. The causative allergen is primine (2-methoxy-6-pentyl-

1,4-benzoquinone) found in the glandular trichomes of leaves.

Airborne Dermatitis

Sometimes dermatitis occurs in areas not covered by clothing, especially the face, neck, presternal region and upper extremities, caused by particles present in the atmosphere. They can be irritating or allergic. The differential diagnosis is established with photodermatoses, but in airborne dermatitis the lesions extend to areas protected from the sun such as the retroauricular region, the eyelids, the submental region and even the scalp (Fig. 12.4). In sensitized people, the evolution to Chronic Actinic Dermatitis (persistent light reaction described by Hawk et Magnus more than 30 years ago) is frequent [24].

Middle-aged men dedicated to agriculture and gardening are the most affected groups, being the Compositae, Frullanias, and Lichen varieties the ones that trigger it most frequently, due to their exposure to pollen or pulverized materials derived from dead plants.

Patients sensitized to sesquiterpene lactones are especially predisposed. In India, the allergy caused by *Parthenium hysterophorus* affects the prevalence of CAD. Due to the intensity of the dermatitis, Verma et al. [25] propose an algorithm for its evaluation. In refractory cases, oral treatment with cyclosporine or azathioprine is used, in addition to topical corticoids and sun protection filters.

Unsuspected vegetables can be the cause of this morphological pattern, for example, the artichoke (*Artichoque thistle*) with allergens in the leaves and yet with few published professional cases.

It is necessary to use the standard markers with Lactonas mix and Compositae mix (see Appendix 1), present in specific series of plants, and to complete the study in specialized units with different portions of the suspect plants contributed by the patient (Fig. 12.5).

Contact Dermatitis due to Spices

Spices are dried and processed variants of barks, roots, seeds, and fruits of different crops. In recent years, large plantations have been developed, mostly in India. Raw spices are subjected to pulverizing, crushing, and sieving procedures to obtain a powdery consistency. These procedures lead to the release of suspended volatiles particles, creating a niche for different possibilities of occupational exposure in the processing industries.

Spices have irritants and pharmacologically active ingredients that can activate the immune response, such as capsaicin, vanilloids in hot spices (black pepper, pepper, cayenne, and chili),

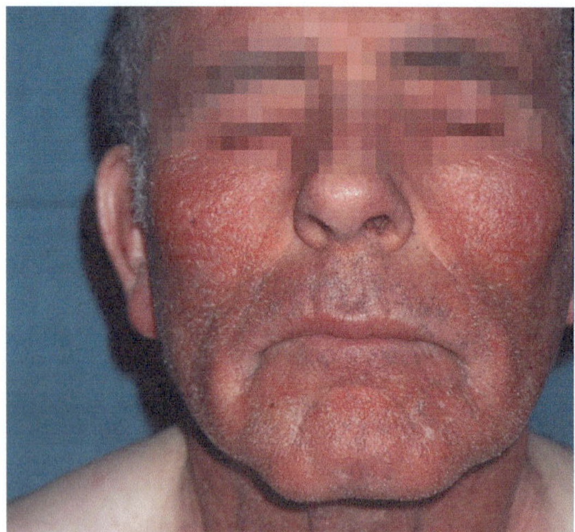

Fig. 12.4 ACD by sesquiterpene lactones. It appears as an airborne dermatitis, eczematous, located in the exposed areas and respecting the palpebral area

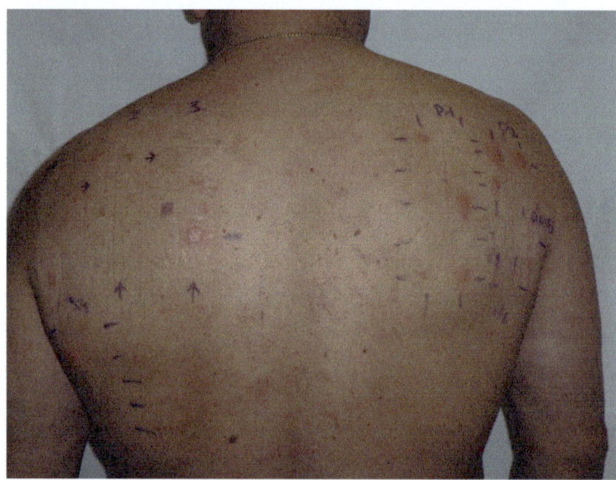

Fig. 12.5 ACD by plants. The image shows the reading after performing the patch tests (labeled 1 to 4) and the plant series (labeled P1 and P2). The positivity manifests in this case as erythema and edema

cinnamic aldehyde, among others. In Europe, laurel has been implicated as the main trigger, while in America pepper, nutmeg, cinnamon, cloves, or vanilla stand out [16].

CD can manifest as contact urticaria (for example, by cinnamic aldehyde), airborne dermatitis, irritant, or allergic contact dermatitis (mainly mediated by the essential oils they contain) [26]. The most frequent clinical manifestation is hand eczema [11].

Protein Contact Dermatitis (PCD)

It is an itchy, eczematous-looking allergic reaction caused by proteins in the region in contact with the plant. A type I hypersensitivity reaction is involved, so the patch test is usually negative, although in some cases, a combination of type I and IV reaction have been described.

It usually affects the upper extremities (hands and feet) shortly after contact with the suspected substance. Amaro and Goossens [27] classify plants, fruits, vegetables, and species in group I, describing the most frequent.

The differential diagnosis has to be made with contact urticaria, although unlike this there is usually no systemic manifestation. For its definitive diagnosis, a prick-test or the prick-by-prick test must be performed.

Non-eczematous Reactions due to Contact with Plants

Other reactions in contact with plants such as **non-immunological contact urticaria** have been described [27–30]. In this case, the lesions appear early and they are characterized by the presence of hives that disappear in a short time. *Urtica dioica* (Urticaceae), rich in histamine, is a representative example.

Immunological contact urticaria (see chap. 4) corresponds to an immediate hypersensitivity reaction, type I, and has been associated with plants such as certain species of Umbelliferae, Liliaceae (asparagus, *Asparagus officinalis*), Coffea, Solanaceae (*Nicotiana tabacum*), derivatives of cinnamic acid - cinnamon - and spices such as pepper (*Capsicum annuum*). Potatoes, kiwi, or apple are more frequent in users.

This type of response is more common in patients with chronic hand eczema and a history of atopic disease. The most affected professions are flower growers, florists, and food handlers. Kanerva et al. [28] associated plants and flowers with 10% of professional-type contact urticarias 25 years ago.

The diagnosis is based on the directed clinical history, prick-test, scratch test and serological studies that confirm positivity for specific IgE. The main differential diagnosis is with Protein Contact Dermatitis.

Another form of non-eczematous adverse reaction produced in this area is **Erythema multiforme-like**. The "on target" papular and erythematous lesions are located in areas not protected by clothing and even around more eczematous reactions and may appear simultaneously or days later. Contact with exotic woods as *Machaerium scleroxylon*, herbal medicine, poison ivy, primine, sesquiterpene lactones and quinolones as well as species (capsicum) are the most described triggers.

Wood Contact Dermatitis

ACD is described in connection with the handling of exotic woods [31]. Its incidence is low even in producing countries such as Central Africa, Asia, and Brazil. The most common allergens are listed in Table 12.4. Forest workers, lumberjacks, carpenters, cabinetmakers, artisans or those engaged in civil construction may be affected.

The minor components of woods such as resins, terpenes, oils, phenols, formic acid and nitrogenous substances [11] are the most sensitizing ones.

Continued trauma without adequate personal protective equipment favors the penetration of the most common allergens, such as alkaloids, glycosides, phenols, flavonoids, saponins and, more frequently, quinones. Allergens are usually found in the heartwood.

Airborne dermatitis is a frequent clinical form in these workers. The hands are affected in the

Table 12.4 Allergic Contac dermatitis: woods

Common name	Species	Family	Alllergen
Red cedar	*Thuja plicata*	Cupressaceae	Tuyaplicina
Ebony	*Diospyrum ebenum*	Ebenaceae	Naphtoquinone
Sucupira	*Bowdichia nítida*	Leguminosae	2–6 Dimethoxybenzoquinone
Pao ferro	*Machaeriuum sclerxylon*		3-4dimethoxyDimethoxidalbergione
Rosewood	*Dalbergia latifolia*		Dalbergiona
Cocobolo	*Dalbergia nigra*		Dimethoxidalbergione
	Dalbergia retusa		Obtusaquinone. 4-methoxidalbergione
Iroko	*Choloforo excelsa*	Moraceae	Chloroforin
Eucalyptus	*Eucaliptus*	Myrtaceae	1,8cineole
			Limonene.
Pine tree	*Pinus pinaster*	Pinaceae	Alphapinene
			Betapinene
			Rosin.
Teak	*Tectonia grandis*	Verbenaceae	Deoxylapacol.
			Lapacol.

first place and progressively spread to the face, neck, and other areas not protected by clothing. Impregnation of clothes can cause generalized eruptions or adopt a pattern of atopic dermatitis. This is due to the fine dust that is generated in the woodworking processes and accumulates on clothing, especially on the neck and in the upper area of the socks.

A marker is not considered in baseline series because of the possibility of active sensitization. It has been proposed to apply as such sawdust from the suspect wood to 10% in pet, to use essential oils (for example, Eucalyptol 2% pet) or extracts in ether at different dilutions, but this requires study in specialized units.

Photodermatosis in the Primary Sector

The term **Photodermatosis** defines an exaggerated response to ultraviolet radiation that interacts with a chemical substance (chromophore) without an immunological basis [32], affecting areas not protected by clothing. It can be due to genetic, metabolic, acquired, and idiopathic causes [32–34].

Phytophotodermatosis is an inflammatory dermatosis caused by interaction between ultraviolet A radiation (UVA: 320 to 400 nanometers) and contact with a specific plant. They are con-

sidered exogenous (due to chemical substances) and can also manifest as **airborne** reactions, either **phototoxic**, which are the most frequent, or **photoallergic**.

Sometimes, this reaction is due to parasites, pesticides and fungicides, present in plants (*Sclerotinia sclerotiorum*) that can present furocoumarins and we call **Pseudophyto-photodermatitis.**

In addition to a complete medical history, knowledge of the workplace, botanical identification and complementary tests to rule out other photodermatoses, a photobiological study that includes photopatch test is necessary [33].

Phytophotodermatosis: Phototoxicity

Phytophotodermatoses present a direct dose-response relationship between the intensity of the reaction, the concentration of furocoumarins (psoralens) and anthraquinone derivatives present in the plant and the amount of radiation of a certain wavelength. Lesions can appear from a few hours after contact to 48 hours later and are characterized by pain and burning.

Different wild species such as *Ammi majus* and *Heracleum sphondylium*, the fig tree (*Ficus carica L*) and many edible vegetables (celery, carrot, and parsley among others) are involved in this type of reaction (Table 12.5). Citrus fruits

Table 12.5 Most frequent plants that produce phytophotodermatosis

Family/ Common name	Species	Reaction
Apiaceae: *Ammi majus* Hercules bush Angelica Celery Carrot Poinsettia Wild plants (wild parsnip) Araliaceae: Common ivy	*Ammi majus L Heracleum sphondyllium L, Angelica archangelicaL L, Apium graveolens L Deucus carotae Euphorbia pulcherrima Pastinaca sativa Hedera helix*	Phototoxic: Psoralen
Rutaceae: Ruda Orange Lime Lemon Bergamot Mokihana White diptamus	*Ruta graveolens Citrus sinensis C. aurantium C. limon C. bergamia Pelea anisata Diptamnus alba L*	Phototoxic: Psoralen ICD ACD
Fabaceae: Crown	*Psoralea coryfolia*	Phototoxic: Psoralen
Moraceae: Fig	*Ficus caricaL*	Phototoxic: Psoralen Photoallergy ICD
Hypericaceae: St. John's wort	*Hypericum perforatum L*	Phototoxic: Hypericin (visible light: 450-600nnm)
Caparidaceae: Caper	*Cleome spinosa*	Phototoxic: Coumarin ICD

also contain psoralens and cases of occupational phototoxicity and in users have been described, affecting the lips after ingestion of orange and / or lemons and subsequent sun exposure. Limonene composition can also cause an allergic and photoallergic reaction, although it is more frequent in the perfumery industry or in the manufacture of liquors.

The most affected workers are farmers, gardeners, florists, cooks, bartenders, and packers [33, 34]. Factors such as damp skin, friction, sweating, and heat can precipitate the appearance of this reaction. Darker-skinned workers are less affected, although they suffer the greatest risk of hyperpigmentation [34].

A **differential diagnosis** must be made in this professional group with allergic contact dermati-

tis, irritant contact dermatitis, bullous impetigo, stings, and burns.

The most common clinical forms are described below.

Dermatitis of the Meadows (Dermatitis Bullosa Pratensis of Oppenheim)

Sun exposure, heat, sweat, or microtrauma intensify the penetration of furocoumarins. It can affect any race. Workers who have more contact with plants, fruits, or vegetables are the most predisposed.

Its symptoms are characteristic and acute −24 hours after sun exposure-: bullous and vesicular lesions on an erythematous surface resembling burns (Fig. 12.6). Its morphology is varied, depending on where the furocoumarins are found, thus linear lesions can be observed, in drops, in plaque. They appear exclusively in contact areas not protected by clothing and they usually present hyperpigmentation.

Berloque Dermatitis

Phototoxic reaction characterized by mottled or linear hyperpigmentation that appears on photo-exposed areas of skin that have been in contact with plants or essential oils. The most affected areas are the sides of the neck, neckline area and wrists. Bergamot oil, rich in 5-methoxyopsoralen, used in the manufacture of fragrances is a representative example [35, 36].

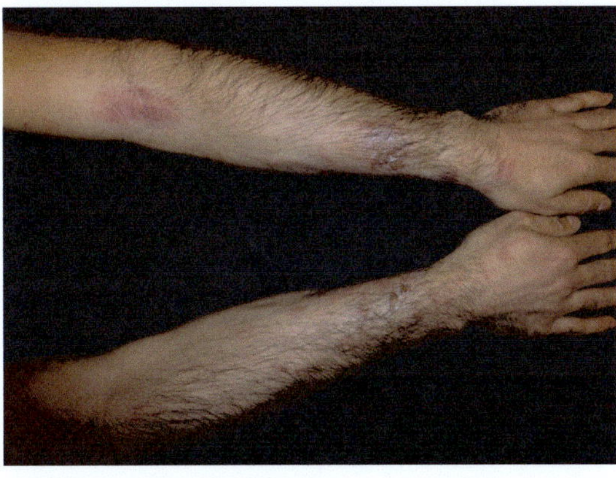

Fig. 12.6 Phytophotodermatosis. It is characterized by the appearance of erythematous, edematous and blistering lesions in the exposed areas

Phytophotodermatosis: Photoallergy

They have been described in relation to species belonging to the Compositae family, especially *Parthenium hysterophorus* and *Rutaceae* (citrus).

There are references of these reactions in growers and processors of oranges in relation to allergens present in their peel such as D-Limonene, Citronellal, or Citral. It is wide used in food, pastry, perfumery, or the manufacture of juices and liquors.

Photosensitivity reactions are also known in farmers with the use of olaquindox, an antibiotic used in the preparation of animal feed (pigs).

Although they are not frequent, photoallergy reactions have been described in contact with wood and sawdust, with carpenters, cabinetmakers, lumberjacks and artisans being the most affected workers. Species of the family Moraceae and Proteaceae, rich in furocoumarins, have been implicated.

Clinically, they are characterized by eczematous reactions or lichenoid papules with a rapid onset after exposure. These lesions can exceed the exposed area and previously affected areas can flare up 1–2 days after exposure.

Photosensitivity may persist, which is called **chronic actinic dermatitis** (CAD) with an intolerance to sunlight (old persistent light reactors) [37]. It essentially affects middle-aged men with a sensitization to sesquiterpene lactones present in the Compositae family and to fragrances.

Diagnosis is made through a detailed medical history and must be completed with patch, photopatch, and photobiological studies.

Given the selective affectation in preferential areas not covered by clothing and of summer presentation, they have to be differentiated from airborne dermatitis, photoaggravation (Methylisothiazolinone), ACD or contact photoallergy by drugs (NSAIDs).

In the case of light-persistent reactors, treatment is difficult. The protocols are varied and topical and systemic corticosteroids, immunosuppressants, and photochemotherapy have been used.

Professional Cancer in the Agricultural Sector

Occupational skin cancer (OSC) is a group of skin neoplasms attributable to exposure to carcinogenic factors in the workplace [38]. We differentiate two groups of skin cancer: melanoma (ICD-10: C43) and non-melanocytic skin cancer (NMSC) (ICD-10: C44). According to the exposoma concept, the profession and other external factors that may influence the appearance of neoplasms must be included.

Ultraviolet radiation (UVR) has been classified as carcinogenic (Group I) in humans since 1992. UVR B has been shown to be the main carcinogen (290–320 nm). Other predisposing factors such as phototype, hours of sunshine, and latitude are essential in epidemiological studies [38]. Other triggers are chemicals present in pesticides, such as paraquat, or naturally in water or in soils such as arsenic and its derivatives. The most predisposed professions are: farmers, ranchers, gardeners, shepherds, foresters, and loggers [38–40].

The early diagnosis of initial lesions such as actinic cheilitis [41–43] or actinic keratoses [39] together with better benefits in terms of prevention and treatment of them pose a therapeutic challenge to reduce their incidence. Nonmelanoma skin cancer [44, 45] (see Chap. 5) is the most common. The increase in the incidence of melanoma [46] in this professional group has been related to actinic exposure and the use of pesticides [47, 48]. Dennis et al. [47], described its relationship with cutaneous melanoma, highlighting the association of sun exposure and use of pesticides, especially Maneb / Mancoceb and Parathion. Sanganelli et al. [48] carried out a systematic review and meta-analysis of the literature on the increase in this tumor and exposure to pesticides.

Contact Dermatitis Diagnose

It is Based on a medical history and botanical identification of the suspected plant and the chemical involved. The patch test of the European and North American standard series contains two mixes: sesquiterpene lactones (alantolactone, costunolide, dehydrocostus lactone) and compositae mix (*Anthemis Nobilis, Chamomilla Recutita, Achillea Millefolium, Tabnacetum Vulgare, Arnica Montana, Parthenolide*), as well as Myroxilon balsamum from Peru, rosin and propolis. It can be completed with specific plant series, different essential oils, fragrances and plant extracts.

Prevention

Protection tips have been published by large organizations such as EHO, US EPA and Crop Life International. In workers in contact with flowers and plants, this requires knowledge of the morphological and botanical characteristics of the plants with which they work, as well as informing workers of this effect, minimizing the time of exposure as necessary. Sun exposure should be avoided with clothing and gloves that protect the skin surface and careful grooming after handling plants with known photosensitizing potential. The photoprotectors to be used must incorporate agents such as titanium or zinc dioxide, which are effective against all wavelengths [49].

The use of gloves is usually indicated (nitrile, rubber, 4H, or Barrier laminated gloves offer the best protection. In the case of Alstroemeriaceae, rubber gloves do not protect workers, but the vinyl ones do. Overalls, aprons, raincoats, gloves, hat, boots, mask and goggles, or face shields are also recommended. In addition, it is important that they are used correctly and that they are properly cleaned. However, in countries with fewer resources, having this protective equipment becomes complicated. Furthermore, in conditions of high humidity or heat it is difficult to be able to work under this equipment.

Diagnose

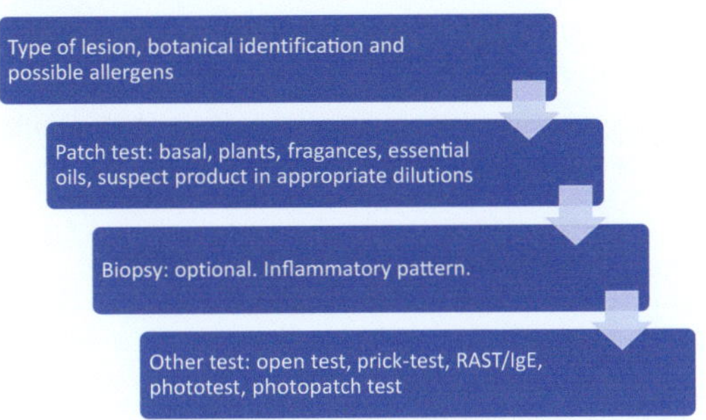

Appendix 1 Standard Allergen Series

Below, we describe the components of the sesquiterpene lactone mix series and compositae mix.

Sesquiterpenic Lactones Mix: 0.1% Pet

Costunolide	0.033% pet
Alantolactone	0.033% pet
Dehydrocostus lactone	0.033% pet

Compositae Mix: 5% or 2.5% Pet

Anthemis nobilis extract	1.2% or 0.6% pet
Chamomilla recutita extract	1.2% or 0.6% pet
Achillea millefolium extract	1.0% or 0.5% pet
Tanacetum vulgare extract	1.0% or 0.5% pet
Arnica Montana extract	0.5% or 0.25%pet
Parthenolide	0.1% or 0.05% pet

Complementary series: plants, fragances, essential oils (www.chemotechnique.com www.smartpractice.com)

Appendix 2 Websites of Interest

- Diagnosis of contact dermatitis due to woods: http//www.fpl.fs.us/research/centers/woodanatomy/
- Diagnosis of contact dermatitis by plants: www.britannica.plant.com

References

1. García-Pérez A, Conde-Salazar L, Giménez-Camarasa JM. Tratado de dermatosis profesionales. Madrid: Eudema; 1987. p. 13.
2. Giménez Camarasa JM. In.Dermatitis de contacto. Madrid: Aula Médica; 1999. p. 283–308.
3. Park H, Sprince NL, Whitten PS, Burmeister LF, Zwerling C. Farm-related dermatoses in Iowa male farmers and wives of farmers: a cross-sectional analysis of the Iowa farm family health and Hazard surveillance project. J Occup Environ Med. 2001;43(4):364–9.
4. Arcangeli G, Traversini V, Tomasini E, Baldassarre A, Lecca LI, Galea RP, et al. Allergic anaphylactic risk in farming activities: a systematic review. Int J Environ Res Public Health. 2020;17(14):4921.
5. Sohrabian S, Maibach H. Contact dermatitis in agriculture. J Agromedicine. 2007;12(1):3–15.
6. Le Coz CJ, Ducombs G, Paulsen E. Plants and plant Products. In: Contact dermatitis. Berlin- Heidelberg: Springer; 2011. p. 873–925.
7. Lidén C. Pesticides. In: Contact dermatitis. Berlin Heidelberg: Springer; 2011. p. 927–36.
8. Kazen C, Bloomer A, Welch R, Oudbier A, Price H. Persistence of pesticides on the hands of some occupationally exposed people. Arch Environ Health. 1974;29(6):315–8.
9. Matsushita T, Nomura S, Wakatsuki T. Epidemiology of contact dermatitis from pesticides in Japan. Contact Dermatitis. 1980;6(4):255–9.
10. Wang B, Tsakiridis EE, Zhang S, Llanos A, Desjardins EM, et al. The pesticide chlorpyrifos promotes obesity by inhibiting diet-induced thermogenesis in brown adipose tissue. Nat Commun. 2021;12(1):5163.
11. DeKoven J, Houle MC. Allergic sensitization to plants. In: Fisher's Contact Dermatitis. BookBaby; 2011. p. 912–1022.
12. Lundh K, Gruvberger B, Persson L, Hindsén M, Zimerson E, et al. Oral provocation of patients allergic to sesquiterpene lactones with German chamomile tea to demonstrate possible systemic allergic dermatitis. Contact Dermatitis. 2020;83(1):8–18.
13. Lovell CR. Phytophototoxic reactions. In: Plants and the skin. Oxford: Blackwell Scientific Publications; 1993. p. 64–95.
14. Frosch PJ, Kügler K. Occupational contact dermatitis. In: Contact dermatitis. Berlin: Springer; 2011. p. 831–9.
15. Lovell CR. Current topics in plant dermatitis. Semin Dermatol. 1996;15(2):113–21.
16. Fernández-Redondo V. Dermatitis de contacto por plantas. In: Dermatitis de contacto. Madrid: Aula Médica; 1999. p. 283–308.
17. Gómez Torrijos E, Gratacós Gómez AR, Gonzalez Jimenez O, Joyanes Romo JB, Cañas AP, et al. Allergic sensitization to the irritant sap of the variegated century plant in a gardener. Contact Dermatitis. 2021;84(3):196–7.
18. Cabanillas M, Fernández-Redondo V, Toribio J. Allergic contact dermatitis to plants in a Spanish dermatology department: a 7-year review. Contact Dermatitis. 2006;55(2):84–91.
19. Worobec SM, Hickey TA, Kinghorn AD, Soejarto DD, West D. Irritant contact dermatitis from an ornamental euphorbia. Contact Dermatitis. 1981;7(1):19–22.
20. Schmidt RJ, Hausen BM, Adams RM, Epstein WL, Mitchell JC. Plants, woods, poison ivy and poison oak, and frullania. Occupational Skin Dis. 1990;2:503–45.
21. Lovell CR. Allergic contact dermatitis due to plants. In: Plants and the skin. Blackwell Scientific Publications Ltd; 1993.
22. Paulsen E, Andersen KE. Contact sensitization to florists' chrysanthemums and marguerite daisies in Denmark: a 21-year experience. Contact Dermatitis. 2020;82(1):18–23.
23. Mei IAF, De Boer EM, Bruynzeel DP. Contact dermatitis in Alstroemeria workers. Occup Med. 1998;48(6):397–404.
24. Hawk JL, Magnus IA. Chronic actinic dermatitis--an idiopathic photosensitivity syndrome including actinic reticuloid and photosensitive eczema [proceedings]. Br J Dermatol. 1979;101:24.
25. Verma KK, Bansal A, Bhari N, Sethuraman G. Parthenium dermatitis severity score to assess clinical severity of disease. Indian J Dermatol. 2017;62(1):85–7.
26. Meding B. Skin symptoms among workers in a spice factory. Contact Dermatitis. 1993;29(4):202–5.
27. Amaro C, Goossens A. Immunological occupational contact urticaria and contact dermatitis from proteins: a review. Contact Dermatitis. 2008;58(2):67–75.
28. Kanerva L, et al. Statistical data on occupational contact urticaria. Contact Dermatitis. 1996;35:229–33.
29. Lukacs, et al. Occupational Contact Urticaria. Contact Dermatitis. 2016;4:195–204.
30. Personen M, Aalto-Korte K. Occupational allergic contact dermatitis and contact urticaria caused by indoor plants in plants keepers. Contact Dermatitis. 2020;83:515–7.
31. Forest Products Laboratory (2021). www.fpl.fs.us/research/centers/woodanatomy/
32. Chang PE. Fitofotodermatitis. In: Fotodermatología. Madrid: Panamericana; 2019. p. 89.

33. DeLeo VA. Photocontact dermatitis. In: Fisher' contact dermatitis. Phoenix: Contact Dermatitis Institute; 1991. p. 633–4.
34. Edward A, Emmett MD. Phototoxicity and photosensitivity reactions. In: Addams' occupational skin disease. Saunders Company; 1990. p. 184–93.
35. Navarro-Maeste M. Dermatosis fotoagravadas In: Fotodermatología Madrid:Panamericana. 2019:99–108.
36. Lovell CR. Phytophototoxic reactions. In: Plants and the skin. Blackwell Scientific Publications Ltd.; 1993. p. 64–95.
37. Wang CX, Belsito DV. Chronic actinic dermatitis revisited. Dermatitis. 2020;31(1):68–74.
38. Zink A, Wurstbauer D, Rotter M, Wildner M, Biedermann T. Do outdoor workers know their risk of NMSC? Perceptions, beliefs and preventive behaviour among farmers, roofers and gardeners. J Eur Acad Dermatol Venereol. 2017;31(10):1649–54.
39. Noels EC, Hollestein LM, van Egmond S, Lugtenberg M, van Nistelrooij LPJ, Bindels PJE, et al. Healthcare utilization and management of actinic keratosis in primary and secondary care: a complementary database analysis. Br J Dermatol. 2019;181(3):544–53.
40. Rocholl M, Ludewig M, John SM, Bitzer EM, Wilke A. Outdoor workers' perceptions of skin cancer risk and attitudes to sun-protective measures: a qualitative study. J Occup Health. 2020;62(1):e12083.
41. Oliveira Silva LV, Arruda JAA, Abreu LG, Ferreira RC, Silva LP, et al. Demographic and Clinicopathologic features of actinic Cheilitis and lip squamous cell carcinoma: a Brazilian multicentre study. Head Neck Pathol. 2020;14(4):899.
42. Rodríguez-Blanco I, Flórez Á, Paredes-Suárez C, Rodríguez-Lojo R, González-Vilas D, et al. Actinic cheilitis prevalence and risk factors: a cross-sectional, multicentre study in a population aged 45 years and over in north-West Spain. Acta Derm Venereol. 2018;98(10):970–4.
43. Trager MH, Farmer K, Ulrich C, Basset-Seguin N, Herms F, et al. Actinic cheilitis: a systematic review of treatment options. J Eur Acad Dermatol Venereol. 2021;35(4):815–23.
44. Bauer A, Haufe E, Heinrich L, Seidler A, Schulze HJ, et al. Basal cell carcinoma risk and solar UV exposure in occupationally relevant anatomic sites: do histological subtype, tumor localization and Fitzpatrick phototype play a role? A population-based case-control study. J Occup Med Toxicol. 2020;15(1):28.
45. Apalla Z, Lallas A, Sotiriou E, Lazaridou E, Vakirlis E, et al. Farmers develop more aggressive histologic subtypes of basal cell carcinoma. Experience from a tertiary Hospital in Northern Greece. J Eur Acad Dermatol Venereol. 2016;30(Suppl 3):17–20.
46. Rushton L, Hutchings SJ. The burden of occupationally-related cutaneous malignant melanoma in Britain due to solar radiation. Br J Cancer. 2017;116(4):536–9.
47. Dennis LK, Lynch CF, Sandler DP, Alavanja MCR. Pesticide use and cutaneous melanoma in pesticide applicators in the agricultural heath study. Environ Health Perspect. 2010;118(6):812–7.
48. Stanganelli I, De Felici MB, Mandel VD, Caini S, Raimondi S, et al. The association between pesticide use and cutaneous melanoma: a systematic review and meta-analysis. J Eur Acad Dermatol Venereol. 2020;34(4):691–708.
49. Gilaberte-Calzada Y. Fotoprotección. In: Fotodermatología. Madrid: Panamericana; 2019. p. 99–108.

Occupational Contact Dermatitis in the Industrial Setting

13

David Pesqué, Cecilia Svedman, and Ana M. Giménez-Arnau

Introduction

The industrial sector, also called secondary sector, is in charge of transforming materials into goods. This sector has been classified into different industries: construction industry, fashion industry, chemical industry, pharmaceutical industry, power, and petroleum industry, automotive industry, electronic industry, food industry and paper industry, among others. In the USA, this economic sector accounted for 20% of the labor force, and, worldwide, 22.7% in 2019 [1].

The relevance of this chapter lies in the important workforce employed in the industrial sector not only in modern industrial countries, but globally, with differences in the specific types of industries. In addition, since this sector is heterogenous, the exposure of workers to irritants and allergens can be significantly different. One aspect to enhance is that irritant contact dermatitis may be common to different industrial jobs, for many entail working under wet conditions, heat, or getting in contact with irritant agents. Furthermore, it should be considered that the resulting final manufactured product usually requires different industrial jobs, thus enhancing the presence of multiple industrial tasks in industrial workplaces.

Table 13.1 summarizes the most characteristic irritants and sensitizers, classified according to the industrial sector.

D. Pesqué
Department of Dermatology, Hospital del Mar –
Institut Mar d'Investigacions Mèdiques, Universitat
Autònoma de Barcelona (UAB), Barcelona, Spain

C. Svedman
Department of Occupational and Environmental
Dermatology, Lund University, Skane University
Hospital, Malmö, Sweden

A. M. Giménez-Arnau (✉)
Department of Dermatology, Hospital del Mar –
Institut Mar d'Investigacions Mèdiques, Universitat
Autònoma de Barcelona (UAB), Barcelona, Spain

Department of Dermatology, Hospital del Mar –
Institut Mar d'Investigacions Mèdiques, Universitat
Pompeu Fabra, Barcelona, Spain

© The Author(s), under exclusive license to Springer Nature Switzerland AG 2023

A. M. Giménez-Arnau, H. I. Maibach (eds.), *Handbook of Occupational Dermatoses*, Updates in Clinical Dermatology, https://doi.org/10.1007/978-3-031-22727-1_13

Table 13.1 Characteristic irritants and sensitizers classified according to the industrial sector

Industrial profession	Irritants	Allergens
Construction workers (including metal workers, cement workers, boat builders, air craft workers, glass workers)	Abrasive hand cleansers Carbon fibers Glass fibers Metal dust Metalworking fluids Sharp metal particles Wet working	Aluminum chloride Cobalt chloride Colophony Epoxy resin Formaldehyde Formaldehyde releasers (e.g., bioban CS-1135®) Methyldiethanolamine Nickel sulfate Polyester resin Potassium dichromate
Fashion industry (including textile workers, leather workers and fur workers)	Acetic acid Caustic soda Ethanol Formic acid Wet working	Disperse dyes (e.g., disperse Brown 1, disperse red 1, etc.) Formaldehyde Reactive dyes (e.g., reactive black 5, reactive blue 21, etc.)
Chemical industry	Exposure to a wide range of possible corrosive and irritant chemicals	Many potential allergens Cobalt chloride Formaldehyde Mercaptobenzothiazole Mercapto mix Nickel sulfate Potassium dichromate Thiuram mix
Cosmetic industry	See chemical industry	2-Bromonitropropanediol 3-Hexylthiophene Methyl heptine carbonate p-toluene diamine
Petrol industry	Barium sulfate Calcium hydroxide Calcium oxide Crude oil Diesel Ilmenite Potassium hydroxide Silicate Zinc bromide	Glutaraldehyde Isothiazolinones Polyamides Resins
Automotive industry	Metal dusts Metalworking fluids Solvents Welding fumes	Epoxy resins Isocyanates Polyvinyl chloride Styrene
Electronic industry	Fiberglass Hydrofluoric acid	Acrylate Cobalt chloride Colophony Epoxy resin Isocyanate Nickel sulfate
Food industry	Detergents and cleaning solutions Enzymes Flavoring agents Spices Sodium chloride Wet working	2-mercaptobenzothiazole Animal proteins Balsam of Perú Carba mix Latex Nickel sulfate Paraphenylenediamine Thiuram mix

Table 13.1 (continued)

Industrial profession	Irritants	Allergens
Paper workers	Ammonia Sodium hypochlorite Wet working	Carba mix Colophony Epoxy resin Formaldehyde Methylchloroisothiazolinone/ methylisothiazolinone Mercapto mix Thiuram mix

Industrial Jobs

Construction Industry

This category includes all those professions linked to infrastructure and industrial construction, which accounts for a significant part of the secondary industry. Examples in this category are metal workers, cement workers, aircraft industry workers, etc.

Metal workers are one of the best-studied groups as there is high risk of irritant hand dermatitis due to exposure to mechanical and chemical irritants or allergens. Prevalence rates of hand dermatitis in metalworking companies may exceed 20%, being frequently irritant contact dermatitis (ICD) [2]. Chemical irritants to be enhanced are cleaning detergents, solvents, and degreasers [3]. Sensitization most commonly occurs to metalworking fluids, which are chemicals used in the metal treatment, but ICD can also occur, being difficult to differentiate. Workers can be exposed through skin contact by splashes and aerosols or when handling parts, tools, and equipment covered with metalworking fluids. The most common causative agents of allergic contact dermatitis (ACD) are antimicrobials, fragrances, formaldehyde, and formaldehyde releasers present in metalworking fluids. Additionally, monoethanolamine, a reported cause of ACD, is used as feedstock in metalworking fluids to stabilize pH or inhibit corrosion. Less commonly, sensitization occurs to specific metals, being nickel, chromium, and copper the most important illustrating examples [4, 5].

There are some specific jobs in the metal industry with specific characteristics, particularly welding workers and grinders of hard metal. The former are in charge of joining metal parts with the use of heat and are exposed to different types of metals due to fume exposure when welding. Metal welding implies the generation of fumes, which can contain metals, and electricity, which generates ultraviolet (UV) radiation, particularly within the UVC region. Sensitizing agents may also be cobalt, chromium, nickel, copper, and aluminum [6]. Despite welders being protected against UV radiation, occasional exposure to UVC has been described, with consequent associated photodamage, exacerbation of previous dermatoses and even photodermatoses. [6]. Figure 13.1 below depicts a case of occupational-induced idiopathic photodermatitis by tungsten welding in a sensitized worker to potassium dichromate.

Grinders use abrasive machining tools to finish workpieces of metal pieces. This process can involve a dry technique, in which workers may be exposed to metals, or a wet process, which requires the use of metalworking fluids. Therefore, grinders may be sensitized to metals (cobalt, chromium, nickel), but also to agents present in metalworking fluids. [7].

Cement workers include a wide range of jobs that are in contact with different forms of cement (mortar or concrete). Bricklayers and concrete workers do not usually wear gloves and are exposed directly exposed to the material, which is a known cause of ICD. [8]. However, there can be ACD to cement, which has a chronic nature and may have a social implication with an

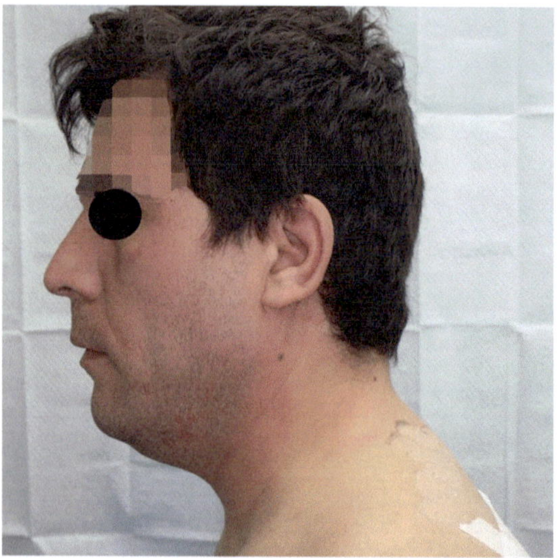

Fig. 13.1 A case of occupational-induced idiopathic photodermatitis by tungsten welding in a sensitized worker to potassium dichromate. A moderate erythema both in face and neck with eczematous patches can be observed

increased job switching. The culprit of allergic cement eczema is chromium, which is present in cement in form of water-soluble hexavalent chromate, Cr (VI). By adding ferrous sulfate to the cement, chromate is reduced from Cr(VI) to Cr(III) with a lower solubility and prevents the occurrence of allergic eczema to chromate. [9]. In addition, these workers also use products containing epoxy resins.

The construction of means of transport is also associated with occupational contact dermatitis. Boat builders deal with a varied exposure to different chemicals and have seldom been object of ICD and ACD. Boats construction require the use of different materials, including plastics, metals, and wood. Therefore, allergens have to be studied depending on the individual exposure. Plastic materials used usually contain polyester resin, epoxy resin, epoxy vinyl ester resins, and acrylates. Wood parts are made of pine or oak wood, and decorations may be made of tropical wood species. Glass fiber or carbon fiber are used as reinforcement. For finishing, waxes, fillers, varnishes, and paints are used. [10].

In contrast, aircraft industry workers present with well-studied occupational contact dermato-

ses, with a significant number of workers affected in different studies [11, 12] ICD can happen when being in contact with metalworking fluids and solvents. ACD are due to the contact with resins, hardeners, coatings, and paintings, with common allergens like epoxy resins, epoxy resin accelerators, chromates, and nickel. In the clinical setting, a picture due to epoxy resin is characterized by dermatitis on the finger pulp spaces, the dorsa and sides of fingers and forearms. In addition, subungual pulpitis by exposure to epoxy resins is specific for the aircraft industry [13].

Wood artisans, such as cabinetmakers, are affected by wood-related contact dermatitis due to direct contact with wood and chemicals used in woodworking (glues, paints, and lacquers). Some woods, particularly tropical woods, contain different sensitizers such as quinones, terpenes, phenols, or stilbenes. A myriad of allergens can be used in woodworking materials (acrylates, epoxy resin, colophony, isothiazolinones) [14].

Glass workers present ICD due to thermal, chemical, and physical trauma during its manufacturing. However, contact allergy is seldom found in literature. Today, the cases of ACD are related to the decoration of glass with cutting fluids, biocides, and glass coating. In these latter products, epoxy resins, silane and polyester resins can be found [15]. In addition, glaziers are exposed to glues and sealants that contain epoxy resins and acrylates [16].

Fashion Industry

Textile contact dermatitis has its particular features. It can occur in an occupational setting, but not necessarily, and it is believed to be more frequently of an allergic background rather than irritant [17]. During the fabrication process, mainly in the stages of dyeing and finishing, workers are exposed to irritants and sensitizers. Exposure to dyes, formaldehyde-containing finishers, rubber compounds, metals, biocides, and smoothers can occur and those are believed to be the main responsible agents for ACD. Disperse dyes with sensitizing potential, which include azo, anthraquinone, and nitro chemical classes, are believed to be the first cause of occupational textile contact dermatitis. Those are used for the coloring of synthetic fibers (polyester, polyamide, acrylic). Reactive dyes (azo, anthraquinone, and phthalocyanine classes) serve to color natural fibers (cotton, silk, and wool) and synthetic polyamides, but these induce contact dermatitis much less frequently. The second most common type of contact dermatitis in these workers are formaldehyde resins, present in the finishing stages. Other occupational textile allergens include p-phenylenediamine, mercaptobenzothiazole, colophony, and isothiazolinones.

The European Union and Japan have already taken initiatives to regulate textile allergens. Such regulations have led, for example, to the production and identification of clothing free from allergenic dyes and high levels of formaldehyde [17] Nevertheless, the prevalence of both occupational textile dermatitis seems to be on the rise, likely as a result of changing textile manufacturing techniques, involving many new substances and potential skin sensitizers, which are probably largely undeclared [18].

Leather industry workers are differently tackled, for the steps of processing leather involves different stages and chemicals. Initially, alkaline leaches and acids are used, and to prevent leather damage, biocides are applied to it. Tanning is performed by using chromium derivates. Afterwards, leather is retanned with synthetic tanning agents, amino resins, and polyacrylate or polymethacrylate solutions. Leather dyeing is based on azo dyes. However, with an increased automation in this field, occupational dermatoses are expected to become less frequent in Europe [19].

Fur industry also holds specific features as it involves storing and chemically or physically processing fur. In this context, workers are not only exposed to dyes, acids, and detergents but also to animal dusts.

Chemical Industry

The diversity of skin-hazardous substances to which workers may be exposed makes difficult to comprehensively analyze the main groups involved. Many chemicals commonly used in the laboratory are corrosive or irritating to the skin, while some are allergenic. In clinical laboratories, automation and encapsulation have importantly led to a reduction of risk of exposure. However, in research and industrial laboratories, the manual handling of hazardous chemicals still poses an important defy.

Occupational dermatoses are normally a consequence of undesired, accidental exposure in the working milieu, such as spillage of a substance on the skin [20]. The working processes that entail a higher risk of skin exposure are synthesis of products and distillation or other purification procedures. Previous literature supports that, normally, the sensitizers are not the final product but intermediate derivates [21].

Allergic occupational chemical dermatitis is reported more frequently than the irritant counterpart. Occupational contact allergic dermatitis has been primarily diagnosed among chemical students and post-graduates [20]. In fact, ACD in chemistry researchers can often be the first clue of a new potential contact sensitizer, clearly depicting that research chemicals often become future laboratory and industrial agents [22].

Chemical burns due to highly corrosive chemicals like concentrated alkalis, concentrated acids, and metal salts can be seen. ICD is frequent in this working group due to frequent hand washing (wet works, soaps, skin disinfectants), use of polymer gloves, organic solvents, and acid and basic liquids [22]. ACD can be secondary to well-known sensitizers, but also even due to rare, new chemicals, making difficult to establish the responsible agent.

Pharmaceutical and Cosmetic Industries

These industries, clearly related to the chemical industry, also present with a burden of occupational dermatoses. Despite in the past, workers in the pharmaceutical industry were considered to present a high risk of irritant and allergic contact dermatitis [23], the current situation may be changing due to an increase of automatization, but occupational contact dermatitis in the pharmaceutical industry is still commonly reported [24]. Occupational dermatoses are usually located at the site of contact, which is generally the hands. However, for this type of industry, a wide spectrum of reactions has been described: airborne reactions on exposed and non-exposed areas, generalized reactions, photosensitivity, urticaria, and fixed drug eruption. Figure 13.2 shows a case of occupational ACD to tetrazepam in a pharmaceutical worker, whose patch tests can be seen below.

The mechanisms of irritancy are homologous to those seen in point 2.3. Chemical industry.

Delayed contact hypersensitivity may be triggered by many different families of drugs: analgesic and anti-inflammatory agents, anthelmintics, antiandrogens, antiarrhythmic agents, antibacterial agents, anti-gout agents, antihypertensive agents, antimalarials, antimuscarinic agents, antineoplastic agents, immunosuppressants, antivirals, neuroleptics, anxiolytics, corticosteroids, dermatology topical agents, diuretics, local anesthetics, among others [24–26].

In the cosmetic industry the burden of ACD is low. However, some occupational allergens have also come to light, as specified in Sect. 4.

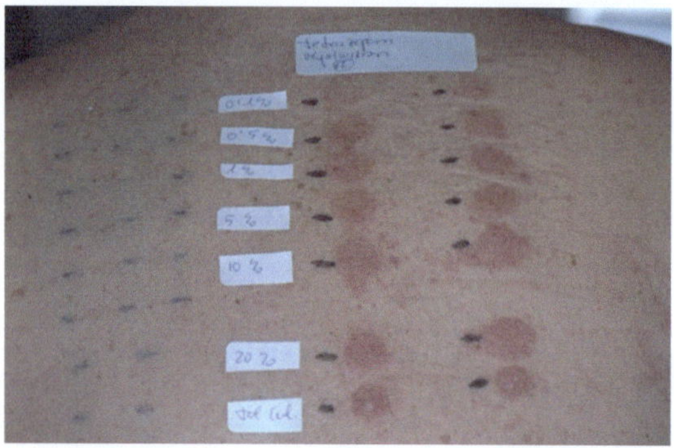

Fig. 13.2 Patch testing of tetrazepam in a pharmaceutical worker. The patient had become sensitized with this product working with the machinery used to manufacture the drug. Patch testing resulted positive on D2 (+++) for the drug "as if," and at different concentrations (from 20% to 0.1%)

Power and Petroleum Industry

The power and petroleum industry sometimes present with occupational contact dermatitis, for example, oil rig workers and workers from the wind energy industry.

Oil rig workers task consists of drilling and maintaining the oil rig. The job categories related to this section are varied. Skin problems are the third largest work-related group of illnesses in the offshore oil industry after noise-induced hearing loss and traumatological problems, according to the Petroleum Safety Authority of Norway [27]. In this section, the focus will be on workers of the drilling operation and maintenance. As it happens with industrial workers, these jobs are characterized by hard physical manual work, unfavorable weather conditions, and exposure to chemical hazardous substances [27].

In the drilling process, drilling fluids are used to ease the process, but these contain hundreds of different types of chemical substances. Drilling fluids are classified depending on whether their primary base is water (called water-based fluids) or oil (oil-based fluids). Experience and reported evidence suggest that oil-based fluids present a further degree of skin damage. ICD of some degree is an expected finding and is almost universally evidenced when prolonged exposure to irritants occurs [27]. Petroleum hydrocarbons may remove the natural lipids from the skin, which can lead to dryness and cracking of the skin, easing latter irritation and sensitization. Different components of drilling fluids can act as irritants and allergens. In addition, working suits may contain epoxy resins, and amines are used in the treatment of hydrocarbons.

The increase in usage of renewable energies is also evidencing the presence of occupational dermatitis. The construction and manufacturing of aerogenerators and turbines in the wind energy industry have increased in Europe in the past decade [28]. Irritant contact dermatitis due to fiberglass can be seen. The use of adhesives, coating, and paints containing epoxy resins, places this allergen as the most commonly evinced in this sector [28].

Automotive Industry

The automotive industry of vehicles includes jobs associated to the production, retailing, and maintenance of vehicles, such as metal and plastic workers, vehicle assemblers, mechanics and car repair workers, etc. Nevertheless, the automotive industry is under constant change due to the use of new fabrication techniques and progressive automotive electrification. Due to this, it should be expected that the automotive industry will present similarities with the electronic industry. Similarly, metal workers of car parts present similar conditions as those seen in metal workers.

Workers in the assemble of vehicle parts and manufacture, deal with some hazardous chemicals, like isocyanates. A common binder used to manufacture sand cores is methylene diisocyanate, which can induce irritation and sensitization. Vehicle repair and maintenance workers are predominantly exposed to cutting fluids, mineral oils, lubricants, and solvents [29].

Electronic Industry

Electronic industry is considered greatly automated, and thus, safe. Notwithstanding the automation, the occurrence of occupational contact dermatitis has been reported. The tasks and materials related to the electronic industry can be summarized in two areas: semiconductor device fabrication and Printed Circuit Board (PCB) fabrication and assembly. The former involves semiconductor device fabrication, chip design, crystal purification and growth, wafer preparation, epitaxy and oxidation, photolithography, doping and type conversion, metallization, and interconnection formation, and encapsulation. Despite the vast size of the electronic industry workforce, there is little information available on how common occupationally related skin disorders in this industry are [30].

Both ICD and ACD appear to be important, mostly due to solvents, metals, soldering flux, epoxy and acrylate resins, oils and coolants, fiberglass, and rubber chemicals.

Food Industry

Contact dermatitis to food is usually related to workers of the primary economic sector, but food industry has also to be taken into account. Broadly speaking, most of these tasks involve wet working, and contact with cleansing and disinfectant agents. Therefore, in all the specific jobs that will be discussed in this section, irritant contact dermatitis may be a common finding. Allergic contact dermatitis related to the food industry is still both underreported and under recognized [31].

Meat industry workers, like slaughterhouse workers or poultry processors, can present with allergic contact dermatitis, mostly to rubber protection materials, and disinfectants or preservatives used in the different processes of meat transformation. In addition, contact urticaria and/or protein contact dermatitis to animal proteins has been described [32].

Cheese makers work daily with milk fat and protein, in the context of a wet work. The most important irritants in cheese dairies include contact with concentrated (20%) sodium chloride solutions and milk proteins [33]. Allergic contact dermatitis to different compounds (particularly antioxidants and allergens in rubber gloves), protein contact urticaria, and protein contact dermatitis have also been described [32].

Baking industry involves the use of flour, yeast, water, and other to produce bread and other products. Allergic contact dermatitis has been described for flours, amylase, wheat, cardamom, and gallates, among others. Contact protein dermatitis has been occasionally described [32].

Confectionery and candymakers work with a wide range of ingredients, flavors, preservatives, and antioxidants. The increased automation in the confectionery industry has led to an overall decrease in the number of occupational contact dermatitis [31]. As with other ranges of food industry, allergic contact dermatitis is a cause of occupational dermatitis, but in this case, flavorings are the most common cause. Some of the flavorings found include balsam of Peru, anethole, cardamom oil, cinnamic alcohol, citral, geraniol, eugenol, ginger, or liquorice, among others. Other allergens may be related to gloves (rubbers) and use of antioxidants, preservatives, sweeteners, or emulsifiers [31].

Paper Industry

Pulp and paper manufacturing are complex processes that involve the use of multiple industrial chemicals. As seen in previous industries, these processes are becoming more automated, which reduces the workers' exposure to hazardous chemicals. Today, contact dermatitis is considered to be rare among pulp and paper workers.

In the process of fabrication, slimicides and their constituents (potent biocides) are used to prevent the growth of different microbes, which would reduce the quality of the paper. Slimicides are the most prominent agents causing allergic contact dermatitis among pulp and paper workers. In line with allergic contact dermatitis, paper dermatitis is also to be considered. Paper dermatitis is defined as allergic contact dermatitis caused by paper, which despite being rare, is a cause of occupational dermatitis. Colophony and formaldehyde are the most important allergens causing paper dermatitis [34].

Prevention and Conclusions

An early diagnosis, workplace exposure assessment and notification of industrial contact dermatitis is of utmost importance. Despite current legislation and policies, there is room for improvement, according to previous studies, in terms of legislation approach, research, and prevention [35]. Occupational risk assessment, as a part of primary prevention, is essential and should be focused on human, technical, and organizational aspects with the aim of reducing exposure to hazardous substances. An improvement in the detection and treatment of early stages of contact allergic dermatitis (secondary prevention) and the treatment of well-established occupational disease (tertiary prevention) are essential to prevent relapses or chronicity, prevent workers from losing their job and promoting social rehabilitation and quality of life in workers.

The growth and development of the industrial sector worldwide, without uniform regulatory policies and surveillance, may pose an important defy with many unmet needs, since workplace assessment and research, as well as secondary and tertiary prevention may differ significantly.

References

1. Employment in industry - The World Bank. https://data.worldbank.org/indicator/SL.IND.EMPL.ZS Assessed 20 Dec 2021.
2. Lima AH, Elsner P. Metal industry. In: John SM, Johansen JD, Rustemeyer T, Elsner P, Maibach HI. Kanerva's occupational dermatology. Springer. 2020; p. 2123–2125.
3. Berndt U, Hinnen U, Iliev D, Elsner P. Hand eczema in metal worker trainees – an analysis of risk factors. Contact Dermatitis. 2000;43:327–32.
4. Foussereau J, Benezra C, Maibach HI. Occupational contact dermatitis: clinical and chemical aspects, vol. 26. Copenhagen: Munksgaard; 1982.
5. Kanerva L, KiilunenM JR, Estlander T, Aitio A. Hand dermatitis and allergic patch test reactions caused by nickel in electroplaters. Contact Dermatitis. 1997;36:137–40.
6. Hindsén M, Bruze M. Welding. In: John SM, Johansen JD, Rustemeyer T, Elsner P, Maibach HI. Kanerva's occupational dermatology. Springer. 2020; p. 2351–2353.
7. Ruokonen EL, Linnainmaa M, Seuri M, Juhakoski P, Söderström KO. A fatal case of hard metal disease. Scand J Work Environ Health. 1996;22:62–5.
8. Avnstorp C. Irritant cement eczema. In: Van Der Valk PGM, Maibach HI, editors. The irritant contact dermatitis syndrome. Boca Raton: CRC Press; 1995. p. 111–9.
9. Bregnbak D, Avnstorp C. Cement. In: John SM, Johansen JD, Rustemeyer T, Elsner P, Maibach HI, editors. Kanerva's occupational dermatology. Springer; 2020. p. 699–711.
10. Aalto-Korte K, Suuronen K. In: John SM, Johansen JD, Rustemeyer T, Elsner P, Maibach HI, editors. Kanerva's occupational dermatology. Springer; 2020. p. 1763–6.
11. Bruze M, Edenholm M, Engström K, Svensson G. Occupational dermatoses in a Swedish aircraft plant. Contact Dermatitis. 1996;34:336–40.
12. Hackett JP. Allergic contact dermatitis in American aircraft manufacture. Am J Contact Dermat. 1999;10:157–66.

13. Isaksson M. Aircraft industry. In: John SM, Johansen JD, Rustemeyer T, Elsner P, Maibach HI, editors. Kanerva's occupational dermatology. Springer; 2020. p. 1701–6.

14. Lobo I, Ferreira M, Silva E, Machado S, Selores M. Contact dermatitis in wood workers. Indian J Dermatol Venereol Leprol. 2008;74:431.

15. Toffoletto F, Cortona G, Feltrin A, et al. Occupational contact dermatitis from amine-functional methoxysilane in continuous-glass-filament production. Contact Dermatitis. 1994;31:320–1.

16. Adams RM. Glaziers. In: Adams RM, editor. Occupational skin disease. WB Saunders: Philadelphia; 1990. p. 628–9.

17. Svedman C, Engfeldt M, Malinauskiene L. Textile contact dermatitis: how fabrics can induce dermatitis. Curr Treat Opt Allergy. 2019;6:103–11.

18. Pesqué D, March-Rodriguez Á, Dahlin J, Isaksson M, Pujol RM, Giménez-Arnau E, et al. Bikini textile contact dermatitis: a Sherlockian approach revealing 2,4-dichlorophenol as a potential textile contact allergen. Contact Dermatitis. 2021;85:679–85.

19. Geier J, Lessmann H. Leather industry. In: John SM, Johansen JD, Rustemeyer T, Elsner P, Maibach HI, editors. Kanerva's occupational dermatology. Springer; 2020. p. 2103–015.

20. Le Coz CJ, Lepoittevin JP. Occupational erythema multiforme-like dermatitis from sensitization to costus resinoid, followed by flare-up and systemic contact dermatitis from β-cyclocostunolide in a chemistry student. Contact Dermatitis. 2001;44:310–1.

21. Dooms-Goossens A, de Boulle K, Snauwaert J, Degreef H. Sensitization to 3,4,6-trichloropyridazine. Contact Dermatitis. 1986;14:64–5.

22. Ezersky A, Maibach HI, Jolanki R. Chemists. In: John SM, Johansen JD, Rustemeyer T, Elsner P, Maibach HI, editors. Kanerva's occupational dermatology. Springer; 2020. p. 1843–9.

23. Sherertz E. Occupational skin disease in the pharmaceutical industry. Dermatol Clin. 1994;12:533–6.

24. Gilissen L, Boeckxstaens E, Geebelen J, Goossens A. Occupational allergic contact dermatitis from systemic drugs. Contact Dermatitis. 2020;82:24–30.

25. Ferran M, Giménez-Arnau A, Luque S, Berenguer N, Iglesias M, Pujol RM. Occupational airborne contact dermatitis from sporadic exposure to tetrazepam during machine maintenance. Contact Dermatitis. 2005;52:17.

26. Goossens A, Hulst KV. Occupational contact dermatitis in the pharmaceutical industry. Clin Dermatol. 2011;29:662–8.

27. Steiner MFC, Ormerod AD. Oil rig workers. In: John SM, Johansen JD, Rustemeyer T, Elsner P, Maibach HI. Kanerva's occupational dermatology. Springer. 2020; p. 2153–2167.

28. Lárraga-Piñones G, Heras-Mendaza F, Conde-Salazar L. Occupational contact dermatitis in the wind energy industry. Actas Dermosifiliogr. 2012;103:905–9.

29. Attwa E, el-Laithy N. Contact dermatitis in car repair workers. J Eur Acad Dermatol Venereol. 2009;23:138–45.

30. Roberts EJ, Smith V, English JSC. Electronic industry. In: John SM, Johansen JD, Rustemeyer T, Elsner P, Maibach HI, editors. Kanerva's occupational dermatology. Springer; 2020. p. 901–17.

31. Alhammadi A, Al-Niaimi FA, Lyon CC. Confectionery and Candymakers. In: John SM, Johansen JD, Rustemeyer T, Elsner P, Maibach HI, editors. Kanerva's occupational dermatology. Springer; 2020. p. 1799–807.

32. Gimenez-Arnau A, Maurer M, De La Cuadra J, Maibach H. Immediate contact skin reactions, an update of contact Urticaria, contact Urticaria syndrome and protein contact dermatitis - "a never ending story". Eur J Dermatol. 2010;20:552–62.

33. Elsner P, Nestle FO. Cheese makers. In: John SM, Johansen JD, Rustemeyer T, Elsner P, Maibach HI, editors. Kanerva's occupational dermatology. Springer; 2020. p. 1839–41.

34. Haeberle M. Pulp and paper workers, and paper dermatitis. In: John SM, Johansen JD, Rustemeyer T, Elsner P, Maibach HI, editors. Kanerva's occupational dermatology. Springer; 2020. p. 2183–202.

35. Alfonso JH, Bauer A, Bensefa-Colas L, Boman A, Bubas M, Constandt L, et al. Minimum standards on prevention, diagnosis and treatment of occupational and work-related skin diseases in Europe - position paper of the COST action StanDerm (TD 1206). J Eur Acad Dermatol Venereol. 2017;31(Suppl 4):31–43.

Occupational Contact Dermatitis in the Service Sector

14

Maria-Antonia Pastor-Nieto
and Maria-Elena Gatica-Ortega

The service (tertiary) sector involves heterogeneous activities producing intangible, short-lasting, non-material benefits that cannot be stored, are inseparable from the individual that provides them and cannot be owned as a property.

There is no exchange of goods, however the buyer receives a benefit, and the service is provided in the presence of the client.

The service sector has increasingly grown as a result of specialization, automatization, globalization, and population expansion. It accounts for an important part of the gross domestic product (GDP), especially in developed countries where it provides employment to almost 60% of the population [1, 2].

The activities included in the service sector are varied including leisure, sports, entertainment business, tourism, hostelry, health care services, beauty business, transport, telecommunication, internet, mass media, financial activities, public administration, estate public services (safety, defense, firefighters, etc.), educational services, technological services, legal departments, etc. [1, 2]

We will hereby discuss the occupational dermatoses resulting from a choice of occupations within the service sector.

Sports

Athletes are prone to irritant contact dermatitis (ICD) and allergic contact dermatitis (ACD) due to a combination of factors (trauma, moist, heat, chemicals, genetic predisposition, etc.) [3].

An important source of dermatoses in sportsmen is their apparel/equipment, especially in atopic patients. More frequent dermatosis from equipment is ICD, although some patients also develop ACD from a variety of allergens, such as rubber additives, dyes, benzoyl peroxide, urea formaldehyde or phenol formaldehyde resins. ACD may also be caused by preservatives, fragrances, antioxidants, sunscreens, etc. in cosmetics and hygiene products. Additionally, athletes often use analgesic, anti-inflammatory, blister preventing, or massage topical preparations with a variety of sensitizing ingredients (e.g., eucalyptus oil, nonsteroidal anti-inflammatory, anesthetics, lanolin, etc.) [3].

M.-A. Pastor-Nieto (✉)
Dermatology Department, Hospital Universitario de Guadalajara, Guadalajara, Spain

Medicine and Medical Specialties Department, Faculty of Medicine, Universidad de Alcalá, Alcala de Henares, Spain

Universidad de Castilla-La-Mancha, Ciudad Real, Spain

M.-E. Gatica-Ortega
Universidad de Castilla-La-Mancha, Ciudad Real, Spain

Dermatology Department, Toledo Hospital Complex, Toledo, Spain

© The Author(s), under exclusive license to Springer Nature Switzerland AG 2023
A. M. Giménez-Arnau, H. I. Maibach (eds.), *Handbook of Occupational Dermatoses*, Updates in Clinical Dermatology, https://doi.org/10.1007/978-3-031-22727-1_14

Water Sports

Allergens may be found in the equipment (goggles, nose clips, ear plugs, elastic swimwear, swim fins, swim caps, footgear, gloves, snorkels, mouthpieces etc.), or pool disinfectants. The anatomical distribution and the temporal relationship are key for the etiological diagnosis [3].

Swimming goggle allergens in the padding (rubber, neoprene), often cause well-demarcated periorbital bilateral reactions, and occasionally, conjunctivitis and leukoderma [3].

Rubber sensitivity in diving masks is currently less common because black rubber has been replaced by other materials [4]. However, outbreaks of ACD ("mask burn") to N-isopropyl-N-phenylpara-phenylenediamine (IPPD) in diving masks have been reported [3].

Neoprene, a synthetic polychloroprene-based rubber, made by polymerization of chloroprene [5], is used in diving gear, wet suits, gloves, socks, mending pieces, knee supports, etc., because of its numerous properties (stretchability, waterproof, chemical-resistance). Chloroprene contains thioureas (diphenylthiourea, diethylthiourea, and dibutylthiourea) used as vulcanization accelerators and antioxidants [6]. Diethylthiourea, the most common in chloroprene, is degraded to ethyl isothiocyanate, a strong sensitizer. Allergy to thioureas may be underdiagnosed as standard series do not include them [5, 6].

ACD due to p-tert-butylphenol-formaldehyde resin (PTBPFR), colophony, zinc diethyl dithiocarbamate and nickel has also been reported in neoprene products [5].

Goggles may cause ACD from other compounds such as phenol-formaldehyde resin and benzoyl peroxide or silprene-30A/B [7]; and photoallergic contact dermatitis to benzophenone [8].

Windsurfers may suffer from ACD from diethylthiourea in wet suits or from the black rubber wishbone (a handle on the sail). "Surf-riders dermatitis" is a type of nipple ICD triggered by sand, seawater, and friction [3].

Sports fishermen may develop ACD to nickel, mercaptobenzothiazole, or IPPD in the fishing rod or azo dyes in baits. Protein contact dermatitis from maggot baits has also been described [3].

Widespread rashes while swimming may be caused by pool disinfectants (chlorinated compounds, halobromo [3], 1-bromo-1-chloro-5.5-dimethylhydantoin) [4]. Chemicals used to disinfect the wet suits (e.g., dodecyl diaminoethyl glycine) may also sensitize [4].

Swimmers, snorkelers, surfers, and divers may develop ICD from seaweed, yellow coral, sponges, sea cucumbers, sea mosses, and plants. The "swimmers' shoulder" is an ICD caused by friction with beard while performing the swim stroke [3].

"Swimmer's itch", caused by a schistosome infesting subtropical water birds and snails, presents with urticarial reactions less evident under a bathing suit, while the "seabather's eruption", caused by jellyfish larva or adult nematocysts stings (*Linuche unguiculata* and *Edwardsiella lineata* in the Caribbean), is mainly located under the bathing suit [4]. Swimmers are also at risk of vesiculobullous *tinea pedis* caused by *T. mentagrophytes* [9].

Athletes and Ball Sports

Runners can develop ACD from clothing or running shoe allergens that are easily released under a moist environment (leather, adhesives, dyes, ethyl butyl thiourea, mercaptobenzothiazole, dibenzothiazyldisulfide, epoxy resin, nickel, etc.) [3]. A jogger became sensitized to palmitoyl hydrolyzed milk protein, palmitoyl collagen amino acids and *Arnica montana* in a cream for blister prevention [4]. Runners may also develop nipple ICD from friction and moist [3].

Basketball players may suffer from ACD to rubber additives and PTBFFR in the ball, tape, or knee guards as well as fingertip ICD from mechanical trauma ("pebble fingers") [3].

Tennis players may develop ACD from isophorone diamine and epoxy resin in rackets or to neoprene splints for epicondylitis [3].

Hockey players may experience ICD from stick fiberglass as well as ACD from epoxy resin in mask adhesives and dyes in gloves [3].

Azetophenone azine is an emerging allergen present in foam shin guards, shoe insoles or flip flops made of ethylene-vinyl acetate (EVA) [10–15]. ACD to it initially presents with a localized vesicular dermatitis that subsequently, becomes widespread. Hyper-eosinophilia and residual depigmentation may also be observed. Most cases affect children yet adult cases have been reported involving two hockey players [13, 14]. Thick socks are not sufficient to avoid ACD from azetophenone azine in shin guards. Polyurethane and leather are safe alternatives [15].

Compounds related to PTBFR in sport gloves have been described to cause hand ACD in one football goalkeeper [16].

Colophony "bags", used by athletes to improve their grips (e.g., rock climbing, gymnastics, weightlifting, bowling, tennis, baseball, handball, cricket), may also cause sensitization in this context. ACD from colophony has also been reported involving a volleyball player who used adhesive tapes to strengthen his fingers [17] as well as a professional football player who wore plasters to tighten his socks [18]. ACD from modified colophony may be underestimated since baseline series use unmodified colophony [17].

Weightlifting may lead to abrasions/lichenification from friction and ACD from metallic weights/bars [3, 19]. Nickel release from equipment in gyms is produced by sweat and may be able to elicit ACD in sensitized subjects. Nickel-sensitized patients should use the dimethyl glyoxime test to avoid contact with nickel-releasing workout devices [20].

Hand and eyelid ACD to epoxy resin in a two-component glue has been reported to involve a golf club repairman who wiped off the excess of the glue with his bare fingers. Golfers may also have palmar eczema from the golf rubber grip or from leather gloves. Epoxy resins permeate latex or rubber gloves, thus, multilayered (4H glove) or heavy-duty vinyl gloves should be used instead [21].

Hand ACD from limonene in a wood bow treated with a paint stripper involving a police archer was reported [22].

Baseball players can suffer from traumatic contusions/abrasions [9], frictional "baseball pitcher's dermatitis" [23], or ACD to the components of the bat (willow, linseed oil wood protectant, phenols, catechol, quinones, saponins, stilbenes, terpenes, metals, rubber), the mitt or the footwear (glutaraldehyde, formaldehyde, potassium dichromate, azo or disperse dyes, PPD, rubber allergens, lanolin) [9].

Shaving, sharing equipment or communal floors, trauma, sweat, heat, occlusive or poorly fitting equipment/garments/footwear, and prolonged activity predisposed to follicular infections, *tinea pedis,* friction blisters, acne *mechanica, talon noir* (syn: calcaneal petechiae, black heel), *tache noir* ("black palm") and "athlete's toenail" (subungual hemorrhage and onycholysis) [9].

Winter Sports

ACD involving skaters may be caused by heterogeneous allergens found in the skate boot (formaldehyde, potassium dichromate, azo or disperse dyes, PPD, PTBFR, thioureas, colophony, epoxy resin, benzoyl peroxide, ethyl acrylate/cyanoacrylate, epicholorhydrin, etc.) or in the blade (nickel, chromium, etc.) [24].

Ice-hockey players may also react to components of the stick (ash, aluminum, fiberglass), face masks (epoxy resin), pads/guards (thioureas), or gloves (thioureas, disperse dyes) [24].

Finally, winter sports can also predispose players to mechanical and cold-induced injuries (chilblains, Raynaud phenomenon, cold panniculitis, frostnip, frostbite, etc.) accelerated by thin garments, rapid speeds, and sweating [24].

Inducible Urticaria

Inducible urticaria (CIndU) provoked by physical stimuli (e.g., exercise, cold, heat, sunlight, water, vibration, or external pressure) is more frequent in athletes than in sedentary individuals [4, 24]. Specific provocation tests should be performed to confirm the diagnosis and determine the activity of the disease.

Cholinergic urticaria was published to be the most common CIndU in athletes aged <30 years [24]. It may be triggered by hot showers, exercise, and sweating.

Cold urticaria may develop while skiing, skating, swimming, etc. Extensive cold exposure in patients with low thresholds can lead to anaphylaxis [24].

Heat-induced urticaria mainly affects basketball and track-and-field athletes; while delayed pressure urticaria is related to swimming, boxing, weightlifting and track-and-field [4].

Vibratory angioedema has been described in a mountain biker (presenting with forearm edema) and in another individual from running, bicycling, and skiing [25–27].

Aquagenic urticaria may result from practicing water sports either by sea or pool water [4].

Exercise-induced anaphylaxis enhanced by food (celery, gluten/wheat, shellfish, snails) or other allergens, occasionally involves runners and other athletes [4]. This disorder may be enabled by exposure to anti-inflammatory drugs (e.g., naproxen, aspirin) [4].

Finally, some sports involving exposure to highly allergenic animal proteins are at risk of contact urticaria (e.g., horse dander or saliva in equestrian sports or maggot baits in fishing) [4]. Anaphylaxis induced by a squash latex-covered racquet has also been described [4].

Music

Musicians are predisposed to ICD and ACD due to close and prolonged contact with the instruments under wet conditions (sweat and saliva). Occlusive and moisture circumstances are not, however, as significant as in other professions [28].

Contact dermatitis is the most prevalent skin disorder in instrumentalists, particularly among string musicians, woodwind players, and brass musicians [29].

German research showed that 8.9% of musicians had occupational skin disease usually involving the hands and lips. The most frequent diagnosis was ACD followed by atopic dermatitis and ICD. The most common sensitizers were nickel, *Myroxylon pereirae*, fragrance mix (FM) I, FM II, and colophony. Surprisingly, there were no cases of sensitization to metals [28].

On the other hand, Italian questionnaire-based research described instrument-related dermatoses in 21% of the participants, most of them being ICD/ callosities with only one case of ACD [30].

Another research emphasized that ACD was more frequent among violinists and violists, while callosities were more frequent among string plucking instrumentalists and brass players [29].

String instrumentalists may develop ACD to unmodified colophony (in wood varnish or string waxing), exotic woods, metals (in strings, and other parts), propolis (in varnish), and PPD (wood or strings). Woodwind players become sensitized to exotic woods and cane reeds; and, brass players to metals. Musicians should be patch tested with baseline and case-specific series as well as the products provided by the patients [28].

Sensitization to colophony in musical instruments may jeopardize the use of many other products (fragranced products, jewelry, adhesive tape, shoes) because of its widespread use. An alternative synthetic hydrocarbon resin (Super-Sensitive Clarity®, Musical String Co., Sarasota, FL, USA), has been proposed to be a safe alternative [31].

One viola player developed submandibular eczema at the areas in contact with the chin-pad metallic bracket. Lesions cleared upon switching to a plastic chin-pad [32].

ACD to acrylates associated to nail dystrophy has been described involving flamenco guitarists who self-apply acrylic nails to strengthen their nails. Onycholysis may be aggravated by trauma from playing the guitar and fungal superinfection [33].

Paronychia, onycholysis, and subungual hemorrhages may also be observed in harpists [28].

Contact with instruments can also induce a variety of ICD (e.g., "fiddler's neck", "cellist's chest", "guitar nipple" and "flautist's chin") [34].

Fiddler's neck involves viola/violin players and results from pressure, friction, poorly fitting chin rest and excessive perspiration [35]. It presents with heterogeneous features including submandibular hyperpigmentation, lichenification, erythema, scaling, cysts, scars and/or pustules [29]. Viola players are more prone to it than violinists because a viola is larger than violin [35].

Lip atrophy or ischemia have been reported in horn/trumpet players [28].

Vibratory angioedema involving a horn player (presenting with lip angioedema), a trumpet professor (upper lip painful edema) and a saxophonist (lower lip edema) have been described [36–38].

Musicians may also develop occupational musculoskeletal/neurological diseases (e.g., tenosynovitis, carpal tunnel syndrome, focal dystonia) [28], dental and respiratory disorders, hearing impairment, reflux laryngitis, and performance anxiety [30].

Stage Artists, Singers, and Dancers

Artists, are often heavily made-up for performances. In addition to conventional cosmetics, artists wear other sensitizing materials such as waxes, liquid plasters as well as adhesives for wigs, false moustaches, eyelashes, and eyebrows. Additionally, female ballet dancers use colophony on their shoes, male ballet dancers use colophony on their hands for lifts and special colophony covering may be laid on the stage. Singers may also be exposed to airborne colophony dust[39, 40].

Swedish research showed that 30% members of an opera company had skin lesions, however, occupational contact dermatitis was rare. More than half reported side effects from cosmetics, but only one dancer experienced intolerance to colophony. Positive patch test reactions to colophony involved 2% and sensitization to perfumes and/or preservatives was related to cosmetic intolerance [40].

Eight choir members were recently published to have experienced skin problems. Five had occupational ICD, ACD, or eye reactions from a blue make-up containing fragrances including linalool [41].

One ballroom dance teacher developed photo-aggravated ACD from ketoprofen transferred to her through the embrace of her partner [42].

Occupational hand ACD to colophony and dancers' colophony has also been published involving a ballet masseuse [43].

Mechanical trauma in dancers can lead to erosions, blisters, onycholysis, callosities, etc., and opera singers may develop acneiform eruptions from heavy oil-based make-up products [39].

Kitchen Workers [44]

Kitchen workers usually develop hand dermatitis from a combination of factors. Thus, patients with atopic backgrounds begin developing ICD from wet work and irritants (raw food, detergents), which subsequently becomes complicated by ACD or protein contact dermatitis (PCD). Most patients initially present with hand dermatitis that, thereafter spreads to other locations (forearms, face, neck), as a result of ectopic or airborne mechanisms [44].

Protein contact dermatitis presents with chronic eczema with episodes of intense pruritus, erythema, edema, wheals, or papules-vesicles, developing within minutes after contact with the culprit food. Food (animal-origin, vegetal-origin, or cereal) or enzymes (in bakery) may potentially cause PCD. PCD rarely presents with generalized urticaria, or systemic symptoms. Immediate IgE-mediated hypersensitivity diagnostic tests should be performed to rule out this frequent condition among food handlers with refractory hand eczema [44].

Gastronomy professionals are exposed to multiple agents with irritant and/or sensitizing properties within a moist environment. Chefs, bakers, and confectioners are more prone to dermatoses. Most frequent dermatoses acquired while working in a kitchen is ICD from exposure to humidity, raw food, and detergents. Atopic background may contribute to ICD. At the same time, ICD is an essential risk factor for both immediate Ig-E-mediated hypersensitivity reactions (contact urticaria and PCD) and delayed reactions (ACD). Often, these disorders may appear simultaneously and/or concomitantly with atopic dermatitis. Accordingly, chefs usually suffer from pathogenetically complex hand eczema difficult to manage and with a significant impairment of their work performance and quality of life [44].

Allergens in this setting are mainly found in food. Other sources of sensitizers are food additives, utensils, furniture, gloves, soaps, disinfectants, etc.

In most ACD cases, hands are involved from direct contact with the culprit agent, but other anatomical sites (wrists, forearms, face, neck, flexures, etc.) can also be affected through a variety of mechanisms, such as ectopic (from contaminated tools, counters, fingers, etc.), airborne (vapors, powders, etc.), or systemic (inhalation of vapors) [44].

An example of ACD in kitchen workers is the hyperkeratotic fingertip ACD from diallyl disulfide in garlic involving the first three fingers of the non-dominant hand [44].

Protein contact dermatitis following exposure to proteins (animal food products, vegetables, cereals, or enzymes) generally occurs without systemic reactions. It usually involves the dorsa of the hands, fingers, periungual skin, wrists, and forearms. The suspicion index for PCD in food-handling professionals should be high in order not to miss the diagnosis [44].

Less often, other reactions (phototoxic and photoallergic reactions, chronic inducible urticaria, fixed food eruptions, infections, vascular stasis dermatitis, rosacea aggravation, acneiform eruptions, cuts, thermal burns, etc.) have been described [44].

Regarding ACD, patch test series should be performed. Open, prick, scratch or rub tests as well as RAST are necessary whenever contact urticaria or PCD are suspected. A stepwise approach is required with precautions to minimize the risk of anaphylaxis. Non-standardized patch testing with food *as is* may induce active sensitization or irritation. Regarding food, semi-open tests, or shorter occlusion periods are preferable. Prick-by-prick with food *as is* is more sensitive than prick tests with commercial food extracts or RAST [44].

Occupational dermatoses involving professionals working in the kitchen may considerably impact patients' quality of life and frequently cause sick leave and loss of jobs. Primary and secondary intervention are not easy but contribute to help patients to continue working and prevent patients from needing complex treatments [44].

Flight and Ground Staff

Ground crew may be exposed to dielectric fluids from electro discharge machining, "prepreg" materials and sealants in aircraft manufacture, aliphatic and aromatic compounds in kerosene (e.g., N-phenyl-1-naph-thylamine) and jet-fuel during refueling and maintenance operations.

Cabin crew may develop ICD from excessive handwashing and the planes low relative humidity; and ACD from gloves, textile dyes [45] or oxygen facemasks.

Pilots have reported less dry skin than other aircrew members although they may be exposed to other irritants during routine aircraft inspections (de-icing agents such as ethyleneglycol, hydraulic fluids, fuel, etc.) [46].

Atopic dermatitis may be exacerbated by environmental dryness and stress and itching may be distracting. Additionally, systemic medications may disqualify pilots from operating in some countries [46].

An atopic airline pilot was diagnosed with chronic actinic dermatosis likely caused by visible light presenting with facial eczema after been exposed to sunlight in the cockpit [47]. The link between UV exposure and skin cancer is less clear [46].

Military Personnel

ICD accounts for 80% of cases of contact dermatitis in the military field. The occupational irritants most frequently reported by military personnel include alcohols, cutting oils, coolants, degreasers, disinfectants, soaps, solvents, and wet work [48].

Contact dermatitis or acneiform eruption from military camouflage creams with castor oil, insect repellents and military uniform/footwear are common dermatological problems. Heat, sweating, and wearing of the uniform aggravate the conditions. Main allergens in military uniforms include formaldehyde resins, chromate, and PTBFFR. The military insect repellent contains DEET (N,Ndiethyl- M-toluamide) which can trigger ICD, contact urticaria, skin necrosis, neurotoxicity, and cardiotoxicity. Fungal foot infection is also common in this setting [49].

Research comparing military personnel and civilians evaluated for suspected shoe and textile dermatitis showed that the atopy rate was significantly higher among military conscripts, yet the patch test reactivity and multiple patch test reactivity and the duration of the dermatitis were lower within the military. Dermatitis seen in the military group tended to be more widely distributed [50].

Military decorative pin dermatitis has been described and pin backs of other materials (rubber, plastic, brass) pin backs have been proposed to prevent it [51].

Unusual dermatoses have been described in military personnel who are deployed worldwide, including sunburn, heat rash, arthropods and venomous bites, phytophotodermatitis, cutaneous *larva migrans*, myiasis, leishmaniasis, leprosy [52], cutaneous melioidosis (*Burkholderia pseudomallei*) [49], "beetle dermatitis" (blister beetles, false blister beetles, rove beetles) [48], "caterpillar dermatitis," [48] self-inflicted (malingering) Agave dermatitis, etc.

Eczema may disqualify the patient from more demanding occupations (aviation, diving, nuclear reactors, or Special Forces) [48].

Health Care Providers

Healthcare workers are at risk of occupational contact dermatitis due to repetitive hand washing, extended use of disinfectants and prolonged exposure to gloves. Sensitization may develop from rubber allergens, fragrances [53, 54], preservatives and corticosteroids [54]. Hand eczema may increase the carriage of pathogenic microbes, including methicillin-resistant *Staphylococcus aureus*, can reduce the compliance with alcohol-based disinfectants [53] and may significantly impact the quality of life.

Hand eczema and facial skin disease associated with hygiene procedures and personal protective equipment (PPE) are more common in the COVID19 units [53, 55]. Healthcare workers tend to use moisturizers instead of corticosteroids to treat it.

Prolonged mask wear, pressure and friction can lead to ICD on the cheeks and nasal bridge as well as acneiform eruptions (*acne mechanica*) especially in vulnerable patients with skin barrier (atopic dermatitis) and/or microbiota dysfunction [56, 57].

On the other hand, ACD or contact urticaria from masks results from sensitization to their components. Prolonged wear, rubbing, and sweating allow transfer of allergens to the skin [56]. Hydrocolloid patches have been recommended to prevent reactions from masks.

Several allergens have been described in masks such as rubber chemicals (carba mix, thiuram mix, tetramethylthiuram disulfide, tetramethylthiuram monosulfide, zinc diethyldithiocarmate, and zinc dibutyldithiocarbamate) in the elastic bands [57], nickel and cobalt in the metal wire [58], formaldehyde releasers [59] or methyldibromo glutaronitrile (in the adhesive beneath the polyester foam) [56].

A doctor experienced ACD to FFP3 masks at work. Patch testing revealed a strong positive reaction to the FFP3 masks, although it was not possible to obtain further information about the mask composition from the manufacturer [58].

The incomplete/absent disclosure of chemicals used in the manufacture of masks often makes investigating relevant allergens difficult.

Reactions localized to the skin covered by masks can also be secondary to allergens in cosmetics or topical medications such as hydrocortisone-17-butyrate [58]. Occlusion, moist, and friction provide an optimal environment for cosmetics to induce ICD or ACD [58].

Accordingly, patch tests with the cosmetics provided by the patient or specific series are advisable.

Interestingly, aquagenic urticaria triggered by intense sweating from wearing disposable gown in a COVID19 ward was reported involving a nurse [60].

Contact with medications can cause occupational ACD in health care providers such as nurses working in geriatric wards who work at crushing drugs with mortars [61]. ACD from handling medications at work may potentially jeopardize their future oral administration to the sensitized patient. Oral tolerance tests with alternative drugs are encouraged.

Thirteen percent of OACD among health care providers were reported to be caused by exposure to drugs. Tetrazepam, a frequent culprit ACD agent in the past, has been withdrawn from the market [61]. Multiple reactions (e.g., benzodiazepines), due to co-sensitization or cross-reactions may be observed [61].

ACD from drugs mainly involve the hands, but airborne facial ACD (from crushing tablets, powders, droplets, aerosols, etc.) or systemic reactions (from inhalation or transcutaneous absorption) may also develop. Women are more frequently involved, due to the higher number of women working in the sector. Physicians are less frequently involved than nurses and pharmacists because they contact less with medications. Damaged skin barrier from daily exposure to irritants facilitates sensitization. Fortunately, a decreasing trend has been observed, due to monitoring, protection measures, ventilation, careful handling, crushing devices, masks, gloves, etc. [61]

Dental Professionals (Dentists, Orthodontists, Technicians, Nurses)

The incidence of occupational skin disease is higher in dental practitioners, particularly dental technicians, and nurses, compared other health care providers [62].

The use of gloves has increased the frequency of ACD to rubber vulcanization accelerators.

Additionally, concerns about potential metal toxicity (amalgam) and demands for cosmetic dentistry have resulted in greater sensitization to (meth)acrylates, urethane acrylates, and epoxy acrylates. Concomitantly, a decrease of allergens that were common in the past (local anesthetics, eugenol, and glutaraldehyde) has been observed [63, 64].

Bonding materials often contain 2-hydroxyethyl methacrylate (2-HEMA) and bisphenol A glycidyl methacrylate (BIS-GMA); composite resins contain bis-GMA and triethyleneglycol dimethacrylate (TREGDMA); and glass ionomers, 2-HEMA and trimethylolpropane trimethacrylate [65]. Dentists and dental nurses are most commonly exposed to 2-HEMA, TREGDMA, and bis-GMA and dental technicians are mainly exposed to methyl methacrylate (MMA) and ethyleneglycol dimethacrylate (EGDMA) [65]. Reactions to bis-GMA, DEGDA, TREGDA, EMA, and EA are also sometimes relevant [65].

Dental technicians and orthodontists manufacture prosthesis and fashioning plates and are more exposed to (meth)acrylate than general dentists [63].

Clinically ACD presents with eczema on the first three fingertips of the dominant hand, paresthesia and pain [63]. Sometimes unusual distribution of the dermatitis occurs because of the unique ways of handling (meth)acrylate materials at work: for example, from wiping off the excessive bonding agent onto the dorsal side of the non-dominant hand [66]. Additionally, airborne (meth)acrylate may cause occupational respiratory disease and conjunctivitis.

ACD to traditional allergens such as eugenol (in dressings or impression materials), colophony (in periodontal dressings and cements), anesthetics used in the past (benzocaine, tetracaine, and procaine), glutaraldehyde (used in the past to sterilize dental materials), metals in restorative work (amalgams of silver, tin, mercury, copper), has decreased [63]. The newer amide anesthetics (lignocaine, mepivacaine, prilocaine, bupivacaine) cause reactions less often, materials are currently sterilized in autoclaves, and metals have been replaced by plastics [63].

Occupational asthma to methacrylates was described to involve a general dentist who operated with prosthesis and fillings. Prick test reactions to methacrylates were negative but the inhalation challenge test with liquid dental methacrylates was positive. Mechanism for occupational asthma induced by methacrylates is unknown since IgE -mediated reactions, to our knowledge, have not been proved. Respiratory disease from methacrylates in the workplace usually leads to a job change. On the other hand, patients with isolated ACD can continue working with adequate protection [67].

Type I allergy to latex in gloves is less frequent than delayed-type hypersensitivity to rubber additives. Anaphylactic reactions from wearing gloves without a primary exposure of mucosae is, however, rare unless latex binds to glove powder and is inhaled. Curiously, the first case of anaphylaxis from natural rubber latex following a gynecological exploration was originally described to involve a young dentist [64].

Patch testing should be performed with the standard series supplemented with dentistry, medicaments, preservatives, rubber series, etc. depending on the clinical history.

Primary prevention involves training dental professionals in the hazards linked to the products they handle at work. Alternative gloves without vulcanization accelerators are polyvinyl chloride, polyurethane, silicone rubber and styrene-based copolymers. They, however, may contain other allergenic chemicals such as plasticizers, stabilizers, ultraviolet absorbers, fungicides, biocides, and colorants [64].

To prevent reactions from methacrylates, a no-touch technique is required. Medical-grade gloves can be permeated by methacrylates. 4H gloves are safe but difficult to find, and too rigid for precise tasks. Nitrile gloves (especially a double layered) may be effective for a few minutes only [66].

Ventilation is crucial to prevent airborne exposure to methacrylates and glutaraldehyde. Powdered latex gloves in the environment should be avoided [64].

Veterinarians

Hand and forearm occupational dermatoses in veterinarians including ICD, CU, and ACD, are triggered by a combination of factors (sweating, wet work, repeated hand washing, occlusion under rubber gloves, animal fluids, antiseptics, medications, insecticides, and atopic skin barrier disruption) [68].

A small animal practice poses a lower occupational hazard than a rural practice where surgical procedures are performed under less hygienic circumstances, colder climate, and difficulties to rinse off disinfectants or animal fluids [68].

Relevant positive patch test reactions have been described to medications (neomycin, ampicillin, benzocaine, tixocortol pivalate, budesonide, triamcinolone acetonide, hydrocortisone, prednisone), as well as other allergens such as propylene glycol, thiuram mix, formaldehyde, phenoxyethanol, animal vaccines, etc.

Contact urticaria may result from exposure to animal products (amniotic fluid during obstetric procedures, saliva, blood, etc.); latex gloves; or animal medication (e.g., penicillin). It usually involves the hands and forearms and occasionally may be associated to systemic symptomatology. During the calving, some vets do not use gloves or use short gloves exposing the bare forearms to the fluids [68].

A veterinarian was reported to develop contact urticaria from dog's milk after performing caesarian sections, examinations of female pregnant dogs or suckling pups. The patient did not react to milk from other species or other dog's fluids [69]. Contact urticaria or PCD are very fluid- and species-specific.

Infectious dermatoses have also been described (including *tinea corporis/manuum*, forearm erysipelas and impetigo of the back of the hands). Mild infectious dermatoses can be underestimated because veterinarians may self-medicate [68].

Skin disease may seriously impact veterinarians' careers. Accurate diagnosis requires performing patch tests and immediate hypersensitivity diagnostic tests with materials/

series determined by the clinical history [68]. Protective equipment to efficiently prevent contact from animal fluids, antiseptics, or medications during obstetric and other procedures should be implemented.

Marine mammal workers (trainers, veterinarians, wildlife rehabilitators, researchers, aquaria and oceanarium workers, etc.) are at risk of occupational disease including traumatic injuries (wounds, cuts, scrapes, bites, needle sticks, scalpel cuts, etc.) often involving the extremities [70] as well as infectious disease such as bacterial infections (including *Clostridium perfringens, Staphylococcus aureus, Mycobacterium marinum, Corynebacter spp., Pseudomonas spp., Vibrio spp., etc.*), viral infections (poxvirus or herpesvirus) or "seal finger" (*Mycoplasma spp.* or *Erysipelothrix rhusiopathiae*) [70].

Additionally, exposure to diseased marine mammals may contribute to the emergence of infectious disease by allowing the flow of pathogens between species. Workers should adhere to safety guidelines (e.g., protective clothing, training, risk evaluation programs, advice on the risks for zoonotic disease, etc.) [70].

Beauty Industry

Hairdressers

Occupational contact dermatitis (OCD) is frequent among hairdressers. Risk factors for irritant damage and skin sensitization in this setting include: wet work and exposure to hair cosmetics, dyes, and detergents without appropriate protection [71, 72].

P-phenylenediamine (PPD) and toluene-2,5-diamine (PTD) in hair dyes, persulfate salts in hair bleaching products and, less often, glyceryl thioglycolate and ammonium thioglycolate in permanent waving agents are important occupational allergens [71, 73]. The Danish Contact Dermatitis Group identified PPD, ammonium persulfate, PTD, m-aminophenol, and p-aminophenol as frequent sensitizers in hairdressers with ACD during 2002–2011 [74]. The

same allergens were detected in Greece and Spain [75, 76].

Following hairdressing chemicals, other allergens relevant for hairdressers' ACD are metals, biocides, rubber additives, and perfumes [72, 77, 78]. Fragrance allergy is more frequently relevant in the beauty industry than in other sectors [77, 79].

Hairdressers/cosmetologists/barbers were reported to be those occupations more frequently associated with nickel allergy (14.3%) in North America [80]. Metallic hairdressing tools are considered a major source of nickel exposure [81].

Hair Dyes

Permanent oxidative hair dye formulations are marketed as two components that should be mixed immediately prior to use. One component contains the dye precursors (PPD, 2,5- diaminotoluene, N,N-bis(2-hydroxymethyl)-p-phenylenediamine, p-aminophenol etc.), the couplers (resorcinol, chlororesorcinol, methyl resorcinol, alpha-naphthol, m-aminophenol, etc.) and an alkaline soap. The other component is a stabilized solution of hydrogen peroxide. The precursors and peroxide diffuse into the hair shaft, where color formation takes place following a cascade of chemical reactions [82].

PPD, a 1,4-substituted benzene derivative, is a key allergen. It may cross-react with chemicals containing an amine group in the benzene ring at the para position, such as black rubber mix, benzocaine group (ester) anesthetics, parabens, paminobenzoic acid (PABA), sulfonamides, p-aminosalicylic acid, thiazides, and azo dyes [75].

Persulfate Salts

Air-bleaching products contain persulfate salts (sodium persulfate, ammonium persulfate, potassium peroxymonosulfate and potassium persulfate). Patch testing with ammonium persulfate is used as a screening diagnostic method for persulfate allergy [83].

Persulfate are highly reactive low-molecular-weight chemicals able to cause ICD, ACD, and immediate reactions (e.g., contact urticaria, rhinitis, asthma, anaphylaxis) [84]. Specific persulfate-IgE has been proved in some cases [85].

Hairdressers are exposed to persulfate salts when mixing bleaching powder with hydrogen peroxide. Dust powder is easily inhaled and transferred to the eye/nasal mucosae [84].

Persulfates salts can also be found in hair coloring products, denture cleansers, pool/hot-tub products, paints, cleaning products and nonskin disinfectants [80, 83].

Permanent Hair Waving Solutions (Thioglycolates and Cysteamine Hydrochloride)

Glyceryl monothioglycolate (GMTG) and ammonium thioglycolate were recognized as the main allergens in permanent waving solutions in the past. The ban of GMTG in Germany in 1997 was followed by a decrease in the frequency of cases [86]. Recently, however, sensitization to it has been observed to involve young females which may indicate continued exposure [87]. On the other hand, thioglycolates were considered an infrequent cause of hairdressers' ACD by other authors [77].

Cysteamine hydrochloride (HCl) has become an emerging permanent waving product allergen in Japan [88]. Several hairdressers in the North of Europe were described to be sensitized to it in the 1990–2000s [89].

Contact dermatitis (both ICD and ACD) is the dermatosis most frequently observed in hairdressers, mainly involving the hands, followed by the forearms.

ICD is more frequent among apprentices from hair washing and mainly involves the dorsal side of hands and fingers as well as interdigital spaces. Palmar atrophy with scales and pronounced skin creasing has also been described.

ACD presents with acute, subacute, or chronic eczema sometimes with dyshidrosiform lesions. Second and third fingers of the non-dominant hand are usually involved from holding the hair with bare fingers (Fig. 14.1). Less often, ectopic, or airborne facial dermatitis, mainly from persulfates, may also be observed [90].

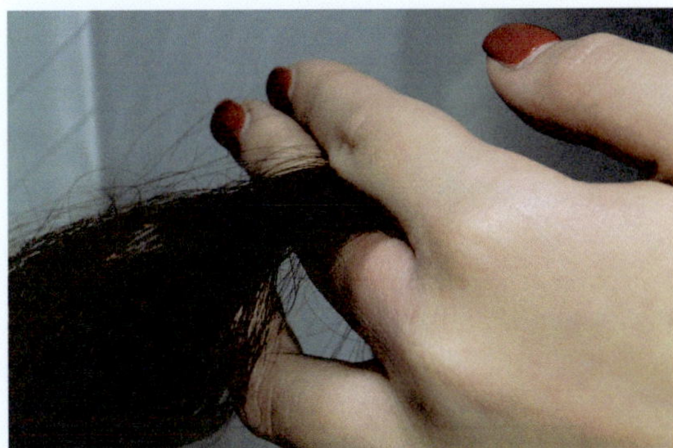
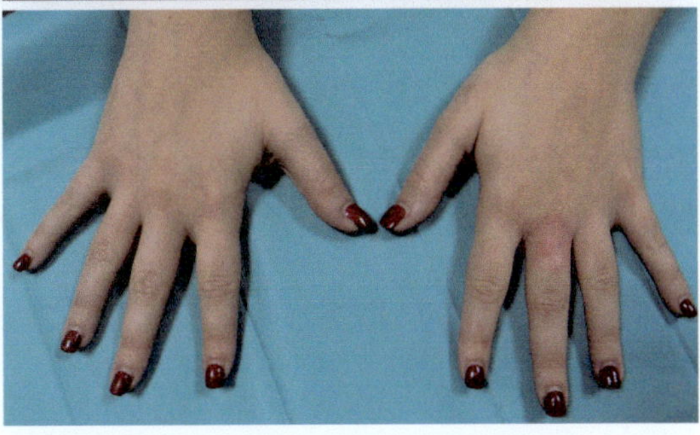

Fig. 14.1 Eczematous lesions at the lateral side of the second and third fingers of the non-dominant hand from holding the dyed hair involving a hairdresser who was sensitized to P-phenylenediamine (PPD)

Persulfates were the most common cause of contact urticaria (CU) in hairdressers [77, 84]. There are scarce reports of asthma, rhinitis, and CU caused by PPD and related compounds [91]. Immediate-type allergies to latex direct hair dye (basic blue 99) have also been published [92–96].

Adequate protective measures and prevention strategies should be emphasized during apprentices training [71, 72, 97].

Disposable gloves while washing hair or handling dyes, bleaching, waving or straightening products should be used. All products should be applied after cutting hair since these substances can long impregnate hair [98]. Gloves should never be reused, regardless of material [98, 99]. The protective efficacy of gloves can be influenced by the nature of the chemicals, the exposure time, occlusion, sweating, stretching, and skin temperature [98].

Nitrile gives good protection against hair dyes [98–100]. Polyvinylchloride (PVC) gloves do not contain rubber allergens and are likely the best choice to minimize the risk of contact allergy from hair dyeing [99]. Latex gloves are discouraged, due to the risk of sensitization.

Avoiding fragrances when they are not essential for function is recommended [79].

Exposure to the persulfate dust can be minimized by switching the powdered hair bleach to granular formulations, wearing protective gloves, providing ventilation, and mixing the products in the designated areas [84, 101]. Patients with asthma caused by persulfate salts are advised to discontinue their work [84].

Nail Beauticians [102]

The popularity and widespread use of semipermanent polishes has caused a progressive increase in the frequency of ACD to (meth)acrylates. HPMA (hydroxypropyl methacrylate), HEMA (hydroxyethyl methacrylate), and THFMA (tetrahydrofurfuryl methacrylate) are the most frequent relevant allergens in ACD to semipermanent polish [102]. The insufficient training of beauticians regarding the risks/preventive measures has contributed to this situation. Additionally, dermatologists occasionally misdiagnose ACD in acrylate-based manicure materials as psoriasis and unnecessarily treat it with immunosuppressants [102].

Beauticians usually combine different techniques and materials. Main techniques include semipermanent (long-lasting) nail polish, gel nails, acrylic nails and preformed nails [102]. Spanish research (2013–2016), showed that 1.82% of the general patch-tested population was sensitized to acrylates in manicure materials (mostly beauticians) [102].

The involvement of the fingertips (especially the first three or four fingers of the dominant hand) is very characteristic (Fig. 14.2). Acute lesions are exudative and itchy, while chronic lesions are painful, hyperkeratotic, and fissured. Lesions on other areas (face, eyelids, lips, neck, forearms) may follow passive transfer through contaminated fingers or objects, or airborne mechanisms [102].

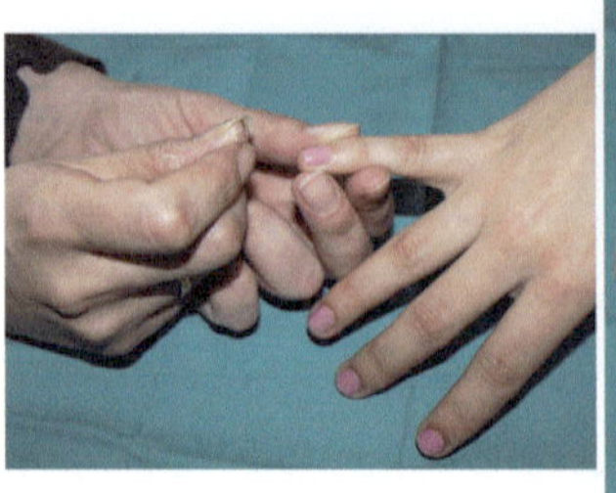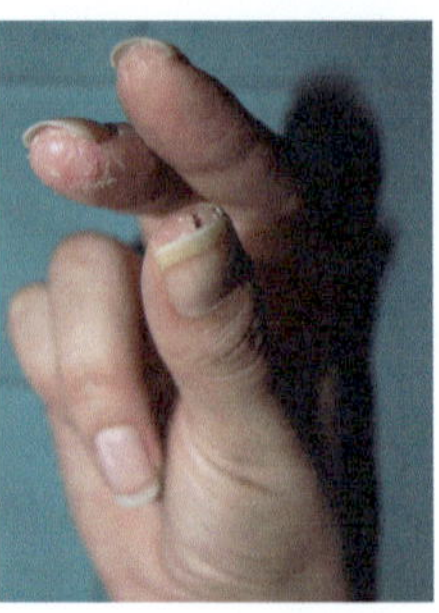

Fig. 14.2 Chronic eczematous lesions involving the fingertips of the first fingers of the dominant hand from holding the nail polish container involving a beautician who was sensitized to several acrylates

Nail dystrophy is frequent including onycholysis, subungual hyperkeratosis, splinter hemorrhages, pseudo-leukonychia, *onychoschizia lamellina* (lamellar splitting), thinning of the nail plate, *pterygium inversum unguis,* or pyogenic granuloma. Acute urticaria and lymphomatoid papulosis-like contact reactions have also been described [102].

Sensitization to acrylates in these merely esthetic procedures, may jeopardize the use of medical devices containing acrylates thereafter. In the European Union manicure products containing acrylates are currently restricted to professional use. Training regarding the risks and preventive measures should be delivered to professionals. 4H gloves are considered the safest option, although they are difficult to find and too rigid to perform fine tasks with dexterity. Nitrile gloves have been proposed as appropriate alternatives for short periods of time, especially when a double layer is used. 4H finger stalls kept in place by wearing nitrile gloves on top have also been recommended. Dermatologists should be trained to manage these patients more efficiently [102].

Conclusions

The typical management strategy for patients, with occupational skin disease within the service sector, relies on an accurate etiological diagnosis. Since the potential etiological factors and sources of exposure are multiple and varied, it is essential to apply individualized specific diagnostic tests according to the clinical history. Patch tests (with baseline and specific series, as well as the personal products provided by the patients), or prick tests, should be tailored to each case to rule out delayed or immediate allergic reactions, respectively.

Secondary prevention of CD involves avoiding the exposure to the agents causing the reaction(s) or switching them over to allergen-free alternatives. Unfortunately, manufacturers do not always provide information regarding the full components of their products. Regulations are urgently needed to compel manufacturers to cooperate in the patch test investigations and to provide transparent information regarding the composition of the products.

Finally, it is crucial to apply effective treatments to lessen the impairment that the disease may have on the professional performance and quality of life of patients.

References

1. Federico J. Caballero Ferrari, 24 de enero, 2016 Sector terciario o servicios. Economipedia.com. https://economipedia.com/definiciones/sector-terciario-servicios.html
2. Sector terciario. https://www.sdelsol.com/glosario/sector-terciario https://www.sdelsol.com/glosario/sector-terciario/
3. Kockentiet B, Adams BB. Contact dermatitis in athletes. J Am Acad Dermatol. 2007;56(6):1048–55.
4. Brooks C, Kujawska A, Patel D. Cutaneous allergic reactions induced by sporting activities. Sports Med. 2003;33(9):699–708.
5. Ramzy AG, Hagvall L, Pei MN, Samuelsson K, Nilsson U. Investigation of diethylthiourea and ethyl isothiocyanate as potent skin allergens in chloroprene rubber. Contact Dermatitis. 2015 Mar;72(3):139–46.
6. Okawa T, Hotta A, Sato M, Takahashi S, Komori J, Aihara M. Allergic contact dermatitis caused by diethyl thiourea in a neoprene-containing wet suit. J Dermatol. 2018;45(3):365–6.
7. Sakuragi Y, Sawada Y, Nakamura M. Leukoderma following allergic contact dermatitis caused by the silicone component silprene-30A/B in swimming goggles. Contact Dermatitis. 2017;77(6):418–9.
8. Melé-Ninot G, Iglesias-Sancho M, Bergendorff O, Lázaro-Simó AI, Quintana-Codina M, Salleras-Redonnet M. Photoallergic contact dermatitis due to benzophenone contained in swimming goggles. Contact Dermatitis. 2020;82(1):59–60.
9. Farhadian JA, Tlougan BE, Adams BB, Leventhal JS, Sanchez MR. Skin conditions of baseball, cricket, and softball players. Sports Med. 2013 Jul;43(7):575–89.
10. Reeder M, Atwater AR. Acetophenone Azine: the 2021 American contact Dermatitis society allergen of the year. Cutis. 2021;107(5):238–40.
11. Raison-Peyron N, Bergendorff O, Bourrain JL, Bruze M. Acetophenone azine: a new allergen responsible for severe contact dermatitis from shin pads. Contact Dermatitis. 2016;75(2):106–10.
12. Raison-Peyron N, Bergendorff O, Du-Thanh A, Bourrain JL, Bruze M. Two new cases of severe allergic contact dermatitis caused by acetophenone azine. Contact Dermatitis. 2017 Jun;76(6):380–1.
13. De Fré C, Bergendorff O, Raison-Peyron N, et al. Acetophenone azine: a new shoe allergen causing severe foot dermatitis. Contact Dermatitis. 2017;77:416–7.
14. Koumaki D, Bergendorff O, Bruze M, Orton D. Allergic contact Dermatitis to shin pads in a hockey player: Acetophenone is an emerging allergen. Dermatitis. 2019;30(2):162–3.
15. Darrigade AS, Raison-Peyron N, Courouge-Dorcier D, Vital-Durand D, Milpied B, Giordano-Labadie F, Aerts O. The chemical acetophenone azine: an important cause of shin and foot dermatitis in children. J Eur Acad Dermatol Venereol. 2020;34(2):e61–2.
16. Aizawa A, Ito A, Masui Y, Sasaki K, Ishimura Y, Numata M, Abe R. A case of allergic contact dermatitis caused by goalkeeper gloves. Contact Dermatitis. 2018;79(2):113–5.
17. Corazza M, Minghetti S, Benetti S, Marchetti N, Borghi A, Virgili A. Allergic contact dermatitis in a volleyball player due to protective adhesive taping. Eur J Dermatol. 2011;21(3):430–1.
18. Corazza M, Musmeci D, Scuderi V, Bernardi T, Cristofaro D, Borghi A. Occupational systemic allergic dermatitis in a football player sensitized to colophonium. Contact Dermatitis. 2018 Nov;79(5):325–6.
19. Ledon JA, Tosti A. CrossFit-associated allergic contact Dermatitis. Dermatitis. 2017;28(6):368.
20. Gumulka M, Matura M, Lidén C, Kettelarij JA, Julander A. Nickel exposure when working out in the gym. Acta Derm Venereol. 2015 Feb;95(2):247–9.
21. Isaksson M, Möller H, Pontén A. Occupational allergic contact dermatitis from epoxy resin in a golf club repairman. Dermatitis. 2008;19(5):E30–2.
22. Tammaro A, Cortesi G, Abruzzese C, Narcisi A, Ermini G, Parisella FR, Persechino S. Archer dermatitis: a new case of allergic contact dermatitis. Occup Environ Med. 2013;70(10):750. https://doi.org/10.1136/oemed-2013-101424. Epub 2013 Jul 19. PMID: 23873984
23. Inui S, Yamamoto S, Ikegami R, Ozawa K, Itami S, Yoshikawa K. Baseball pitcher's friction dermatitis. Contact Dermatitis. 2002;47(3):176–7.
24. Tlougan BE, Mancini AJ, Mandell JA, Cohen DE, Sanchez MR. Skin conditions in figure skaters,

ice-hockey players and speed skaters: part II - cold-induced, infectious and inflammatory dermatoses. Sports Med. 2011;41(11):967–84.

25. M.A. Pastor-Nieto, L. Vergara-de-la-Campa, M.E. Gatica-Ortega, Giménez-Arnau A. Angioedema vibratorio adquirido (nofamiliar), ACTASDermo-Sifiliográficas. https://doi.org/10.1016/j.jad.2021.06.005.

26. Mathelier-Fusade P, Vermeulen C, Leynadier F. Vibratory angioedema. Ann Dermatol Venereol. 2001 Jul;128(6–7):750–2.

27. Pressler A, Grosber M, Halle M, Ring J, Brockow K. Failure of omalizumab and successful control with ketotifen in a patient with vibratory angiooedema. Clin Exp Dermatol. 2013;38(2):151–3.

28. Kraft M, Schubert S, Geier J, Worm M, IVDK. Contact dermatitis and sensitization in professional musicians. Contact Dermatitis. 2019 May;80(5):273–8.

29. Gambichler T, Uzun A, Boms S, Altmeyer P, Altenmüller E. Skin conditions in instrumental musicians: a self-reported survey. Contact Dermatitis. 2008;58(4):217–22.

30. Patruno C, Napolitano M, La Bella S, Ayala F, Balato N, Cantelli M, Balato A. Instrument-related skin disorders in musicians. Dermatitis. 2016;27(1):26–9.

31. Vandebuerie L, Aerts C, Goossens A. Allergic contact dermatitis resulting from multiple colophonium-related allergen sources. Contact Dermatitis. 2014;70(2):117–9.

32. Alves PB, Todo-Bom A, Regateiro FS. Viola duet: a rare case of double sensitization to contact allergens in a professional musician. Contact Dermatitis. 2020 Dec;83(6):523–4.

33. Alcántara-Nicolás FA, Pastor-Nieto MA, Sánchez-Herreros C, Pérez-Mesonero R, Melgar-Molero V, Ballano A, De-Eusebio E. Allergic contact dermatitis from acrylic nails in a flamenco guitarist. Occup Med (Lond). 2016;66(9):751–3.

34. Okoshi K, Minami T, Kikuchi M, Tomizawa Y. Musical instrument-associated health issues and their management. Tohoku J Exp Med. 2017 Sep;243(1):49–56.

35. Jue MS, Kim YS, Ro YS. Fiddler's neck accompanied by allergic contact Dermatitis to nickel in a Viola player. Ann Dermatol. 2010 Feb;22(1):88–90.

36. Guarneri F, Guarneri C, Marini HR. Amitriptyline and bromazepam in the treatment of vibratory angioedema: which role for neuroinflammation? Dermatol Ther. 2014;27:361–4.

37. Sarmast SA, Fang F, Zic J. Vibratory angioedema in a trumpet professor. Cutis. 2014;93:10–1.

38. Patruno C, Ayala F, Cimmino G, Mordente I, Balato N. Vibratory angioedema in a saxophonist. Dermat Contact Atopic Occup Drug. 2009;20:346–7.

39. Fisher AA. Dermatitis in actors, dancers, singers, and circus performers. Cutis. 1999;63(2):62.

40. Färm G, Karlberg AT, Lidén C. Are opera-house artistes afflicted with contact allergy to colophony and cosmetics? Contact Dermatitis. 1995 May;32(5):273–80.

41. Isaksson M, Linauskiene K, Dahlin J. Skin problems in an opera choir. Contact Dermatitis. 2020;83(3):244–5.

42. Gallo R, Paolino S, Marcella G, Parodi A. Consort allergic contact dermatitis caused by ketoprofen in a tango dancer. Contact Dermatitis. 2010;63(3):172–4.

43. Aberer W. Allergy to colophony acquired backstage. Contact Dermatitis. 1987;16:34–6.

44. Pastor-Nieto MA, Giménez-Arnau AM. Immediate and delayed hypersensitivity reactions occurring in the kitchen: the hazards related to being a chef or kitchen staff. In: John S, Johansen J, Rustemeyer T, Elsner P, Maibach H, editors. Kanerva's occupational dermatology. Cham: Springer; 2018. https://doi.org/10.1007/978-3-319-40221-5_214-1.

45. Khanna M, Sasseville D. Occupational contact dermatitis to textile dyes in airline personnel. Am J Contact Dermat. 2001;12(4):208–10.

46. Leggat PA, Smith DR. Dermatitis and aircrew. Contact Dermatitis. 2006 Jan;54(1):1–4.

47. Yones SS, Palmer RA, Hextall JM, Hawk JL. Exacerbation of presumed chronic actinic dermatitis by cockpit visible light in an airline pilot with atopic eczema. Photodermatol Photoimmunol Photomed. 2005;21(3):152–3.

48. Dever TT, Walters M, Jacob S. Contact dermatitis in military personnel. Dermatitis. 2011;22(6):313–9.

49. Chong WS. Dermatology in the military field: what physicians should know? World J Clin Cases. 2013;1(7):208–11.

50. Slodownik D, Reiss A, Mashiach Y, Ingber A, Sprecher E, Moshe S. Textile and shoe allergic contact dermatitis in military personnel. Dermatitis. 2018;29(4):196–9.

51. Limone BA, Jacob SE. Military decorative pin Dermatitis: prevention for nickel allergy among service members. Dermatitis. 2018;29(1):46–7.

52. Bailey MS. Tropical skin diseases in British military personnel. J R Army Med Corps. 2013 Sep;159(3):224–8.

53. Hamnerius N, Pontén A, Bergendorff O, Bruze M, Björk J, Svedman C. Skin exposures, hand eczema and facial skin disease in healthcare workers during the COVID-19 pandemic: a cross-sectional study. Acta Derm Venereol. 2021;101(9):adv00543.

54. Huang C, Greig D, Cheng H. Allergic contact dermatitis in healthcare workers. Occup Med (Lond). 2021;71(6–7):294–7.

55. Erdem Y, Inal S, Sivaz O, Copur S, Boluk KN, Ugurer E, Kaya HE, Gulsunay IE, Sekerlisoy G, Vural O, Altunay IK, Aksu Çerman A, Özkaya E. How does working in pandemic units affect the risk of occupational hand eczema in healthcare workers during the coronavirus disease-2019 (COVID-19) pandemic: A comparative analysis with nonpandemic units. Contact Dermatitis. 2021; https://doi.org/10.1111/cod.13853.

56. Yu J, Chen JK, Mowad CM, Reeder M, Hylwa S, Chisolm S, Dunnick CA, Goldminz AM, Jacob SE, Wu PA, Zippin J, Atwater AR. Occupational dermatitis to facial personal protective equipment in health care workers: a systematic review. J Am Acad Dermatol. 2021;84(2):486–94.

57. Navarro-Triviño FJ, Merida-Fernández C, Ródenas-Herranz T, Ruiz-Villaverde R. Allergic contact dermatitis caused by elastic bands from FFP2 mask. Contact Dermatitis. 2020;83(2):168–9.

58. Schwensen JFB, Simonsen AB, Zachariae C, Johansen JD. Facial dermatoses in health care professionals induced by the use of protective masks during the COVID-19 pandemic. Contact Dermatitis. 2021;85(6):710–1.

59. Aerts O, Dendooven E, Foubert K, Stappers S, Ulicki M, Lambert J. Surgical mask dermatitis caused by formaldehyde (releasers) during the COVID-19 pandemic. Contact Dermatitis. 2020;83(2):172–3.

60. Alves PB, Alves MP, Todo-Bom A, Regateiro FS. Concomitant allergic contact dermatitis and aquagenic urticaria caused by personal protective equipment in a healthcare worker during the COVID-19 pandemic. Contact Dermatitis. 2021;85(4):471–2.

61. Gilissen L, Boeckxstaens E, Geebelen J, Goossens A. Occupational allergic contact dermatitis from systemic drugs. Contact Dermatitis. 2020;82(1):24–30.

62. Larese Filon F, Pesce M, Paulo MS, Loney T, Modenese A, John SM, Kezic S, Macan J. Incidence of occupational contact dermatitis in healthcare workers: a systematic review. J Eur Acad Dermatol Venereol. 2021;35(6):1285–9.

63. Rubel DM, Watchorn RB. Allergic contact dermatitis in dentistry. Australas J Dermatol. 2000;41(2):63–9. quiz 70–1

64. Hamann CP, DePaola LG, Rodgers PA. Occupation-related allergies in dentistry. J Am Dent Assoc. 2005;136(4):500–10.

65. Aalto-Korte K, Alanko K, Kuuliala O, Jolanki R. Methacrylate and acrylate allergy in dental personnel. Contact Dermatitis. 2007 Nov;57(5):324–30.

66. Prasad Hunasehally RY, Hughes TM, Stone NM. Atypical pattern of (meth)acrylate allergic contact dermatitis in dental professionals. Br Dent J. 2012;213(5):223–4.

67. Lindström M, Alanko K, Keskinen H, Kanerva L. Dentist's occupational asthma, rhinoconjunctivitis, and allergic contact dermatitis from methacrylates. Allergy. 2002;57(6):543–5.

68. Bulcke DM, Devos SA. Hand and forearm dermatoses among veterinarians. J Eur Acad Dermatol Venereol. 2007;21(3):360–3.

69. Foti C, Antelmi A, Mistrello G, Guarneri F, Filotico R. Occupational contact urticaria and rhinoconjunctivitis from dog's milk in a veterinarian. Contact Dermatitis. 2007;56(3):169–71.

70. Hunt TD, Ziccardi MH, Gulland FM, Yochem PK, Hird DW, Rowles T, Mazet JA. Health risks for marine mammal workers. Dis Aquat Organ. 2008;81(1):81–92.

71. Goebel C, Diepgen TL, Blömeke B, Gaspari AA, Schnuch A, Fuchs A, Schlotmann K, Krasteva M, Kimber I. Skin sensitization quantitative risk assessment for occupational exposure of hairdressers to hair dye ingredients. Regul Toxicol Pharmacol. 2018;95:124–32.

72. Carøe TK, Ebbehøj NE, Agner T. Occupational dermatitis in hairdressers - influence of individual and environmental factors. Contact Dermatitis. 2017;76(3):146–50.

73. Chu C, Marks JG Jr, Flamm A. Occupational contact Dermatitis: common occupational allergens. Dermatol Clin. 2020;38(3):339–49.

74. Schwensen JF, Johansen JD, Veien NK, et al. Occupational contact dermatitis in hairdressers: an analysis of patch test data from the Danish contact dermatitis group, 2002-2011. Contact Dermatitis. 2014;70(4):233–7.

75. Gregoriou S, Mastraftsi S, Hatzidimitriou E, et al. Occupational and non-occupational allergic contact dermatitis to hair dyes in Greece. A 10-year retrospective study. Contact Dermatitis. 2020;83(4):277–85.

76. Valks R, Conde-Salazar L, Malfeito J, Ledo S. Contact dermatitis in hairdressers, 10 years later: patch-test results in 300 hairdressers (1994 to 2003) and comparison with previous study. Dermatitis. 2005;16(1):28–31.

77. Pesonen M, Koskela K, Aalto-Korte K. Hairdressers' occupational skin diseases in the Finnish register of occupational diseases in a period of 14 years. Contact Dermatitis. 2021;84(4):236–9.

78. Piapan L, Mauro M, Martinuzzo C, Larese F. Characteristics and incidence of contact dermatitis among hairdressers in North-Eastern Italy. Contact Dermatitis. 2020;83(6):458–65.

79. Montgomery RL, Agius R, Wilkinson SM, Carder M. UK trends of allergic occupational skin disease attributed to fragrances 1996–2015. Contact Dermatitis. 2018;78(1):33–40.

80. Warshaw EM, Schlarbaum JP, DeKoven JG, et al. Occupationally related nickel reactions: a retrospective analysis of the north American contact dermatitis group data 1998-2016. Dermatitis. 2019;30(5):306–13.

81. Symanzik C, John SM, Strunk M. Nickel release from metal tools in the German hairdressing trade - a current analysis. Contact Dermatitis. 2019;80(6):382–5.

82. European Commission Scientific Committee on Consumer Products (SCCP). Updated recommended strategy for testing oxidative hair dye substances for their potential mutagenicity/genotoxicity. 2006. https://ec.europa.eu/health/ph_risk/committees/04_sccp/docs/sccp_s_02.pdf. Accessed 10 Feb 2022.

83. Dean O, Somers K. Persulfate-containing consumer products in the United States market. Contact Dermatitis. 2022;86:1–5. https://doi.org/10.1111/cod.14028.

84. Hougaard MG, Menne T, Sosted H. Occupational eczema and asthma in a hairdresser caused by hair-bleaching products. Dermatitis. 2012;23(6):284–7.

85. Aalto-Korte K, Mäkinen-Kiljunen S. Specific immunoglobulin E in patients with immediate persulfate hypersensitivity. Contact Dermatitis. 2003;49(1):22–5.

86. Uter W, GeierJ LG, SchnuchIs A. Is contact allergy to glyceryl monothioglycolate still a problem in Germany? Contact Dermatitis. 2006;55(1):54–6.

87. Uter W, Gefeller O, John SM, Schnuch A, Geier J. Contact allergy to ingredients of hair cosmetics-a comparison of female hairdressers and clients based on IVDK 2007-2012 data. Contact Dermatitis. 2014;71(1):13–20.

88. Nishioka K, Koizumi A, Takita Y. Allergic contact dermatitis caused by cysteamine hydrochloride in permanent wave agent—a new allergen for hairdressers in Japan. Contact Dermatitis. 2018;80(3):174–5.

89. Isaksson M, van der Walle H. Occupational contact allergy to cysteamine hydrochloride in permanent-wave solutions. Contactact Dermatitis. 2007;56(5):295–6.

90. Valdés-Morales KL, Alonzo-Romero L. Occupational allergic contact dermatitis from ammonium persulfate in a hairdresser. Contact Dermatitis. 2021;1–2:362.

91. Helaskoski E, Suojalehto H, Virtanen H, Airaksinen L, Kuuliala O, Aalto-Korte K, Pesonen M. Occupational asthma, rhinitis, and contact urticaria caused by oxidative hair dyes in hairdressers. Ann Allergy Asthma Immunol. 2014;112(1):46–52.

92. Valks R, Conde-Salazar L, Cuevas M. Allergic contact urticaria from natural rubber latex in healthcare and non-healthcare workers. Contact Dermatitis. 2004;50(4):222–4.

93. Davari P, Maibach H. Contact urticaria to cosmetic and industrial dyes. Clin Exp Dermatol. 2011;36(1):1–5.

94. Jagtman BA. Urticaria and contact urticaria due to basic blue 99 in a hair dye. Contact Dermatitis. 1996;35(1):52.

95. Wigger-Alberti W, Elsner P, Wuthrich B, et al. Immediate-type allergy to the hair dye basic blue 99 in a hairdresser. Allergy. 1996;51(1):64–5.

96. BroeckeK V, Bruze M, Persson L, Deroo H, Goossens A. Contact urticaria syndrome caused by direct hair dyes in a hairdresser. Contact Dermatitis. 2014;71(2):108–28.

97. Brans R, Schröder-Kraft C, Skudlik C, John SM, Geier J. Tertiary prevention of occupational skin diseases: prevalence of allergic contact dermatitis and pattern of patch test results. Contact Dermatitis. 2018;80(1):35–44.

98. Lind M-L, Johnsson S, Lidén C, Meding B, Boman A. The influence of hydrogen peroxide on the permeability of protective gloves to resorcinol in hairdressing. Contact Dermatitis. 2015;72(1):33–9.

99. Antelmi A, Ewa Young A, Svedman C, ZimerssonE EM, Foti C, Bruze M. Are gloves sufficiently protective when hairdressers are exposed to permanent hair dyes? An in vivo study. Contact Dermatitis. 2015;72(4):229–36.

100. Havmose M, Thyssen JP, Zachariae C, Johansen JD. Use of protective gloves by hairdressers: a review of efficacy and potential adverse effects. Contact Dermatitis. 2020;83(2):75–82.

101. Warshaw EM, Ruggiero JL, DeKoven JG, Pratt MD, Silverberg JI, Maibach HI, Zug KA, Atwater AR, Taylor JS, Reeder MJ, Sasseville D, Fowler JF Jr, Fransway AF, Belsito DV, DeLeo VA, Houle MC, Dunnick CA. Patch testing with ammonium persulfate: the north American contact Dermatitis group experience, 2015-2018. J Am Acad Dermatol. 2021;S0190-9622(21):02289–1.

102. Gatica-Ortega ME, Pastor-Nieto MA. The present and future burden of contact Dermatitis from acrylates in manicure. Curr Treat Options Allergy. 2020;7:291–311. https://doi.org/10.1007/s40521-020-00272-w.

Medicolegal Implications and the Importance of the Medical Report

Peter Elsner

P. Elsner (✉)
Dermatology, Allergology, Dermatopathology, SRH Wald-Klinikum Gera, Gera, Germany

Prof. Dr. Peter Elsner & Rolf-Peter Dröge, Solicitors, Hamburg, Germany

The Concept of "Occupational Disease" in the Legal Sense

For many dermatologists, occupational dermatology represents a sub-area of our field that is difficult to understand, not because there is a lack of medical knowledge, but because two realities of life and science meet in it. From a medical point of view, occupational dermatology is environmental dermatology; it deals with the specific effects of the environment - the occupational one - on the human skin and the diseases caused by these effects. That physical, chemical, and biological noxae may affect the human organism and may lead to specific and non-specific damage is a fact that medical students learn early on in their training. The medical term of occupationally caused skin disease therefore encounters hardly any difficulties in understanding, as it is an internal definition of medical science. The problems of understanding begin where the term "occupational disease" is not defined medically but legally and is not congruent with the medical term. The situation may become even more complicated since occupational diseases are differently defined in different jurisdictions. A condition that may legally qualify for an occupational disease in one jurisdiction may not so in another one; this is even true in the European Union due to the different health and social systems. For obvious practical reasons, this work will thus focus on the concept of "occupational disease" based on German legislation and jurisdiction.

In Germany, occupational diseases are legally defined in §9 Para. 1 SGB (Social Code) VII as "diseases which the Federal Government designates as occupational diseases by statutory order with the consent of the Federal Council and which the insured suffer as a result of an activity that justifies the insurance cover according to § 2, 3 or 6." Not every disease that a dermatologist diagnoses as an occupational skin disease is therefore an occupational disease; rather, these must be listed in the statutory ordinance mentioned - the Occupational Diseases Ordinance (BKV). The Federal Government cannot arbitrarily decide which diseases to include in the regulation; instead, Section 9 (2) SGB VII stipulates that these must be diseases "which, according to the findings of medical science, are caused by special effects to which certain groups of people are exposed to a significantly higher degree than the rest of the population through their insured activity." The Federal Government "can determine that the diseases are only occupational diseases if they were caused by activities in certain hazardous areas or if they led to the omission

© The Author(s), under exclusive license to Springer Nature Switzerland AG 2023
A. M. Giménez-Arnau, H. I. Maibach (eds.), *Handbook of Occupational Dermatoses*, Updates in Clinical Dermatology, https://doi.org/10.1007/978-3-031-22727-1_15

of all activities that were the cause of the development, aggravation or recurrence of the disease or could be."

Occupational diseases of the skin in the legal sense are therefore only the diseases listed in Annex 1 to the BKV, which are provided with numbers:

- 5101: Severe or repeatedly recurring skin diseases
- 5102: Skin cancer or skin changes with a tendency towards cancer formation due to soot, crude paraffin, tar, anthracene, pitch or similar substances
- 5103: Squamous cell carcinoma of the skin or multiple actinic keratoses due to natural UV radiation

Further occupational diseases may cause skin symptoms, such as No. 1108 "Diseases caused by arsenic or its compounds" or diseases caused by infectious agents or parasites and tropical diseases (BK 3101, 3102, and 3104); furthermore, §9 Para. 2 SGB also contains an "opening clause" for "like-occupational diseases."

Even if the definitions of the above mentioned occupational diseases appear to be easy to understand, there are many guidelines from case law for their precise interpretation and application to individual cases, which an occupational dermatological expert should be familiar with.

The Occupational Skin Disease No. 5101 According to German Law

The importance of medicolegal definitions in occupational dermatology may be well demonstrated by the development of the occupational skin disease No. 5101. As a dermatological occupational disease, BK 5101 ("severe or repeatedly relapsing skin diseases") is, in terms of numbers, of the greatest importance. Examples of conditions fulfilling the definition of BK 5101 are given in Table 15.1.

This occupational skin disease was first mentioned in the second Ordinance on Occupational Diseases in 1929, when it was defined as "chronic

Table 15.1 Skin diseases fulfilling the definition of the German Occupational Disease No. 5101

Contact dermatitis (mostly on the hands)
• Allergic
• Irritative/subtoxic cumulative
• Protein contact dermatitis
Exacerbation of an endogenous dermatosis
• (Hand-)Eczema
• Psoriasis
• Lupus erythematosus
• Genodermatoses (e.g., Darier's disease).
Other skin diseases
• Contact urticaria
• Cold-induced skin damage (e.g., chilblains)
• Heat-induced skin damage
• Photodermatoses
• Acne (due to work with tar, pitch, oils, fats, organic chlorine compounds)

and chronic recurrent skin diseases" due to "electroplating" or "tropical timber" [1]. In the third Ordinance on Occupational Diseases dating from 1936, the definition was changed to "severe or recurrent occupational skin diseases that have forced the patient to change the occupation or to give up any gainful employment." This change of definition was intended to include more causes of dermatitis beyond mere "electroplating" and "tropical timber" on the one hand, on the other hand, the obligation to cease an occupation was included in order to compensate only those diseases that were chronic and severe enough to significantly impair the affected persons. Mild and temporary illnesses should be excluded from compensation.

The definition of occupational disease No. 5101 as "severe or repeatedly recurrent skin disease having forced to refrain from all activities which were or may be the cause of the development, aggravation or recurrence of the disease" had been in effect until January 1, 2021, when with the "Seventh Act amending the Fourth Book of the German Social Code (SGB) and other Laws," an amendment to the Occupational Diseases Law, came into force, with which the obligation to cease work was abolished. The reason for this decision of the German Parliament was that while nearly 20,000 suspected cases of occupational disease No. 5101 had been notified each year, only less than 500 cases were recognized since the condition of "ceasing the occupation" was only rarely met by the affected workers.

Duty to Notify an Occupational Disease

The statutory occupational accident insurance was introduced in Germany already in 1884, originally to guarantee the care of insured individuals in case of work accidents, and it was extended to the coverage of occupational diseases in 1925. However, the insurance companies will be unaware of cases requiring their services unless notified by physicians treating patients with occupational accidents and diseases, or by affected workers or their employers. In order to inform the insurance companies as early as possible, physicians are obliged by law to report the suspected diagnosis of an occupational disease to the accident insurance company or to the state authority responsible for medical occupational health and safety (Para. 202 SGB VII). However, this notification legally only applies when an occupational disease is already present, thus wasting valuable time for the prevention of an occupational disease.

The Dermatologist's Procedure as an Early Intervention with the Intention to Prevent the Occurrence of an Occupational Skin Disease

As early as in the 1970s, it was realized that many cases of occupational skin diseases were preventable by technical measures or improvement of skin protection at the workplace. At that time, the accident insurance companies were required by law to engage in the early prevention of occupational diseases according to §3 the Occupational Diseases Ordinance (BKV) ("If there is a risk for insured persons that an occupational disease will develop, revive or worsen, the accident insurance institutions shall counteract this risk by all appro-

priate means."). In order to enable early prevention of occupational skin diseases, the "dermatologist's procedure" was established based on §§ 41–43 of the "Contract between physicians and accident insurers" [2]. Upon presentation of the dermatologist's report by the dermatologist, measures of secondary individual prevention are implemented by the accident insurer, including out-patient and/or in-patient dermatological treatment, seminars on skin protection for prevention training of the insured person, and optimization of protective measures at work [3]. Only if these measures proved unsuccessful, the medical-objective obligation to refrain from risky work activities in the case of severe or repeatedly recurrent skin diseases could be confirmed; in this case, the dermatologist was obliged to submit a notification of occupational disease pursuant to Para. 202 SGB VII as above. Cases for which the obligation to refrain from risky work activities was confirmed already at first diagnosis, such as severe airborne contact dermatitis due to epoxy resin, were rare.

The Occupational Skin Diseases No. 5102 and 5103 According to German Law

As mentioned above, occupational skin disease No. 5102 refers to skin cancer due to soot, crude paraffin, tar, anthracene, pitch or similar substances and No. 5103 to squamous cell carcinoma of the skin or multiple actinic keratoses due to natural UV radiation. While skin cancers due to polyaromatic hydrocarbons have become rare following better hygienic conditions at work places, skin cancer due to natural UV radiation, which was only introduced as an occupational disease in 2015, is of increasing importance with more than 7000 cases acknowledged each year [4]. However, for occupational skin cancers no early prevention program as for the occupational skin disease No. 5101 has been established. The recognition of these skin cancers as occupational skin diseases thus requires a notification based on § 202 SGB VII to the statutory accident insurance.

The Expert Opinion in Occupational Dermatology

Medicine and law come together in an occupational dermatological expert opinion, which is required by the statutory accident insurance or the courts to evaluate whether a medical fact can be assigned to a legal term - "subsumed" in legal language. This requires expert knowledge of medicine, which a statutory accident insurance institution as a corporation under public law or a social court usually lack. The task of the dermatological expert is ultimately to "translate" his medical findings about an insured person into legally usable statements. In order for him to succeed in this, he must understand the legal issues addressed to him.

Qualifications and Duties of the Occupational Dermatological Expert

For occupational dermatological expert opinions, the qualification as a specialist in dermatology will be required [5]; if allergological questions are to be processed, as is often the case with BK 5101, the additional qualification "allergology" is necessary. In order to support dermatologists in acquiring expert-specific knowledge, an "occupational dermatology" certificate in the 1990s [6], which provides an interdisciplinary introduction to expert work. By participating in regularly offered quality circles, experts can always keep their knowledge up to date. Of course, the diagnostic methods required for the expert questions must be available to the expert, for example, the spectrum of allergological test methods with regard to BK 5101 (Table 15.1). In addition to qualifications, occupational dermatological experts have special obligations that deviate from the usual curative medical work. While medical ethics dictates that the patient's well-being must be the primary concern of the physician, the medical expert is not primarily committed to the "well-being" of the insured person, but to an objective determination of the medical facts in accordance with the expert opinion order. This may lead to conflicts of interest if a dermatologist simultaneously takes care of an insured person as his physician and, on the other hand, acts as an expert for accident insurance or a court. In order to be able to fulfill his function as "assistant of the accident insurance or the court," an expert must be independent, i.e., he may not represent the interests of either the accident insurance nor the person to be examined.

The Preparation of an Occupational Dermatological Expert Opinion in Practice [5]

The prerequisite for the preparation of an occupational dermatological expert opinion is always an order of an insurance or a court, usually accompanied by a more or less extensive file, to the dermatologist.

The order describes which person is to be examined with which legal questions to be answered. The expert should study this letter of engagement carefully and check whether he can fulfill the assignment. If this does not fall within his area of expertise, he must return the assignment immediately, and if he realizes that additional assessments from other areas of expertise are required, he should also inform the insurance or the court of this in a timely manner.

In most cases, an occupational dermatological export - with the exception of opinions based on files only - requires a personal examination of the insured person. The insured person is therefore to be summoned to this examination. Sufficient time should be planned for this, as experience has shown that taking history and dermatological assessment and the necessary documentation are time-consuming. Photographic documentation of the findings at the time of the examination is useful.

Expert opinions on BK 5101 often require additional investigations; these may be laboratory assessments, biopsies, or patch testing. Especially if a patch test is planned, it will usually be necessary to arrange additional appointments with the insured person. For the testing of own substances, these must be procured and checked for their testability or prepared accordingly. In the case of expert opinions on BK 5102/5103, dermatohistological examinations, for example, to clarify whether an actinic keratosis is present or whether a lesion is a squamous cell carcinoma, and thus tissue removal may be necessary, which the insured person must of course give their legally valid informed consent. The person to be examined does not have to tolerate invasive examinations, but if they are necessary and still rejected, a possible deterioration of the legal position may be the consequence.

If all the necessary information for the expert opinion - legal question, file extract, history, examination, results of diagnostic tests - is available, this must be processed in the expert opinion. The usual style of expert opinion presents the information to be evaluated in the order mentioned, in order to then carefully work through the questions in a section "expert assessment and discussion," possibly using scientific literature, and finally in a last section to answer the questions to the expert. To support occupational dermatological experts and to ensure quality in occupational dermatology expert opinions, the Working Group for Occupational and Environmental Dermatology has been publishing assessment recommendations ("Bamberg Recommendations") for over 20 years, which were last updated and published in 2017 [7].

References

1. Elsner P. Abolition of the obligation to cease an occupation for acknowledgment of an occupational skin disease: backgrounds and perspectives. J Dtsch Dermatol Ges. 2021;19:679. https://doi.org/10.1111/ddg.14337.
2. Schwantes H, Schliemann S, Elsner P. Rehabilitation bei Berufsdermatosen. Hautarzt. 2010;61:323–31.
3. Elsner P. The "dermatologist's procedure" after the abolition of the obligation to refrain from risky work activities in occupational disease law. Hautarzt. 2021;72:509. https://doi.org/10.1007/s00105-021-04776-7.
4. Diepgen TL, Drexler H, Elsner P, Schmitt J. UV-irradiation-induced skin cancer as a new occupational disease. Hautarzt. 2015;66:154–9.
5. Elsner P. Expert opinions in dermatology. J Dtsch Dermatol Ges. 2019;17:810–23.
6. Diepgen TL, Elsner P. Zertifikat "Berufsdermatologie". Aktuelle Derm. 2018;44:516–9.
7. Bamberger Empfehlung (2017). http://abd.dermis.net/content/e03abd/e08FormulareLeitlinien/PDFs/BambergerEmpfehlungen10196.pdf.

© The Editor(s) (if applicable) and The Author(s), under exclusive license to Springer Nature Switzerland AG 2023
A. M. Giménez-Arnau, H. I. Maibach (eds.), *Handbook of Occupational Dermatoses*, Updates in Clinical Dermatology, https://doi.org/10.1007/978-3-031-22727-1

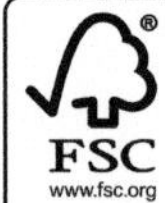

MIX
Papier aus verantwortungsvollen Quellen
Paper from responsible sources
FSC® C105338

FSC
www.fsc.org

If you have any concerns about our products,
you can contact us on
ProductSafety@springernature.com

In case Publisher is established outside the EU,
the EU authorized representative is:
Springer Nature Customer Service Center GmbH
Europaplatz 3, 69115 Heidelberg, Germany

Printed by Libri Plureos GmbH
in Hamburg, Germany